Autism and Child Psychopathology Series

Series Editor

Johnny L. Matson, Department of Psychology
Louisiana State University, Baton Rouge, LA, USA

Brief Overview

The purpose of this series is to advance knowledge in the broad multidisciplinary fields of autism and various forms of psychopathology (e.g., anxiety and depression). Volumes synthesize research on a range of rapidly expanding topics on assessment, treatment, and etiology.

Description

The **Autism and Child Psychopathology Series** explores a wide range of research and professional methods, procedures, and theories used to enhance positive development and outcomes across the lifespan. Developments in education, medicine, psychology, and applied behavior analysis as well as child and adolescent development across home, school, hospital, and community settings are the focus of this series. Series volumes are both authored and edited, and they provide critical reviews of evidence-based methods. As such, these books serve as a critical reference source for researchers and professionals who deal with developmental disorders and disabilities, most notably autism, intellectual disabilities, challenging behaviors, anxiety, depression, ADHD, developmental coordination disorder, communication disorders, and other common childhood problems. The series addresses important mental health and development difficulties that children and youth, their caregivers, and the professionals who treat them must face. Each volume in the series provides an analysis of methods and procedures that may assist in effectively treating these developmental problems.

More information about this series at http://www.springer.com/series/8665

Russell Lang • Peter Sturmey
Editors

Adaptive Behavior Strategies for Individuals with Intellectual and Developmental Disabilities

Evidence-Based Practices Across the Life Span

Springer

Editors
Russell Lang
College of Education
Texas State University
San Marcos, TX, USA

Peter Sturmey
City University of New York
Queens College
Flushing, NY, USA

ISSN 2192-922X ISSN 2192-9238 (electronic)
Autism and Child Psychopathology Series
ISBN 978-3-030-66440-4 ISBN 978-3-030-66441-1 (eBook)
https://doi.org/10.1007/978-3-030-66441-1

This Springer imprint is published by the registered company Springer Nature Switzerland AG
The registered company address is: Gewerbestrasse 11, 6330 Cham, Switzerland

Preface

People living with intellectual and developmental disabilities often experience difficulty learning skills necessary for daily living. Often referred to as adaptive behavior, these functional life skills range from basic hygiene (e.g., bathing, brushing teeth, and dressing) to more complex skills such as driving. Skills related to recreation, play and leisure and those necessary to remain safe in community settings (e.g., abduction prevention skills for children) are also considered paramount for independence and autonomy. Despite the widely recognized importance of adaptive daily-living skills and the tremendous corpus of peer-reviewed research in this area, there is a surprising lack of books devoted to the topic. Although many textbooks used in graduate courses devoted to the education and treatment of people with intellectual and developmental disabilities have chapters on adaptive behavior, we are aware of no recent books providing the depth and breadth of coverage proposed here. This book will present nine chapters focused exclusively on adaptive behavior and daily-living skills. Furthermore, as opposed to limiting the coverage to a specific phase of development (e.g., childhood), this volume includes adaptive behavior interventions across the life span.

This book begins with a chapter from Tasse that presents a conceptual analysis of adaptive behavior, a review of measurement and assessment issues, and some comprehensive assessments of adaptive behavior. The second chapter by Penrod, Silbaugh, Page, and Moseman presents a systematic review of recent work on teaching a very basic adaptive behavior – feeding skills – which also includes work on food refusal and selectivity. Chapter 3 by McLay, van Deurs, Gibbs, and Whitcombe-Dobbs reviews research on teaching hygiene skills such as dressing, oral hygiene, menstrual care, handwashing, bathing, grooming, and toileting. Communication is another important adaptive behavior. Over the years teaching communication skills has undergone a revolutionary change with the adoption of a functional approach based on Skinner's *Verbal Behavior*. Sigafoos's chapter provides an in-depth review of this continuously developing technology. Chapter 5 by Kim, Lory Kim, Gregori, and Rispoli reviews approaches to teach academic skills. Long excluded from education, individuals with intellectual and developmental disabilities now receive an education, but school services are challenged as how to teach them effectively. This chapter illustrates the evidence available to guide practice in this area. Access to the community often does not occur, merely by being located in a community setting. Chapter 6 by Ayres, Tyson, White, and Herrod reviews one important aspect of enhancing the community presence of individuals with intellectual and developmental disabilities using an ecological framework. Chapter 7 by Didden, Jonker, Delforterie, and Nijman systematically reviews research on teaching community safety skills, such as responding to lures, being lost in the community, road safety, bullying, first aid, and putting out a fire, which are essential as people live in community settings. Teaching adaptive behavior on the scale needed to impact the lives of many people with intellectual and developmental disabilities cannot and perhaps should not be done by a few experts and professionals in clinics and centers. Thus, the chapter by Hansen, DeMarco, and Etchison reviews a relatively and surprisingly sparse literature on training family members and community staff to do so in community settings, such as families. We are living in a new age of web-based technologies that have transformed everyone's lives, including the lives of individuals with intellectual and developmental disabilities. Thus, in the final chapter Wehmeyer, Tanis, Davies, and Stock provide a comprehensive review of teaching this technology thoughtfully framed within a disability rights perspective.

We hope that this book will be suited for graduate students and professionals in the fields of clinical child, school, and developmental psychology, family studies, behavior analysis, special education, developmental disability, and public health interested in both practical and applied aspects as well as theoretical implications and scientific processes inherent to teaching life skills and supporting adaptive behavior in people with intellectual and developmental disabilities. We thank the chapter authors for their work on this volume. We chose them because of their high level of expertise and international reputations in this field: We were not disappointed.

San Marcos, TX, USA — Russell Lang
Flushing, NY, USA — Peter Sturmey

Contents

Contributors

Kevin M. Ayres is a professor of Special Education at The University of Georgia and co-director of the Center for Autism and Behavioral Education research. He specializes in school-based applications of behavior analysis for improving learning outcomes.

Daniel K. Davies is the founder and president of AbleLink Smart Living Technologies. He has been closely associated with issues important to individuals with disabilities and their families all his life, as his oldest brother John lived with severe intellectual disability, and several significant physical disabilities. He has been actively involved in research and development of assistive technology for individuals with cognitive and other disabilities and has authored over 75 journal articles, book chapters, and reports specifically on the use of assistive technology for individuals with cognitive disabilities and is an invited presenter at conferences nationally and internationally.

Monique Delforterie is a senior researcher at Trajectum, a treatment facility for adults with mild intellectual disabilities and severe behavioral and mental health problems.

Jessica DeMarco is a doctoral student at Georgia State University. Her research interests include early intervention, applied behavior analysis, reducing challenging behaviors in school settings, and language development.

Jenna van Deurs is a Registered Child and Family Psychologist in Christchurch, New Zealand. Her research interests include the assessment and treatment of sleep problems in adolescents on the autism spectrum, adolescent-led interventions, and child and adolescent mental health.

Robert Didden is Professor of Intellectual Disability, Learning and Behavior at the Behavioural Science Institute of the Radboud University at Nijmegen, the

Netherlands. As a researcher, he is also affiliated with Trajectum, a treatment facility for adults with mild intellectual disabilities at Zwolle.

Hannah Etchison is a doctoral student at Georgia State University. Her research interests include early intervention in low-resource settings, applied behavior analysis, and theory and pedagogy in special education.

Rosina Gibbs is an experienced Early Childhood Educator and a Postgraduate student in Child and Family Psychology at the College of Education, Health and Human Development, University of Canterbury. She provides support for researchers in investigating the effectiveness of behavioral sleep interventions for children with autism and rare genetic disorders.

Emily Gregori is an Assistant Professor in the Department of Special Education at the University of Illinois at Chicago. Her works examine the assessment and treatment of challenging behavior for adults with developmental disabilities, and methods for training direct care staff and other natural change agents to implement behavioral programming.

Sarah G. Hansen is an assistant professor of early childhood special education, Georgia State University. Her research focuses on assessment, intervention, and training of natural change agents on early and pivotal social communication skills for children with autism spectrum disorder and other developmental disabilities and preparing natural change agents to support children with special needs to succeed in the preschool classroom and other natural environments.

Jessica L. Herrod is a doctoral student studying special education at the University of Georgia. Her areas of interest include applied behavior analysis and classroom interventions for individuals with intellectual and developmental disabilities.

Femke Jonker is a clinical psychologist at Pro Persona, a psychiatric hospital in The Netherlands. She also works as a diagnostician for The Netherlands Institute for Forensic Psychology and Psychiatry. She is currently conducting a PhD study on adaptive skills in individuals with mild intellectual disabilities.

Soo Jung Kim is a doctoral student of Special Education at the College of Education, Purdue University. Her work focuses on mathematics education and the use of technology for children with disabilities.

So Yeon Kim recently received a PhD from the College of Education, Purdue University. Her research focuses on teaching reading skills to students with developmental disabilities and using technology as an instructional tool.

Russell Lang is an associate professor of Special Education and a Board Certified Behavior Analyst (BCBA-D). He has published over 100 peer-reviewed research papers and multiple book chapters concerning the education and treatment of people with intellectual and developmental disabilities. His primary research interest is in the treatment of challenging behaviors and the acquisition of play and leisure skills in children with autism spectrum disorders.

Catharine Lory is a doctoral student of Special Education at the College of Education, Purdue University. Her work focuses on applied behavior analysis, teacher and staff training, and challenging behavior in children with autism and developmental disabilities.

Laurie McLay is an associate professor in the School of Health Sciences at the University of Canterbury. She specializes in the assessment and treatment of sleep problems in children and adolescents with developmental disabilities, and she leads the Good Nights Programme at the University of Canterbury. Her research interests also include interventions for toilet training and other adaptive living skills.

Melissa Moseman is a graduate student, under the advisement of Dr. Becky Penrod, at California State University, Sacramento. Her research and applied interests include pediatric feeding behavior, parent and teacher training, and verbal behavior.

Henk Nijman is Professor of Forensic Psychology at the Behavioural Science Institute of the Radboud University in Nijmegen, The Netherlands. He is also senior researcher at the forensic psychiatric institute, Fivoor, The Netherlands.

Scott V. Page is a doctoral student in applied behavior analysis at Utah State University. His research interests include the use of computer and internet-based technologies to change health behaviors, the assessment and treatment of feeding problems, multitiered systems of support, and evidence-based procedures in schools.

Becky Penrod is a professor of Psychology and Director of the Pediatric Behavior Research Laboratory at California State University, Sacramento. She specializes in applied behavior analysis with an emphasis on the assessment and treatment of pediatric feeding disorders.

Mandy Rispoli is a professor in the Department of Educational Studies at Purdue University. Her work examines functional behavior assessment and intervention implemented by natural change agents with young children with autism and other developmental disabilities.

Jeff Sigafoos is a professor in the School of Education at Victoria University of Wellington and an adjunct Professor at James Madison University in Virginia, USA. He has authored numerous journal articles, book chapters, books describing the results of his research on educational and behavioral interventions for individuals with developmental and physical disabilities. He is co-editor-in-chief of

Evidence-Based Communication Assessment and Intervention. His current research includes using iPad technology to promote communication and social skills in children with autism spectrum disorders, enhancing the communication skills of children with autism and intellectual disability, and augmentative and alternative communication intervention for children with developmental and physical disabilities.

Bryant C. Silbaugh is Director of Research and Development at Empower Behavioral Health in San Antonio, Texas. He specializes in applied behavior analysis, with an emphasis on the assessment and treatment of children with autism and pediatric feeding disorders.

Steven E. Stock is at AbleLink Smart Living Technologies. He has published widely on assistive technology, self-determination, and inclusion.

Peter Sturmey, PhD is Professor of Psychology at the Graduate Center and Queens College, City University of New York. He has published over 220 articles, 80 chapters, 25 books, and over 300 presentations mostly in the areas of developmental disabilities and applied behavior analysis.

Shea Tanis is the director for Policy and Advocacy at the Coleman Institute for Cognitive Disabilities at the University of Colorado and is also on the faculty of the Department of Psychiatry at the University of Colorado. Her research interests include the definition of intellectual disability, measurement of adaptive behavior and support need, the construct of self-determination, federally funded supports and services for people with intellectual and developmental disabilities, and their families, and self-directed employment strategies, applied cognitive technology supports, cognitive accessibility, and advancing the rights of people with cognitive disabilities to technology and information access.

Marc J. Tassé, PhD is Professor in the Department of Psychology and in the Department of Psychiatry and Behavioral Health, and Director of the Ohio State Nisonger Center, The Ohio State University. He has published over 155 articles in peer-reviewed journals, book chapters, and books in the area of intellectual disabilities, autism spectrum disorders and other neurodevelopmental disorders and given over 275 scientific and professional presentations. He has been involved in the development of a number of standardized assessment tests for people with ID/ASD, including *Diagnostic Adaptive Behavior Scale, Supports Intensity Scale for Children, Supports Intensity Scale for Adults, Nisonger Child Behavior Rating Form, and the Quebec Adaptive Behavior Scale.*

Kelsie M. Tyson is a doctoral student in the special education program at the University of Georgia. Her areas of interest include applied behavior analysis and early intervention for young children with autism spectrum disorder.

Michael L. Wehmeyer is the Ross and Marianna Beach Distinguished Professor in Special Education at the Schiefelbusch Institute for Life Span Studies, University of Kansas. He has directed externally funded projects totaling in excess of $33 million pertaining to the education and support of youth and adults with intellectual and developmental disabilities. He is the author or co-author of 385 peer-reviewed journal articles or book chapters and has authored, co-authored, edited, or co-edited 36 books on disability and education related issues, including issues pertaining to self-determination, positive psychology and disability, transition to adulthood, the education and inclusion of students with severe disabilities, and technology use by people with cognitive disabilities.

Sarah Whitcombe-Dobbs is a Registered Psychologist and lecturer in Child and Family Psychology at the School of Health Sciences, University of Canterbury. Her research focuses on assessment and intervention with families who have involvement with Child Protection Services. She also specializes in developmental and mental health assessment and intervention with children and adolescents who have histories of trauma and complex needs.

Emily N. White is a doctoral student in the special education program at The University of Georgia. Her areas of interest include applied behavior analysis and communication interventions for preschool-aged children with intellectual and developmental disabilities.

Chapter 1
Adaptive Behavior and Functional Life Skills Across the Lifespan: Conceptual and Measurement Issues

Marc J. Tassé

1.1 Definition and History

Adaptive behavior involves skills that people learn throughout their life and put forth to meet the demands and expectations of their environment and society at large. Adaptive behavior is a broad construct that encompasses practical skills (e.g., self-care, toileting, cooking, cleaning, caring for one's home, money concepts, and work skills), social skills (e.g., interpersonal skills, managing one's emotions), and conceptual skills (e.g., functional academics, communication skills, concept of time, money management, and self-direction; American Psychiatric Association, 2013; Schalock, Luckasson, & Tassé, 2021; Tassé et al., 2012). The complexity of the adaptive behavior increases with chronological age and the onset of diverse social roles and responsibilities (e.g., going to school, participating in sports and leisure activities, maintaining friendship, dating, independence/interdependence, financial responsibilities, following rules, social responsibilities, employment, and raising children).

Impairment in adaptive behavior is a crucial diagnostic criterion for a number of neurodevelopmental disorders, including autism spectrum disorder (American Psychiatric Association, 2013) and intellectual disability (APA, 2013; Schalock et al., 2021; World Health Organization, 1992). The presence of deficits in adaptive behavior is also present in a number of other conditions, including attention deficit/hyperactivity disorder, emotional and behavioral disorders, hearing and motor impairments, communication disorders, and learning disabilities (Harrison & Oakland, 2003). Research has shown that the strength of adaptive skills is a strong predictor of success of post-high school outcomes for students with disabilities (Dell'Armo & Tassé, 2019). Conversely, the loss of adaptive skills in aging adults is

M. J. Tassé (✉)
Nisonger Center, The Ohio State University, Columbus, OH, USA
e-mail: Tasse.1@osu.edu

R. Lang, P. Sturmey (eds.), *Adaptive Behavior Strategies for Individuals with Intellectual and Developmental Disabilities*, Autism and Child Psychopathology Series, https://doi.org/10.1007/978-3-030-66441-1_1

an early indicator of age-related decline (Takata et al., 2013) and the onset of dementia in persons with Down syndrome (Zigman, Schupf, Urv, & Silverman, 2009; Zigman, Schupf, Urv, Zigman, & Silverman, 2002).

Deficits in adaptive behavior are attributable to a number of independent and overlapping variables. Some of these factors include: (a) opportunities to develop/learn a skill/behavior, (b) opportunities to perform or practice a learned skill, (c) intrinsic or extrinsic motivation to perform a learned skill when called upon, (d) the awareness that a particular skill or behavior is needed in a particular situation, (e) physical or mental health problems, and/or (f) brain disease or impairment. One's context also influences significantly a person's adaptive behavior, situationally (e.g., in a demand setting where the person is rewarded for emitting a specific adaptive behavior) or permanently (e.g., growing up in a severely impoverished environment where there was a paucity of opportunities to learn adaptive skills).

Although the concept of adaptive behavior has evolved over time, it remains remarkably similar to the definition initially proposed by the American Association on Intellectual and Developmental Disabilities (AAIDD) more than 50 years ago (see Heber, 1959). Heber (1959) first proposed introducing this concept into the diagnostic criteria of intellectual disability in a draft version of the American Association on Mental Deficiency's (now AAIDD) terminology and classification manual. Heber defined this second diagnostic criterion as deficits in at least one of the following: "maturation, learning, and social adjustment" (see Heber, 1959; p. 3). After receiving feedback and comments from the field, Heber (1961) revised slightly the AAIDD diagnostic criteria for intellectual disability proposed in 1959 and formally introduced in the definition of intellectual disability the concept of "adaptive behavior." Heber described the concurrent impairments in adaptive behavior as consisting of deficits in one of the three previously mentioned domains: maturation, learning, and/or social adjustments (see Heber, 1961; p. 3). The Diagnostic and Statistical Manual for Mental Disorders (DSM) incorporated AAIDD's (Heber, 1961) proposed construct of adaptive behavior in its revision of the DSM, published in 1968 (DSM-II; American Psychiatric Association, 1968).

Fast forward 50 years, and our current diagnostic definitions of intellectual disability look surprisingly similar to these two earlier definitions of AAIDD (Heber, 1961) and DSM-II (American Psychiatric Association, 1968); (see Tassé, Luckasson, & Schalock, 2016). The current AAIDD definition (see Schalock et al., 2021) and DSM-5 (APA, 2013) both require the presence of significant impairments in adaptive behavior when diagnosing intellectual disability and operationalize it as the presence of deficits in one or more of the following: conceptual (aka learning), social (aka social adjustment), and/or practical adaptive skills (aka maturation).

1.2 Disorders Associated with Deficits in Adaptive Behavior

There are a number of conditions and situations in which the assessment and teaching of adaptive behavior is a critical and essential component of the clinician's or educator's responsibility. Before we discuss some of these specific conditions, it is important to point out that the presence of problem behavior may at times coexist in a person who has deficits in adaptive behavior. First, we much mention that problem behavior (e.g., aggression, stereotypy, and elopement) are not necessarily "maladaptive" or purposeless, nor are problem behavior and adaptive behavior on opposite ends of the same construct. Problem behavior can, in fact, be very "adaptive" and serve as an effective response to the person's environment and the contingencies in the environment (e.g., scream to get someone's attention and hit a teacher to get out of a task). Problem behaviors most often serve a function (e.g., get something, avoid something, communicate a desire, and sensory regulation), and a function-based intervention will use teaching and reinforcing of alternative behaviors to replace the problem behavior. Often, these alternative behaviors are adaptive skills. For example, if the function of a student's problem behavior of slapping a classmate is motivated by a desire to escape the demands of the classroom by being removed from the classroom contingently on the aggressive behavior, perhaps an alternative behavior to this aggression might be to teach the student to ask for help, or communicate (e.g., words, picture/symbol, and sign language) more effectively when he/she is feeling overwhelmed by a task or demand that is too difficult.

Incorporating the teaching of alternative adaptive skills should be considered an essential component of all behavior change interventions. Research has shown that conducting parent training that focuses on enhancing adaptive behavior and behavior management strategies results in improved adaptive behavior and a reduction in challenging behaviors (Scahill et al., 2012, 2016). There is a growing body of research that has shown that poor adaptive behavior in childhood is a barrier to achievements in social relationships, inclusion, independence, and employment (Bruininks, Hill, & Morreau, 1985; Papazoglou, Jacobson, & Zabel, 2013).

1.2.1 Developmental Disabilities

Developmental disabilities is an administrative definition at the federal level that defines a level of human functioning that determines individuals eligible for federal and state disability benefits (e.g., early intervention, waiver services for community-based services, social security supplemental income). The definition for developmental disabilities is found in US legislation entitled Developmental Disabilities Assistance and Bill of Rights Act (DD Act, 2000) that is operationalized based on the person's level of functioning rather than on the presence of specific conditions or disorders (meaning it is largely based on the person presenting certain prescribed functional deficits). Developmental disability is not a condition defined in either the DSM (DSM-5; American Psychiatric Association, 2013) or the International Classification of Diseases (ICD-10; World Health Organization, 1992). The DD Act (2000) defines developmental disabilities as follows:

(A) "… a severe, chronic disability of an individual that:

- (i) Is attributable to a mental or physical impairment or combination of mental and physical impairments;

(ii) Is manifested before the individual attains age 22;
(iii) Is likely to continue indefinitely;
(iv) Results in substantial functional limitations in 3 or more of the following areas of major life activity:

1. Self-care.
2. Receptive and expressive language.
3. Learning.
4. Mobility.
5. Self-direction.
6. Capacity for independent living.
7. Economic self-sufficiency; and

(v) Reflects the individual's need for a combination and sequence of special, interdisciplinary, or generic services, individualized supports, or other forms of assistance that are of lifelong or extended duration and are individually planned and coordinated.

(B) Infants and young children. An individual from birth to age 9, inclusive, who has a substantial developmental delay or specific congenital or acquired condition, may be considered to have a developmental disability without meeting 3 or more of the criteria described in clauses (i) through (v) of subparagraph (A) if the individual, without services and supports, has a high probability of meeting those criteria later in life." (DD Act, 2000; pp. 1683–1684)

It is important to note that a person's cognitive ability is not a criterion in diagnosing a developmental disability. Rather, its determination rests largely on the presence of deficits in adaptive behavior, or what is called "areas of major life activity" in the DD Act.

1.2.2 Autism Spectrum Disorder

Autism spectrum disorder is a life-long neurodevelopmental disorder that has an onset during early childhood. It is characterized by significant deficits in social communication skills and the presence of restrictive and repetitive behavior and/or interests (American Psychiatric Association, 2013). Deficits in social communication include skills such as social and emotional reciprocity, interpersonal skills, emotion recognition and sharing, nonverbal communication skills, eye contact, and friendship and relationship skills. Deficits in social skills and communication deficits are core features of autism spectrum disorder (see DSM-5).

People with autism spectrum disorder present with varying levels of severity in symptoms and functioning across the social and communication skills continuum as well as the severity of their stereotypic behavior, behavioral rigidity, restrictive interests and activities, and sensory behaviors. The DSM-5 proposed three levels of severity of autism spectrum disorder, based on the intensity of supports needed around the person's social communication deficits and their restricted and repetitive behaviors. Hence, interventions almost always focus on teaching and enhancing these adaptive skills to impact the core features of autism spectrum disorder and directly reduce the severity of the condition and ameliorate the prognosis.

1.2.3 Intellectual Disability

Adaptive behavior is perhaps best associated as a core feature of intellectual disability. The condition of intellectual disability has long been conceptualized as consisting of problems in adapting to societal demands and expectations, along with deficits in intellectual abilities. Adaptive behavior has been an essential diagnostic criterion of intellectual disability for more than 50 years (see American Psychiatric Association, 1968; Heber, 1961). Even before adaptive behavior was included as a diagnostic criterion, Tredgold (1937; p. 4) described it as follows: "*[Intellectual disability] is a state of incomplete mental development of such a kind and degree that* ***the individual is incapable of adapting himself to the normal environment of his fellows*** *in such a way to maintain existence independently of supervision, control or external support.*" [emphasis mine]. Edouard Seguin as early as the mid-1800s differentiated the severity levels of intellectual disability on the basis of a combination of deficits in intellectual ability and adaptive functioning (see Scherenberger, 1983).

An important assumption that is defined as essential to the application of the definition of intellectual disability put forth by AAIDD stipulates the following: "With appropriate personalized supports, the life functioning of the person with intellectual disability will improve" (Luckasson et al., 2002; Schalock et al., 2010; Schalock, Luckasson, & Tassé, 2021). We argue that the most important form of ongoing support is lifelong instruction. People with intellectual disability, as well as any other disability, are capable of learning new adaptive skills throughout their life.

1.2.4 Relation Between Adaptive Behavior and Intellectual Functioning

It is not surprising that the exact relationship between intelligence and adaptive behavior is misunderstood and erroneously confounded as causal. In fact, earlier definitions of intelligence incorporated elements in its definition that included terms such as "adaptation" or "one's ability to respond to their environment's expectations and demands" (see Binet & Simon, 1905; Sternberg et al., 2000; Thorndike, 1920). Nonetheless, in a study of the relationship between adaptive behavior and intelligence, Keith and his colleagues (Keith, Fehrman, Harrison, & Pottebaum, 1987) tested three hypotheses of the relationship between these two constructs: (a) separate but related constructs, (b) completely independent constructs, or (c) different facets of a unitary construct. Based on their findings, they concluded that adaptive behavior and intelligence are related but separate constructs. This finding has been supported over the years by a number of research studies examining the correlational relationship between adaptive behavior and intelligence that has consistently reported that the correlation between FSIQ and composite adaptive behavior score is moderate (De Bildt, Kraijer, Sytema, & Minderaa, 2005; Harrison, 1987; Harrison & Oakland, 2003; McGrew, 2012; Papazoglou, Jacobson, McCabe, Kaufmann, & Zabel, 2014; Sabat, Tassé, & Tenorio, 2019). The correlation between IQ and adaptive behavior is strongest between the full-scale IQ score and conceptual adaptive skills and to a lesser extent with social and practical adaptive skills (Carpentieri & Morgan, 1996; Sabat et al., 2019).

There may be concern that the correlation coefficients may be attenuated between these two constructs on account of range restrictions of scores on the intelligence and adaptive behavior tests. Alexander and Reynolds (2020) in a large meta-analytic study of 148 samples containing a total of 16,464 participants, after correcting for range restriction and attenuation, reported an estimated population correlation coefficient = 0.51. These results confirmed an overall moderate relationship between intelligence and adaptive behavior. Alexander also reported that moderator analyses confirmed that the correlation coefficients between IQ and adaptive behavior were strongest as the IQ score decreased; hence, it is ever more crucial to consider adaptive behavior measures as intellectual abilities increase.

Meyers, Nihira, and Zetlin (1979) eloquently summarized the differences between these two related but separate psychological constructs as follows: "(a) adaptive behavior emphasizes everyday behavior, whereas intelligence emphasizes thought processes; (b) adaptive behavior focuses on common or typical behavior whereas intelligence focuses on maximum performance; and (c) adaptive behavior stresses non-abstract, non-academic aspects of life, whereas intelligence stresses those aspects that are abstract and academic." (pp. 433–434).

1.2.5 Importance of Adaptive Behavior

The importance of adaptive behavior has only grown over the last century of research and intervention in the field of intellectual disability. A person's functioning in terms of adaptive behavior and intellectual skills must be weighed equally and considered jointly when diagnosing intellectual disability (Tassé et al., 2016). In fact, both AAIDD and DSM have moved to place equal, if not more, importance on adaptive behavior than intellectual functioning in their conceptualization of intellectual disability. For example, the DSM-5 has abandoned the use of IQ scores in defining the severity of a person's intellectual disability and has replaced IQ with the person's level of adaptive behavior (American Psychiatric Association, 2013). Hence, the determination of severity of intellectual disability (mild, moderate, severe, profound) is best determined on the basis of the severity of deficits in adaptive behavior rather than intellectual functioning, the reason being that deficits in adaptive behavior are a better correlate with intensity of support needs than deficits in intellectual functioning (American Psychiatric Association, 2013; Simões, Santos, Biscaia, & Thompson, 2016), and, equally important, research has shown that higher levels of adaptive behavior are strongly correlated with improved quality of life (Claes et al. 2012; Nota et al. 2007; Simões et al., 2016).

There is a growing consensus on the importance of focusing our interventions and treatments on increasing the learning and performance of adaptive behavior. This book has, to that end, several chapters that present different interventions and approaches to teaching adaptive behavior and functional skills across the lifespan. In this chapter, we will present the important elements related to the concepts and assessment of adaptive behavior, which are a critical first step to the identification of strengths and areas of needed intervention. We will present some of the tools that exist that can aide in assessing the outcomes and effectiveness of an intervention.

1.3 Assessment of Adaptive Behavior

Coulter and Morrow (1978) observed that the field's interest in the assessment of adaptive behavior falls into two primary purposes. Adaptive behavior assessment continues to be driven essentially by these two goals: (1) establish a diagnosis/determine eligibility (i.e., does the person present with significant deficits in adaptive behavior) and (2) identify areas of deficits and relative strengths that can inform intervention objectives and strategies (i.e., individual education plan, individual support plan, identify strengths and weaknesses).

Edgar Doll (1936) was the first person to recognize the importance of adaptive behavior and develop a standardized measure, called the *Vineland Social Maturity Scale*. Since the first publication of the *Vineland Social Maturity Scale*, more than 200 measures of adaptive behavior and functional skills have been identified (Reschly, Myers, & Hartel, 2002; Schalock, 1999). Some of these instruments might consist of a brief inventory, checklist, or questionnaire dealing with a very specific skill area (e.g., social skills, communication, motor skills, vocational skills) and most of these 200 assessments are not comprehensive measures of adaptive behavior. Some are direct measures, while others are created to assess the person's adaptive behavior by getting input from a third-party respondent (e.g., parent, caregiver, teacher, direct support professional, etc.). Almost all rating scales are designed to allow the respondent to complete the scale on their own by entering their ratings directly onto the form. A few more rigorous standardized scales, predominantly developed for diagnostic purposes, rely more heavily on a semi-structured interview procedure between a trained professional and the respondent (e.g., parent/caregiver, teacher or direct support staff, etc.).

Although there was a time when the validity and psychometric properties of adaptive behavior scales were viewed with skepticism (see Witt & Martens, 1984;

Zigler, Balla, & Hodapp, 1984), this has changed over the last couple of decades. There are currently several existing standardized adaptive behavior scales that have been robustly developed and have strong psychometrically properties that rely on comprehensive norm-based evaluations of adaptive behavior across the lifespan and include well-written items that encompass all three critical domains: conceptual (i.e., communication, functional academics, self-direction, budgeting/paying bills), social (i.e., interpersonal skills, emotion regulation, social problem solving, wariness, following rules and laws), and practical (i.e., self-care, domestic skills, money and time concepts, vocational/work skills) adaptive skills. These are several of these instruments that are considered examples of "gold standard" measures of adaptive behavior and include: *Adaptive Behavior Assessment System*, third edition (Harrison & Oakland, 2015); *Adaptive Behavior Diagnostic Scale* (Pearson, Patton, & Mruzek, 2016); *Diagnostic Adaptive Behavior Scale* (Tassé et al., 2019); and *Vineland Adaptive Behavior Scales*, third edition (Sparrow, Cicchetti, & Saulnier, 2016). We do not include in this list, the *Scales of Independent Behavior, Revised* (SIB-R; Bruininks et al., 1996). Despite being a highly respected, well-constructed, and psychometrically robust measure of adaptive behavior, the SIB-R has become somewhat outdated since its last revision and re-norming in 1996 (i.e., almost 25 years ago). Unlike with tests of intelligence, aging norms on scales of adaptive behavior do not cause a spurious rise in adaptive behavior scores (i.e., the Flynn effect). It remains, nonetheless, important to periodically revise item content and refresh normative data on these tests. Item content on measures of adaptive behavior needs to be periodically refreshed to keep up with changing societal norms and expectations. For example, more current adaptive behavior scales may include more technology items such as using a cell phone or microwave and should have deleted outdated items such as using a pay phone or using a telephone book to find a phone number. We will briefly present these four aforementioned standardized adaptive behavior instruments.

1.3.1 Adaptive Behavior Assessment System: Third Edition

The *Adaptive Behavior Assessment System: Third Edition* (ABAS-3; Harrison & Oakland, 2015) is in its third edition, having been first published in 2000. The ABAS-3 was the first comprehensive norm-referenced measure of adaptive behavior to offer standard scores for the three adaptive behavior domains: conceptual, social, and practical adaptive skills. The ABAS-3 can be used for multiple purposes, including: (1) making the determination of intellectual disability, developmental disabilities, learning disability, and behavioral and emotional disorders; (2) identifying functional limitations of people with autism spectrum disorder, attention deficit/hyperactivity disorder, and Alzheimer disease; (3) establishing an individual's eligibility for services and supports under Individuals with Disabilities Education Act (IDEA), social security administration benefits, and intensity of need for other types of supports and services; (4) identifying and measuring intervention goals and progress in adaptive behavior and functional limitations interventions, and (5) being used as an outcome measure in program evaluations and interventions. It has robust norms drawn from the general population and it can be used to assess adaptive behavior across the lifespan, including the ages of 0–89 years.

The ABAS-3 consists of five distinct survey forms:

- **Parent or Primary Caregiver Form** (0–5 years old): appropriate for the assessment of adaptive behavior in infants and preschoolers in the home. The respondent providing adaptive behavior information on this form is the child's parent or other primary caregiver.
- **Teacher or Daycare Provider Form** (2–5 years old): used for the assessment of adaptive behavior in toddlers and preschool-aged children in daycare, preschool, and other similar setting. The respondent for the Teacher or Daycare Provider Form is typically the child's daycare or preschool teacher or teacher's aide or some other childcare or preschool personnel.
- **Parent Form** (5–21 years old): appropriate for the assessment of adaptive behavior in children and adults and having been observed at home and other community settings. The respondent completing the Parent Form is generally the child's parent or other caregiver who lives with the child or adult.
- **Teacher Form** (5–21 years old): used to assess adaptive behavior in children or adults in the context of the classroom and school (Kindergarten to 12th grade). The respondent for this form is generally the student's teacher, teacher's aide, and other school personnel.
- **Adult Form** (16–89 years old): appropriate for the assessment of adaptive behavior in adolescents and adults in the context of their home and across community settings. The respondent on the Adult Form is most often a parent/caregiver or other family member but can also be completed, when the respondent has sufficient knowledge of the person's adaptive behavior, a spouse/significant other, co-worker, work supervisor, friend, or other knowledgeable person who has good familiarity with the individual's everyday functioning. The ABAS-3 Adult Form is the only adaptive behavior form that has been developed and normed for self-report by the individual him or herself. Self-reported adaptive behavior information is most valuable for the identification and prioritization of teaching and training goals targeting adaptive skills.

Although the ABAS-3 User's Manual (Harrison & Oakland, 2015) indicated that the administration time is approximately 15–20 minutes, a more realistic time of administration is probably closer to 30–40 minutes to complete the adult form. The ABAS-3 continues to be the only standardized adaptive behavior scale that provides a self-report administration and norms for self-reported adaptive behavior using the Adult Form.

The ABAS yields standard scores (Mean = 100; standard deviation = 15) presenting an overall assessment of adaptive behavior (i.e., General Adaptive Composite [GAC]) and the three adaptive behavior domains: conceptual, social, and practical skills. The ABAS-3 forms also provide more discrete standard scores (mean = 10 and standard deviation = 3) across the following 10 subscales: (1) communication,

(2) functional academics, (3) self-direction, (4) leisure, (5) social, (6) community use, (7) home/school living, (8) health & safety, (9) self-care, and (10) work (completed only when assessed person has a part-time or full-time job). These subscale scores are probably the most informative sources of measurement when looking to assess adaptive behavior/functional limitations for the purpose of intervention planning and evaluation.

The ABAS-3 has been in use for more than two decades and has good psychometric properties (Henington, 2017; Wu, 2017). Harrison and Oakland (2015) reported internal consistency for the ABAS-3 GAC Cronbach alphas ranging from 0.96 to 0.99 and from 0.85 to 0.99 for conceptual, social, and practical domains. Harrison and Oakland also reported very good score stability for the ABAS-3 average GAC correlation coefficient of $r = 0.86$, average correlation coefficients of $r = 0.76$ for the domain standard scores, and an average $r = 0.70$ across the 10 adaptive skill areas.

1.3.2 Adaptive Behavior Diagnostic Scale

The *Adaptive Behavior Diagnostic Scale* (ABDS; Pearson et al., 2016) is one of the newer standardized adaptive behavior scales. Although an entirely new adaptive behavior scale, the ABDS was developed by Pro-Ed and is a replacement for the *Adaptive Behavior Scale: School Edition* (Lambert, Nihira, & Leland, 1993) and *Adaptive Behavior Scale: Residential and Community* (Nihira, Leland, & Lambert, 1993).

The ABDS is an interview-based scale that assesses adaptive behavior with robust general population norms for individuals from 2 to 21 years. This instrument was specifically developed using the conceptual model of adaptive behavior domains, including conceptual, social, and practical skills. The ABDS consists of a total of 150 items, with 50 discrete adaptive skill items across each of the three domains. Administration of this instrument is approximately 15–20 minutes. The results of the ABDS yield standard scores (mean = 100 and standard deviation = 15) for each of the three domains: conceptual, social, and practical, as well as an overall Adaptive Behavior Index.

Pearson et al. (2016) reported excellent psychometric properties, including internal consistency coefficients for all domain and overall index standard scores above 0.90. Pearson et al. reported sensitivity coefficient of 0.85 (accuracy of ABDS to correctly identify people with intellectual disability) and specificity coefficient of 0.99 (accuracy of ABDS to correctly identify people who do not have intellectual disability).

1.3.3 Diagnostic Adaptive Behavior Scale

The *Diagnostic Adaptive Behavior Scale* (DABS; Tassé et al., 2017) is the newest of the comprehensive adaptive behavior scales available. Like the ABDS, the DABS was developed and refined to accurately measure adaptive behavior according to the conceptual model adopted by AAIDD (Schalock et al., 2010) and the DSM-5 (American Psychiatric Association, 2013). The DABS construction used item response theory (IRT) to select and include the most precise and relevant items/skills that inform about a person's adaptive behavior across the ages of 4–21 years (Tassé et al., 2016, 2017). The DABS's item pool includes items that are often missing from more traditional adaptive behavior scales, items measuring concepts of higher order social skills, such as gullibility, vulnerability, and social naiveté.

The DABS consists of the fewest number of total items among all the comprehensive standardized adaptive behavior scales described in this chapter. It consists of a total of 75 items across all three adaptive behavior domains: conceptual, social, and practical skills (25 items per domain). The DABS is administered via a semi-structured interview between a professional (i.e., DABS interviewer) and a respondent (e.g., parent, grandparent, caregiver, teacher, etc.). The time needed to administer the DABS is generally estimated to be approximately 20 minutes. Because the DABS uses IRT to score the responses and yield individualized standard error or measurement, the scoring of the DABS can only be done via online computerized scoring (see https://aaidd.org/dabs). This scoring provides standard scores (mean = 100 and standard deviation = 15) for each of the three domains (conceptual, social, and practical) as well as Overall or Total Adaptive Behavior score.

The DABS was standardized on a large national sample of the general US population between the ages of 4 and 21 years (Tassé et al., 2017). The authors of the DABS (Balboni et al., 2014; Tassé et al., 2017; Tassé et al., 2016) have published several studies reporting strong psychometric properties, including robust validity and reliability. Tassé, Schalock, et al. (2016) reported good to excellent concurrent validity between the DABS and the *Vineland-II* ranging from $r = 0.70$ to 0.84. They also reported strong DABS test score stability, as measured using test–retest reliability coefficients, ranging from $r = 0.78$ to 0.95 and good interrater concordance as measured by intraclass correlation coefficients that ranged from 0.61 to 0.87. Balboni et al. (2014) reported on the DABS sensitivity and specificity. The DABS sensitivity (correctly identifying someone who has intellectual disability) ranged from 81% to 98% and specificity (correctly identifying someone who does not have intellectual disability) ranged from 89% to 91%.

1.3.4 Vineland Adaptive Behavior Scale, Third Edition

The *Vineland Adaptive Behavior Scale, 3rd Edition* (Vineland-3; Sparrow et al., 2016) is the oldest and probably best known comprehensive standardized adaptive behavior scale. The Vineland-3 has its roots in the *Vineland Social Maturity Scale* (VSMS; Doll, 1936) and has gone through several revisions since its first edition. The Vineland-3 measures adaptive behavior in individuals from 0 through 90 years old and consists of three forms: (1) Interview Form (0 through age 90), (2) Parent/Caregiver Form (0 through age 90), and (3) Teacher Form (3–21 years old). All three forms have two versions, depending on the purpose of the evaluation, including the Domain-level Form and a longer version called the Comprehensive Form. The Comprehensive Form is used for the purpose of providing more detailed skill information needed for intervention planning and evaluation. It yields standard scores (mean = 100 and standard deviation = 15) for: (a) Composite Score and (b) three domain scores (daily living skills, communication, socialization). It also provides standard scores on a scale of mean = 10 and standard deviation =3 for nine subdomain scores: personal, domestic, community, receptive communication, expressive communication, written communication, interpersonal relationships, play and leisure time, and coping skills. The Domain-level Form is shorter and provides standard scores (mean = 100 and standard deviation = 15) across the three VABS-3 domains: daily living skills, communication, and socialization (as well as the optional domain of motor skills) and is most useful for the purpose of making diagnostic determinations.

The Vineland-3 can be administered via a semi-structured interview using the Interview Form or be given directly to the parent or caregiver who completes the instrument directly on their own (i.e., Parent/Caregiver Form). These different forms consist of approximately comparable number of items but have slightly different item stem wordings. The Comprehensive Form consists of 502 items and Domain-Level Form consists of 195 items on the interview form and 180 items on the parent/caregiver form. The Teacher Form is not usually used in isolation but instead is often used in conjunction with the Interview Form or the Parent/Caregiver Form. The Teacher Form: Comprehensive Form consists of 333 items and Teacher Form: Domain-level Form consists of 149 items. Below is a brief description of the different Vineland-3 forms:

- Interview Form (0–90 years old): The Interview Form is administered via a semi-structured interview between a professional and the respondent (parent or caregiver). The Vineland-3 uses an interview procedure that encourages the interviewer to engage in a conversation with the respondent about the assessed person's adaptive behavior and encourages the interviewer to avoid directly eliciting ratings from the respondent on the individual item stems but rather instructs the interviewer complete the item ratings at the end of the interview with the respondent. The Interview Form has two versions: Comprehensive Form (502 items) or Domain-level Form (195 items). According to the Vineland-3 User's

Manual, the time of administration is 25 minutes for the Domain-level Form (195 items) and 40 minutes for the Comprehensive Form (502 items).

- Parent/Caregiver Form (0–90 years old): This form is completed directly by the parent or caregiver much like a rating scale. The respondent rates the assessed person's performance on each of the adaptive skill items. The Parent/Caregiver Form has two versions: Comprehensive Form (502 items; identical items that are included on the Interview Form) or Domain-level Form (180 items). The Vineland-3 User's Manual lists the time of administration for the Domain-level Form at 15 minutes and the Comprehensive Form at 40 minutes.
- Teacher Form (3–21 years old): Similar to the Parent/Caregiver Form, the Teacher Form is completed directly by the teacher, teacher's aide, or a daycare staff member who assesses the student's observed performance on each of the adaptive skill items. The Teacher Form also consists of two forms: (1) Comprehensive Form (333 items) and (2) Domain-Level Form (149 items). The Vineland-3 User's Manual reports the administration time for the Teacher Form: Domain-Level version (149 items) at approximately 10 minutes and the Teacher Form: Comprehensive version (333 items) necessitating approximately 25 minutes to complete.

The Vineland-3 domains are slightly different from the other comprehensive standardized scales (e.g., ABAS-3, ABDS, and DABS) and not consistent with the recommended domains in the AAIDD (Schalock et al., 2021) and DSM-5 (American Psychiatric Association, 2013).

The Vineland-3 provides its items and standard scores (mean = 100 and standard deviation = 15) aggregated across the following four domains: daily living skills, communication, socialization, and motor skills (optional domain for children under 6 years old). These Vineland-3 domain names are the same domain names used in original Vineland scale, and the authors have chosen to maintain these domain names despite their lack of alignment with the current tripartite model of adaptive behavior (conceptual, social, and practical) used by the existing diagnostic systems (e.g., AAIDD, *DSM-5*).

The Vineland-3 has robust and representative norms of the general population. It has good to excellent psychometric properties, including internal consistency, score stability as measured by test–retest reliability, and inter-respondent concordance (Pepperdine & McCrimmon, 2017). Sparrow et al. (2016) reported excellent internal consistency coefficients across all domains, with Cronbach alphas ranging from 0.90 to 0.98. The test–retest reliability of the Vineland-3 scores ranged from $r = 0.80$ to 0.92 for the adaptive behavior composite standard score. Inter-respondent concordance was reported at $r = 0.79$ for the adaptive behavior composite and ranging from 0.70 to 0.81 for the different domains.

1.3.5 Other Means and Measures

An important source of information about a person's skills and functional abilities can be obtained from direct observations of the person or via semi-structured clinical interviews with people who have lived with, worked with, or had the opportunity to observe the person on a regular basis and seen how they function at home, school, work, and/or play. These semi-structured interviews do not need to be based on a standardized measure and can consist of tailored questions that focus on the skill areas of interest or at the center of an intervention (e.g., self-care, cooking, home living skills, money concepts, work skills, social skills).

There exists also a number of school, medical, or other personal records that might provide valuable information, either as a primary source or as a supplemental use, to corroborate adaptive behavior or functional skills information obtained through other means. These records include social and family history, medical records, school performance, individual education plans, educational, psychological, or neuropsychological evaluations, work records, social security administration evaluations, etc.

There are a number of other comprehensive standardized measures that are more focused on specific adaptive skills or functional skills that can provide useful information about a person's skill levels. These can also serve well to inform on specific skill or domain areas. Following are a couple of good examples of such instruments.

1.3.6 Social Skills Improvement System: Rating Scales

The *Social Skills Improvement System: Rating Scales* (SSIS; Gresham & Elliott, 2008) is a revision of the popular *Social Skills Rating System* (SSRS; Gresham & Elliott, 1990). The SSIS is a suite of rating scales that are used to measure the social skills as well as problem behaviors of children and adolescents between the ages of 3 and 18 years old. The SSIS is particularly focused on social skills and problem behavior that the authors have identified as especially relevant for school success (Doll & Jones, 2010).

The SSIS can be completed directly by student on a self-report form or completed by a third-party respondent (e.g., parent form or teacher form). Students, parents, and teachers provide an individual rating of the frequency and perceived importance of each social skill item. The student self-report form consists of 46 items, whereas the parent/teacher forms consist of 46 social skill items and an additional 33 items identifying problem behaviors for the parent to rate or 30 additional items identifying problem behaviors for the teacher to rate. The administration time of the SSIS ranges from 10 to 25 minutes.

The SSIS can be scored by hand or using a computerized scoring system. The scoring of the SSIS yields standard scores (mean = 100, standard deviation = 15) and a criterion-based evaluation (well-above average, above average, average, below average, well below average) across: social skills, problem behaviors, and academic competence (teacher ratings only). Perhaps the most practical information comes in the form of a series of suggested actions and interventions objectives derived from the results from the SSIS ratings.

In terms of psychometric properties for the SSIS, they are good (Crosy, 2011). The social skills assessment across all three forms provides practical and psychometrically sound information (Doll & Jones, 2010) and a useful screening tool to aide teachers in planning interventions targeting social skills (e.g., the accompanying intervention guide; Crosy, 2011; Lee-Farmer & Meikamp, 2010).

1.3.7 Texas Functional Living Scale

The *Texas Functional Living Scale* (TFLS; Cullum, Weiner, & Saine, 2009) is a brief performance-based individually administered screening measure that assesses independent living skills in the areas of time, money concepts and calculations, communication, and memory. The focus of the TFLS items is on the abilities that might be most impacted by age-related cognitive decline. Although initially developed to assess functional living skills in older adults with dementia, the FTLS was normed on a larger sample of the general population aged from 16 to 90 years old in the hopes of expanding its utility to include individuals across the lifespan with other disabilities (e.g., intellectual disability, traumatic brain injury, and schizophrenia; Lindsay-Glenn, 2010).

The TFLS consists of 24 items that are administered directly to the assessed person and requires either a verbal or written response. The total administration time requires less than 15 minutes. The TFLS yields t-scores (mean = 50, standard deviation = 10) which are typically more complicated for most practitioners to use and understand than the more traditional normative scores with a mean = 100 and a standard deviation = 15. The TFLS has shown some utility in identifying intervention goals as well as measuring treatment outcomes and effectiveness in the defined independent living skill areas that it assesses.

The psychometric properties of the TFLS are adequate for a screening instrument (Lindsay-Glenn, 2010; Strang, 2010). The internal consistency reliability ranges from 0.65 to 0.81 and reportedly good test score stability. Its validity evidence was measured using a comparison between the TFLS and the ABAS, second Edition. These correlation coefficients assessing its concurrent validity were in the range of 0.41–0.80. Overall, the range of skills assessed is limited but the TFLS has shown to be a useful screening tool that can inform on performance across the limited number of functional skills its measures: time, money and calculations, communication and memory (Lindsay-Glenn, 2010).

1.3.8 Teaching Adaptive Behavior

A person's level of adaptive behavior is an indicator of how well an individual typically functions in everyday life, which is also highly predictive of positive life outcomes and has important implications for intervention (Farley et al., 2009; Kanne et al., 2011). Teaching and promoting the acquisition of adaptive behavior should be an essential goal of any intervention. Gresham and colleagues have described the importance of social skills as academic enablers and problem behaviors as academic disablers (Gresham, 2015; Gresham & Elliott, 2008). The outcome of increasing a person's adaptive behavior will often lead to greater independence, personal autonomy, likelihood of being in an inclusive setting, self-direction, overall quality of life, as well as a reduced perception among laypeople that the person has a disability. The DSM-5 (American Psychiatric Association, 2013) embraced using the person's level of adaptive functioning as the determinant of severity of intellectual disability, because adaptive behavior is a better indicator of the person's overall functioning and intensity of needed supports. With the proper level of instruction and supports, people with intellectual disability can learn new adaptive skills throughout their life, and as a result, their overall functioning will generally improve (Schalock et al., 2021).

Henry Leland, a pioneer in the field of intellectual disability, once said that it was a person's adaptive behavior deficits that made others in their community take notice of them and identify them as a person with a disability. Once exited from school, one's intellectual functioning plays a lesser role than their adaptive functioning in predicting successful life outcomes. A good illustration of this is what was once called the "6-hour retarded student." These were students who, when in school, were identified as having an intellectual disability and received special education services but when out of school, they were seen by others in their neighborhood as a regular kid largely because of their adaptive behavior (President's Committee on Mental Retardation, 1970).

A fundamental assumption is that with proper instruction and supports, people with intellectual disability can and will learn new adaptive skills throughout their lifetime, and their functioning will improve (Schalock et al., 2021).

1.4 Summary and Conclusions

Adaptive behavior is a separate and independent construct of intellectual functioning and equally essential in making the determination of intellectual disability. Adaptive behavior is a complex construct that includes skills in domains such as conceptual, social, and practical skills. It is an important aspect of human functioning such that deficits in adaptive behavior are a core feature of a number of conditions. There are a number of robust and reliable assessment instruments available to assist clinicians in determining intervention goals geared at increasing adaptive skills. The presence of adaptive behavior has been shown to be associated with fewer challenging behaviors, enhanced opportunities across settings and throughout the lifespan as well as being related to improved overall quality of life. With person-centered interventions and supports, a person can learn and improve their adaptive skills and ability to meet the expectations and demands. Teaching and promoting the acquisition of adaptive behavior should be an essential goal of any intervention. It is important to remember that anyone can learn new adaptive behaviors and functional living skills, no matter their ability/disability level and these new skills, if selected appropriately, can contribute to improved functioning, enhanced independence, and overall quality of life.

References

Alexander, R. M. & Reynolds, M. R. (2020). The relation between intelligence and adaptive behavior: A meta-analysis. *School Psychology Review, 49*, 85–110. https://doi.org/10.1080/2372966X.2020.1717374.

American Psychiatric Association. (1968). *Diagnostic and statistical manual of mental disorders (2nd edition; DSM-II)*. Washington, DC: American Psychiatric Association.

American Psychiatric Association. (2013). *Diagnostic and statistical manual of mental disorders (5th edition; DSM-5)*. Arlington, VA: American Psychiatric Publishing.

Balboni, G., Tassé, M. J., Schalock, R. L., Borthwick-Duffy, S. A., Spreat, S., Thissen, D., Widaman, K. F., Zhang, D., & Navas, P. (2014). The Diagnostic Adaptive Behavior Scale: Evaluating its diagnostic sensitivity and specificity. *Research in Developmental Disabilities, 35*, 2884–2903.

Bruininks, R. H., Woodcock, R., Weatherman, R., & Hill, B. (1996). Scales of Independent Behavior—Revised. Chicago, IL: Riverside.

Binet, A., & Simon, T. (1905). Méthodes nouvelles pour le diagnostic du niveau intellectuel des anormaux. *L'Année Psychologique, 11*, 191–244. https://doi.org/10.3406/psy.1904.3675

Carpentieri, S., & Morgan, S. B. (1996). Adaptive and intellectual functioning in autistic and nonautistic retarded children. *Journal of Autism and Developmental Disorders, 26*, 611–620. https://doi.org/10.1007/BF02172350

Claes, C., van Hove, G., Vandevelde, S., van Loon, J., & Schalock, R. L. (2012). The influence of support strategies, environmental characteristics, and client characteristics on quality of life-related outcomes. *Research in Developmental Disabilities, 33*(1), 96–103. https://doi.org/10.1016/j.ridd.2011.08.024.

Coulter, W. A., & Morrow, H. W. (1978). A contemporary conception of adaptive behavior within the scope of psychological assessment. In W. A. Coulter & H. W. Morrow (Eds.), *Adaptive behavior: Concepts and measurements* (pp. 3–20). New York, NY: Grune and Stratton.

Crosy, J. W. (2011). Test review. *Journal of Psychoeducational Assessment, 29*, 292–296.

Cullum, C. M., Weiner, M. F., & Saine, K. C. (2009). *Texas functional living scale: Examiner's manual*. San Antonio, TX: Pearson Assessment.

De Bildt, A., Kraijer, D., Sytema, S., & Minderaa, R. (2005). The psychometric properties of the Vineland Adaptive Behavior Scales in children and adolescents with mental retardation. *Journal of Autism and Developmental Disorders, 35*, 53–62.

Developmental Disabilities Assistance and Bill of Rights Act (2000). Amendments of 2000, Pub. L. No. 106-402, 114 Stat. 1677-1740.

Dell'Armo, K. A., & Tassé, M. J. (2019). The role of adaptive behavior and parent expectations in predicting post-school outcomes for young adults with intellectual disability. *Journal of Autism and Developmental Disorders, 49*, 1638–1651. https://doi.org/10.1007/s10803-018-3857-6.

Doll, E. (1936). Preliminary standardization of the Vineland social maturity scale. *American Journal of Orthopsychiatry, 6*, 283–293.

Doll, B., & Jones, K. (2010). Test review of social skills improvement system rating scales. In R. A. Spies, J. F. Carlson, & K. F. Geisinger (Eds.), *The eighteenth mental measurements yearbook* (pp. 561–565) Retrieved from http://marketplace.unl.edu/buros/.

Farley, M. A., McMahon, W. M., Fombonne, E., Jenson, W. R., Miller, J., Gardner, M., … Coon, H. (2009). Twenty-year outcome for individuals with autism and average or near-average cognitive abilities. *Autism Research, 2*(2), 109–118.

Gresham, F. M. (2015). Evidence-based social skills interventions for students at risk for EBD. *Remedial and Special Education, 36*, 100–104.

Gresham, F. M., & Elliott, S. N. (1990). *Social skills rating system*. Minneapolis, MN: Pearson, Inc..

Gresham, F. M., & Elliott, S. N. (2008). *Social skills improvement system-rating scales*. Minneapolis, MN: Pearson Assessments.

Harrison, P. L. (1987). Research with adaptive behavior scales. *The Journal of Special Education, 21*(1), 37–68. https://doi.org/10.1177/002246698702100108.

Harrison, P. L., & Oakland, T. (2003). *Adaptive behavior assessment system second edition: Manual*. San Antonio, TX: Harcourt Assessment.

Harrison, P. L., & Oakland, T. (2015). *Adaptive behavior assessment system, third edition (ABAS-3): Manual*. San Antonio, TX: Harcourt Assessment.

Heber, R. (1959). A manual on terminology and classification in mental retardation: A monograph supplement. *American Journal of Mental Deficiency, 64*, 1–111.

Heber, R. (1961). A manual on terminology and classification in mental retardation: A monograph supplement. *American Journal of Mental Deficiency, 64*, 1–111.

Henington, C. (2017). Test review of the adaptive behavior assessment system. In J. F. Carlson, K. F. Geisinger, & J. L. Johnson (Eds.), *The twentieth mental measurement yearbook* (3rd ed.) Retrieved from http://marketplace.unl.edu/buros/.

Kanne, S. M., Gerber, A. J., Quirmbach, L. M., Sparrow, S. S., Cicchetti, D. V., & Saulnier, C. A. (2011). The role of adaptive behavior in autism spectrum disorders: Implications for functional outcome. *Journal of Autism Developmental Disorders, 41*, 1007–1018.

Keith, T. Z., Fehrman, P. G., Harrison, P. L., & Pottebaum, S. M. (1987). The relation between adaptive behavior and intelligence: Testing alternative explanations. *Journal of School Psychology, 25*, 31–43.

Lambert, N., Nihira, K., & Leland, H. (1993). *Adaptive behavior scale—School, 2nd edition (ABS-S: 2)*. Austin, TX: Pro-Ed.

Lee-Farmer, J., & Meikamp, J. (2010). Test review of social skills improvement system rating scales. In R. A. Spies, J. F. Carlson, & K. F. Geisinger (Eds.), The eighteenth mental measurements yearbook. Retrieved from http://marketplace.unl.edu/buros/.

Lindsay-Glenn, P. (2010). Test review of Texas functional living scale. In R. A. Spies, J. F. Carlson, & K. F. Geisinger (Eds.), *The eighteenth mental measurements yearbook*. Retrieved from http://marketplace.unl.edu/buros/.

Luckasson, R., Borthwick-Duffy, S., Buntinx, W. H. E., Coulter, D. L., Craig, E. M., Schalock, R. L., … Tassé, M. J. (2002). *Mental retardation: Definition, classification, and systems of supports* (10th ed.). Washington, DC: American Association on Mental Retardation.

McGrew, K. S. (2012). What is the typical IQ and adaptive behavior correlation? *IAP Applied Psychometrics 101 Brief Report # 11*. Retrieved on 4-13-2018 from http://www.iqscorner.com/search?q=adaptive+behavior.

Meyers, C. E., Nihira, K., & Zetlin, A. (1979). The measurement of adaptive behavior. In N. R. Ellis (Ed.), *Handbook of mental deficiency- Psychological theory and research* (2nd ed., pp. 215–253). Hillsdale, NJ: Erlbaum.

Nihira, K., Leland, H., & Lambert, N. (1993). *Adaptive behavior scale-residential and community, 2nd edition (ABS-RC: 2)*. Austin, TX: Pro-Ed.

Nota, L., Ferrari, L., Soresi, S., & Wehmeyer, M. (2007). Self-determination, social abilities and the quality of life of people with intellectual disability. *Journal of Intellectual Disability Research, 51*(11), 850–865.

Papazoglou, A., Jacobson, L. A., McCabe, M., Kaufmann, W., & Zabel, T. A. (2014). To ID or not to ID? Changes in classification rates of intellectual disability using DSM-5. *Mental Retardation, 52*(3), 165–174.

Papazoglou, A., Jacobson, L. A., & Zabel, T. A. (2013). More than intelligence: Distinct cognitive/behavioral clusters linked to adaptive dysfunction in children. *Journal of International Neuropsychological Society, 19*, 189–197. https://doi.org/10.1017/S1355617712001191

Pearson, N. A., Patton, J. R., & Mruzek, D. W. (2016). *Adaptive behavior diagnostic scale: Examiner's manual*. Austin, TX: PRO-ED.

Pepperdine, C. R., & McCrimmon, A. W. (2017). Test Description: Vineland Adaptive Behavior Scales (3rd Edition). *Canadian Journal of School Psychology 33*(2), 157–163. https://doi.org/10.1177/0829573517733845.

President's Committee on Mental Retardation. (1970). *The six-hour retarded child*. Washington, DC: US Government Printing Office.

Public Law 106-402. (2000, October). *Developmental disabilities assistance and bill of rights act: 106th United States Congress*. Washington, DC.

Reschly, D. J., Myers, T. G., & Hartel, C. R. (Eds.). (2002). *Mental retardation: Determining eligibility for social security benefits*. Washington, DC: National Academy Press.

Sabat, C., Tassé, M. J., & Tenorio, M. (2019). Adaptive behavior and intelligence in Down syndrome: An exploratory investigation. *Intellectual and Developmental Disabilities, 57*, 79–94. https://doi.org/10.1352/1934-9556-57.2.79

Scahill, L., Bearss, K., Lecavalier, L., Smith, T., Swiezy, N., Aman, M. G., … Levato, L. (2016). Effect of parent training on adaptive behavior in children with autism spectrum disorder and disruptive behavior: Results of a randomized trial. *Journal of the American Academy of Child & Adolescent Psychiatry, 55*(7), 602–609.

Scahill, L., McDougle, C. J., Aman, M. G., Johnson, C., Handen, B., … for the Research Units on Pediatric Psychopharmacology Autism Network. (2012). Effects of risperidone and parent training on adaptive functioning in children with a pervasive developmental disorders and serious behavioral problems. *Journal of the American Academy of Child & Adolescent Psychiatry, 51*, 136–146.

Schalock, R. L. (1999). The merging of adaptive behavior and intelligence: Implications for the field of mental retardation. In R. L. Schalock (Ed.), *Adaptive behavior and its measurement: Implications for the field of mental retardation* (pp. 43–59). Washington, DC: American Association on Mental Retardation.

Schalock, R. L., Buntinx, W. H. E., Borthwick-Duffy, S., Bradley, V., Craig, E. M., Coulter, D. L., … Yeager, M. H. (2010). *Intellectual disability: Definition, classification, and systems of supports* (11th ed.). Washington, DC: American Association on Intellectual and Developmental Disabilities.

Schalock, R. L., Luckasson, R., & Tassé, M. J. (2021). *Intellectual disability: Definition, diagnosis, classification, and systems of supports* (12th ed.). Washington, DC: American Association on Intellectual and Developmental Disabilities.

Scheerenberger, R.C. (1983). A history of mental retardation. Baltimore, MD: Paul H. Brookes.

Simões, C., Santos, S., Biscaia, R., & Thompson, J. (2016). Understanding the relationship between quality of life, adaptive behavior and support needs. *Journal of Developmental and Physical Disabilities, 28*(6), 849–870. https://doi.org/10.1007/s10882-016-9514-0

Sparrow, S. S., Cicchetti, D. V., & Saulnier, C. A. (2016). *Vineland adaptive behavior scales* (3rd ed.). Minneapolis, MN: Pearson Assessments.

Sternberg, R. J., Forsythe, G. B., Hedlund, J., Horvath, J., Snook, S., Williams, W. M., … Grigorenko, E. L. (2000). *Practical intelligence in everyday life*. New York, NY: Cambridge University Press.

Strang, J. M. (2010). Test review of Texas functional living scale. In R. A. Spies, J. F. Carlson, & K. F. Geisinger (Eds.), *The eighteenth mental measurements yearbook*. Retrieved from http://marketplace.unl.edu/buros/.

Takata, Y., Ansai, T., Soh, I., Nakamichi, I., Akifusa, S., Goto, K., … Sonoki, K. (2013). High-level activities of daily living and disease-specific mortality during a 12-year follow-up of an octogenarian population. *Clinical Interventions in Aging, 8*, 721–728.

Tassé, M. J., Balboni, G., Navas, P., Luckasson, R. A., Nygren, M. A., Belacchi, C., … Kogan, C. (2019). Identifying behavioral indicators for intellectual functioning and adaptive behavior for use in the ICD-11. *Journal of Intellectual Disability Research, 63*, 386–407. https://doi.org/10.1111/jir.12582

Tassé, M. J., Luckasson, R., & Schalock, R. L. (2016). The relation between intellectual functioning and adaptive behavior in the diagnosis of intellectual disability. *Intellectual and Developmental Disabilities, 54*(6), 381–390. https://doi.org/10.1352/1934-9556-54.6.381

Tassé, M. J., Schalock, R. L., Balboni, G., Bersani, H., Borthwick-Duffy, S. A., Spreat, S., … Zhang, D. (2012). The construct of adaptive behavior: Its conceptualization, measurement, and use in the field of intellectual disability. *American Journal on Intellectual and Developmental Disabilities, 117*, 291–303. https://doi.org/10.1352/1944-7558-117.4.291

Tassé, M. J., Schalock, R. L., Balboni, G., Bersani, H., Borthwick-Duffy, S. A., Spreat, S., … Zhang, D. (2017). *Diagnostic adaptive behavior scale: Manual*. Washington, DC: American Association on Intellectual and Developmental Disabilities.

Thorndike, E. L. (1920). Intelligence and its use. *Harper's Magazine, 140*, 227–335.

Tredgold, A. F. (1937). *Mental deficiency*. Baltimore, MD: Williams and Wilkins.

Witt, J. C., & Martens, B. K. (1984). Adaptive behavior: Tests and assessment issues. *School Psychology Review, 13*, 478–484.

Wu, T. C. (2017). Test review of the adaptive behavior assessment system. In J. F. Carlson, K. F. Geisinger, & J. L. Johnson (Eds.), *The twentieth mental measurement yearbook* (3rd ed.) Retrieved from http://marketplace.unl.edu/buros/

World Health Organization. (1992). *International statistical classification of diseases and related health problems, 10th Edition (ICD-10)*. Geneva, Switzerland: Author.

Zigler, E., Balla, D., & Hodapp, R. (1984). On the definition and classification of mental retardation. *American Journal of Mental Deficiency, 89*, 215–230.

Zigman, W. B., Schupf, N., Urv, T., Zigman, A., & Silverman, W. (2002). Incidence and temporal patterns of adaptive behavior change in adults with mental retardation. *American Journal on Mental Retardation, 107*, 161–174.

Zigman, W. B., Schupf, N., Urv, T. K., & Silverman, W. (2009). Adaptive behavior change and dementia in down syndrome: Case classification using the adaptive behavior scale. In *Neuropsychological assessments of dementia in Down syndrome and intellectual disabilities* (pp. 90–105). London, UK: Springer.

Chapter 2
Interventions to Support Feeding in People with Intellectual and Developmental Disabilities

Becky Penrod, Bryant C. Silbaugh, Scott V. Page, and Melissa Moseman

2.1 Eating and Feeding

Adequate nutritional intake is essential for physical growth and development, as well as sustaining life. Furthermore, eating, drinking, and other adaptive mealtime behaviors play a significant role in developing and maintaining relationships with friends and family. Eating and drinking are adaptive skills to the extent that they help the individual function independently in their environment (Farmer, Swineford, Swedo, & Thurm, 2018).

As typically developing children grow and contact changes in mealtime environments, more complex eating skills develop and adapt with repeated practice, progressing from liquid feeding to accepting, mouthing, and chewing a variety of increasingly higher textured solid foods. As viewed through a behavior analytic lens, increasingly higher textured foods acquire reinforcing properties and evoke a behavior chain beginning with mastication (Silbaugh, Swinnea, & Penrod, 2017). Mastication alternates with lateralization of the food to form a bolus. The formation of the bolus reinforces mastication and lateralization. The bolus also evokes a sequence of additional responses such as movement of the bolus to the pharynx (Rudolph & Link, 2002) and ultimately transfer of the bolus to the stomach. In the stomach, the post-ingestive effects of swallowing maintain the chain by producing or modulating private stimuli (Skinner, 1945) and altering the effects of external

B. Penrod (✉) · M. Moseman
Department of Psychology, California State University, Sacramento, Sacramento, CA, USA
e-mail: penrodb@csus.edu

B. C. Silbaugh
Empower Behavioral Health, San Antonio, TX, USA

S. V. Page
Utah State University, Logan, UT, USA

R. Lang, P. Sturmey (eds.), *Adaptive Behavior Strategies for Individuals with Intellectual and Developmental Disabilities*, Autism and Child Psychopathology Series, https://doi.org/10.1007/978-3-030-66441-1_2

terminal reinforcers (e.g., an empty plate) depending on the individual's learning history.

In contrast to eating, feeding refers to when an individual (i.e., feeder) evokes eating by preparing and presenting food to the child's mouth. One essential role of the feeder is to provide the child with the nourishment necessary for healthy development and well-being. Because children initially depend on effective feeders for successful eating, another essential role of the feeder is to ensure that the contingencies associated with eating are reinforcing. The latter of which is highly relevant to designing effective interventions for feeding problems. The emergence of increasingly complex mealtime skills of typically developing children ultimately learning to self-feed can be viewed as "progressive changes in interactions between the behavior of an individual and the people, objects, and events in the environment" (Bijou, 1993, p. 12). The emergence of the typical self-feeder across a variety of nutritive foods and drinks, settings, and people coincides with the development of, and their involvement in, mealtime routines (e.g., dinnertime) and rituals (e.g., birthday parties), and cultural practices around food and drink that provide stability in times of stress and transition, promote healthy and happy family functioning, social cohesion, interpersonal harmony, and feelings of belonging and closeness (Fiese et al., 2002).

When feeders provide frequent opportunities to practice eating a variety of foods, this facilitates not only the development of complex eating skills but preferences for a range of nutritive foods and liquids. Changes in food and drink preferences are produced through repeated taste exposure, Pavlovian pairing, and post-ingestive effects of foods (Birch, 1999). Ultimately, if the contingencies associated with the process of eating are reinforcing, children are more likely to continue to eat.

2.1.1 Picky Eating

Picky eating, occasionally skipping a meal, and changes in food preference are common transient characteristics of typically developing children who successfully transition to self-feeders across a wide variety of foods and fall outside the classification of a feeding disorder (Kerzner et al., 2015). A widely accepted definition of picky eating, also known as "fussy" eating, is lacking and prevalence estimates vary widely across cultures and instruments. Yet, it is useful still to characterize this pattern of behavior as consisting of avoidance of familiar and new foods, a lack of dietary variety, especially fruits and vegetables, and a strong preference for certain foods (Taylor, Wernimont, Northstone, & Emmett, 2015). When characterizing one's behavior as "picky eating" based on a lack of dietary variety, it is important to consider cultural norms in the part of the world where the individual lives as well as what is customary for the individual's family unit. That is, we might say dietary variety is limited when an individual refuses to eat meat, but this would only be true if the individual lives in a place where meat is abundantly available and widely consumed within their family unit. Typical feeding guidelines, which are believed to mitigate common picky eating, include eliminating distractions such as technology at mealtimes, modeling neutral or pleasant affect during the meal, limiting mealtime duration to 30 min, arranging for four to six meals and snacks per day with only water between meals, providing age-appropriate foods, gradually introducing new foods (8–15 times before expecting the child to enjoy and readily consume the food), reinforcing self-feeding, and tolerating a mess commensurate with the child's age (Kerzner et al.). However, it is important to note that some of these practices may not be easily adopted across cultures. For example, it is common for people in Southern Italy to enjoy a meal over the course of 90 min or more, in which case, recommending that meals be limited to 30 min may not be appropriate. Alternatively, we might simply recommend that foods be limited outside of scheduled mealtimes, allowing flexibility in the duration of mealtime and number of meals offered throughout the day to align with cultural and contextual norms.

2.1.2 Disabilities and Persistent Feeding Problems

Unfortunately for the large majority of children with developmental disorders (up to 89%; Ledford & Gast, 2006) or intellectual and developmental disabilities (IDD) (Gale, Eikeseth, & Rudrud, 2011) show picky eating; delays or deficits in the development of self-feeding skills; and co-morbid medical factors (e.g., gastroesophageal reflux disease; GERD) which tend to interact with respondent and operant mechanisms across mealtime experiences ultimately resulting in clinically significant feeding problems. Results of several studies have suggested that children with autism spectrum disorders (ASD) up to 12 years of age, in particular, demonstrate more problematic feeding, sometimes associated with gastrointestinal dysfunction, than children without ASD (Badalyan & Schwartz, 2012; Bandini et al., 2017). Common indicators of significant feeding problems include prolonged (e.g., exceeding cultural and contextual norms in duration), disruptive and stressful mealtimes, difficulties swallowing, sudden cessation of feeding after a traumatic event, failure to thrive, and failure to advance to higher textures. Ultimately, if the caregiver says there is a problem, there often is a problem (Kerzner et al., 2015). Significant feeding problems adversely affect the child's health and development (Kedesdy & Budd, 1998), decrease the quality of social interactions, negatively impact mealtime routines and rituals, and exacerbate chronic caregiver stress (Curtiss & Ebata, 2019).

2.1.3 A Continuum of Pediatric Feeding Disorders

Like picky eating, consensus on a precise definition of pediatric feeding disorders and a universally adopted diagnostic system are still lacking (Goday et al., 2019). Although a new diagnostic category, "Avoidant/Restrictive Food Intake Disorder" (ARFID) was recently established in the *Diagnostic and Statistical Manual of Mental Disorders, 5th Edition* (DSM-5; American Psychiatric Association, DSM 5 Task Force, 2013), distinguishing between feeding disorders (i.e., ARFID) and eating disorders (i.e., anorexia nervosa, bulimia nervosa, binge-eating disorder, rumination, pica), diagnostic criteria fail to address the heterogeneity of feeding disorders because the criteria exclude children who consume a highly limited variety of nutritive food and exhibit persistent inappropriate mealtime behavior (IMB) yet continue to maintain adequate growth and nutrition and exhibit normal energy levels.

Based on current trends in the literature, aligned with a highly prescriptive behavior analytic approach to assessment and treatment sensitive to the full continuum of pediatric feeding disorders, we conceptualize pediatric feeding disorders as clinically significant learned biobehavioral conditions characterized by medical, feeding skill, nutritional, and psychosocial factors (Goday et al., 2019) ranging in severity from food selectivity (i.e., moderate) to food refusal (i.e., severe) (Silbaugh et al., 2016). For the purposes of this chapter, we define mild cases of *food selectivity* (FS) as consumption of a limited variety of nutritive foods that are restricted by type, texture, or other food dimensions (e.g., color, brand) in the absence of biomedical factors that would necessitate medical intervention, such as nutritional deficiency and failure to thrive, and *food refusal* (FR) as the rejection of all or most foods or liquids requiring medical intervention to prevent or remediate nutritional and/or growth deficiencies, including placement of a gastrostomy tube or use of nutritionally complete oral supplements.

2.1.4 Common Behavioral Deficits and Excesses

Severe cases of FS and FR, including those which persist into adulthood may include co-morbid oral motor problems (e.g., Matson, Fodstad, & Boisjoli, 2008), self-feeding difficulties (e.g., Jenkins, LeBlanc, & Lambert, 2017; Mansell, Ashman, Macdonald, & Beadle-Brown, 2002), and IMB (e.g., Piazza et al., 2003). These problems can be broadly conceptualized as behavioral deficits and excesses, respectively.

2.1.4.1 Behavioral Deficits

Swallowing disorders, such as dysphagia and oral motor problems, have been well-documented among individuals with IDD (Ball et al., 2012; Matson et al., 2008). Exact oral motor deficits can be isolated to specific muscles (e.g., Obicularis oris, the muscle responsible for sealing of the lips), muscular groups, or broadly categorized as weaknesses in mouth and lip closure (e.g., pursing and suckling); tongue movement (e.g., thrusting, lateralizing, curling); and chewing (e.g., inability/lack of and incomplete). Of most concern, difficulty in preparing food for swallowing (e.g., chewing and tongue coordination) or in successfully moving the bolus from mouth to stomach can place individuals at increased risk of choking and aspiration (Matson et al.). Furthermore, poor motor control of the mouth and throat can also result in failure to advance texture (Troughton & Hill, 2001).

Difficulty completing the specific behaviors required to bring food to the mouth to feed one's self (i.e., self-feeding) constitute another class of deficits considered to be among one of the greatest areas of need for individuals with IDD (Matson et al., 2008). Deficits related to self-feeding include trouble preparing foods for delivery and using utensils such as a fork, spoon, knife, cup, or napkin (Mansell et al., 2002), which can negatively impact one's autonomy and result in social stigma.

2.1.4.2 Behavioral Excesses

Individuals with IDD may also demonstrate a number of excesses, often categorized as IMB (Piazza et al., 2003). Within the behavioral feeding literature IMB is a term used to describe several response topographies, including but not limited to: head turns, batting at the spoon, throwing food or utensils, negative vocalizations, self-injury, aggressive behavior, expulsion, packing, gagging, and vomiting. IMB was recently conceptualized as consisting of two general topographically defined response classes: (a) "developmentally inappropriate behavior other than oral motor behavior that prevents or delays the onset, pace, or completion of meals" (Silbaugh et al., 2016, p. 348) called *mealtime challenging behavior*, such as batting at the spoon or crying, and (b) "deficient or developmentally inappropriate oral motor behavior that disrupts chewing and/or swallowing food or liquids, or formation and ingestion of the bolus such as vomiting, packing, gagging, or expulsion" (Silbaugh et al., 2016, p. 348), called *disordered feeding*.

2.1.4.3 The Development and Maintenance of Feeding Problems

In addition to obstacles experienced during eating that may arise through a combination of medical and physical factors (Rommel, De Meyer, Feenstra, & Veereman-Wauters, 2003), feeding disorders may also develop or worsen as a result of environmental variables (Piazza, Milnes, & Shalev, 2015; Volkert, Patel, & Peterson, 2016), including caregiver–child interactions and environmental arrangements related to mealtime structure and routine. Specifically, an individual may acquire learned behaviors that have been previously reinforced by the removal of food and/or caregiver attention (Peterson & Ibañez, 2018). Previous research has demonstrated that IMBs are functionally related to escape or attention (Piazza et al., 2003). Likewise, caregiver responses to IMBs may be negatively reinforced when IMB ceases to occur contingent upon the caregiver removing nonpreferred foods and/or delivering attention. As a result of this interaction, caregivers may stop presenting nonpreferred foods because it enables them to avoid IMB.

Lack of mealtime structure (e.g., unrestricted access to food, irregular meals), continual exposure to developmentally inappropriate textures, or parental modeling of inappropriate eating habits (Sanders, Patel, Le Grice, & Shepherd, 1993) can also further influence the development and persistence of feeding problems. For example, grazing on food throughout the day and maintaining satiation with preferred foods can function as an abolishing operation, making food less reinforcing during mealtimes and abating consumption (Vollmer & Iwata, 1991). Furthermore, when a caregiver models refusal of a novel food, it is less likely that their child will subsequently accept that food (Berlin, Davies, Lobato, & Silverman, 2009).

2.1.5 *Evidence-Based Treatment*

Due to the complexity of pediatric feeding disorders (i.e., medical, feeding skill, nutritional, and psychosocial factors; Goday et al., 2019) an interdisciplinary approach to treatment is ideal (Silverman, 2010). However, because feeding problems are learned behaviors, they are likely to persist even after initial precipitating events have been addressed (Clawson & Elliott, 2014). Furthermore, the leading empirically supported approach to treating clinically significant feeding problems is behavioral intervention using applied behavior analysis (ABA; Silbaugh et al., 2016; Volkert & Piazza, 2012). As such, we focus the remainder of the chapter on behavior analytic interventions to address feeding disorders.

Although there are multiple current reviews of behavioral interventions for pediatric feeding disorders (Bachmeyer, 2009; Ledford & Gast, 2006; Marshall, Ware, Ziviani, Hill, & Dodrill, 2014; Matson & Fodstad, 2009; Seubert, Fryling, Wallace, Jiminez, & Meier, 2014; Sharp, Jaquess, Morton, & Herzinger, 2010; Silbaugh et al., 2016), none have examined variations in participant characteristics, study characteristics, and the certainty of the evidence supporting behavioral intervention for feeding problems across age groups. Thus, the purposes of the current chapter are: (a) to review recent behavioral intervention feeding research across the life span, and (b) suggest practice guidelines for using evidence-based practices in ABA to support feeding in individuals with IDD.

2.2 Method

2.2.1 *Search Procedures*

Articles for inclusion in the review were identified in a three-stage search and screening process. In the first stage, the first author searched Academic Search Complete, PsycINFO and the Cumulative Index of Nursing and Allied Health Literature (CINAHL) Plus with Full Text through the Sacramento State University Library to identify peer-reviewed journal articles written in English and published between 2008 and 2018. The search terms entered into the database search fields were: food refusal, or food selectivity, or feeding problem, not eating disorder; and intellectual disability, or developmental disability, or autism, or autism spectrum disorder; and behavioral intervention, or applied behavior analysis, or feeding therapy, or treatment. Initially, the search yielded 147 articles. After exact duplicates were removed, 90 articles remained, of which only empirical studies evaluating behavior analytic treatments focused on problems related to feeding occurring in the context of a mealtime, using a within-subject research design, and including one or more participants with IDD, learning disability, or ASD were included in the review. Articles for inclusion were determined by both the first and second author scanning titles and abstracts and 26 studies were retained. After data extraction began, one study was excluded due to the absence of procedural detail sufficient to enable coding. Thus, a total of 25 studies from this initial search were included.

In the second stage, the first author conducted a second search using the same databases listed above to identify additional peer-reviewed empirical studies evaluating interventions for adolescents and adults. The search terms were: feeding problems, or food refusal, or food selectivity; and adults, or adolescents, or young adults; and intellectual disability, or developmental disability, or autism, or autism spectrum disorder. The search yielded an initial 26 results, of which two additional studies were included after titles and abstracts were scanned by the first and second author to identify articles meeting inclusion criteria.

In the final stage, we scanned the titles of all references of included studies for additional studies meeting our inclusion criteria. We identified eight additional studies, the titles of which were then entered into Google Scholar. For each of the eight additional studies, we reviewed titles and abstracts of citing studies listed in Google Scholar which resulted in the identification of 15 additional studies that were included in the review. Thus, a total of 50 studies were included in the review (i.e., 27 from electronic databases; 8 from review of references of included studies; and 15 from Google Scholar). Studies included in this review are denoted by an asterisk in the reference section.

2.2.2 *Inclusion and Exclusion Criteria*

We included studies that: (a) evaluated a behavior analytic intervention; (b) addressed any problem related to feeding that occurs in the context of a mealtime; (c) utilized a single subject research design and included a graphical display of data; and (d) included at least one participant with a developmental disability, intellectual disability, learning disability, or ASD. We excluded studies that: (a) addressed problems that occur independent of mealtimes (e.g., rumination, operant vomiting), or (b) used an A-B or sequential design with no replication.

2.2.3 *Data Extraction and Interobserver Agreement*

A coding guide developed by the first and second authors was used to extract data on participant and study characteristics. Participant information included: (a) total number of participants in the study; (b) type of diagnoses represented; (c) number of participants across infant, toddler, preschool, school-age, adolescent, and adult age groups; (d) reported skill sets (e.g., language, IQ, and imitation skills); (e) reported medical conditions of a physical nature other than developmental delays (e.g.,

GERD, congenital heart failure, and dysphagia); (f) feeding and mealtime problems and feeding-related diagnoses (e.g., FS, FR, ARFID, packing, gagging, expulsion, chewing and swallowing problems, inappropriate volume [too much or too little], and IMB); (g) sex; (h) ethnicity; (i) bodyweight status; (j) dietary information; and (k) treatment history specific to feeding and mealtime problems. Study characteristics included: (a) setting; (b) interobserver agreement; (c) treatment integrity; (d) dependent variables; (e) pretreatment assessments; (f) intervention agent(s); (g) maintenance; (h) generalization; (i) social validity data; (j) certainty of evidence; (k) treatment components and parameters of treatment (e.g., treatment package, component analysis, and comparative analysis), and (l) effective treatment conditions.

Interobserver agreement (IOA) was calculated by dividing the number of agreements by the total number of agreements plus disagreements then multiplying by 100 to obtain a percentage. For most coded variables, an agreement was recorded only if there was exact correspondence between the first and second author. For example, for the number of participants in each age group, the same number had to be recorded for all six age groups for that section of the coding guide to be counted as an agreement. For sections of the coding guide that had several line items (i.e., feeding and mealtime problems; pretreatment assessments; certainty of evidence; and treatment components and parameters of treatment), each line item was counted as an agreement if there was exact correspondence between the first and second author.

For each study, mean IOA was determined separately for each coding guide section (i.e., participant information and study characteristics). Mean IOA scores were then summarized across studies and divided by the total number of studies to yield an overall mean IOA score for participant information and study characteristics. After IOA was calculated for each study, the first and second author compared and discussed data until reaching 100% agreement. Mean IOA before complete agreement reached was 85.5% (range, 71–100%) for participant information, and 88.2% (range, 71–98%) for study characteristics.

2.2.4 Classification of Certainty of Evidence

Following procedures described by Verschuur, Didden, Lang, Sigafoos, and Huskens (2014), certainty of evidence from each study was classified as suggestive, preponderant, or conclusive. Certainty of evidence was classified as: (a) *suggestive* if the study did not evaluate the intervention using an experimental design (e.g., used an A-B design only) and/or did not meet the other criteria to be classified as preponderant; (b) *preponderant* if the study used an experimental design, had adequate IOA and treatment fidelity data (i.e., measured at least 30% of sessions with at least 80% agreement and fidelity), included operational definitions for dependent variables, and provided sufficient details for replication; or, (c) *conclusive* if the study included all of the attributes of a preponderant classification and also provided at least some control for alternative explanations for treatment outcomes (i.e., threats to internal validity can be ruled out by the design).

2.3 Results

We begin by providing an overarching view of the synthesized literature and conclude by reporting results aggregated by age group to: (a) more directly address the question of what the research reveals about the effects of behavioral interventions on feeding problems for each age group, and, (b) promote practitioners' access to relevant information in their search for the best available evidence in the evidence-based practice of ABA when treating feeding problems.

We report the results in terms of studies, participants, and experiments based on the dependent variable on which we report so as to maintain precision and highlight the most important findings. We use the term "study" to refer to individual articles as some studies consisted of multiple experiments.

2.3.1 Participant Characteristics

The studies included a total of 86 participants with IDD, learning disabilities, or ASD. Over the past decade, the rate at which researchers published behavioral interventions in these populations steadily increased. Figure 2.1 shows that researchers evaluated behavioral interventions in preschool-age children at a faster rate than all other age groups, and almost no participants were adolescents or adults. Specifically, there were no infants (0–1-year-old), one participant was an adult, three were adolescents (12–17-years-old), 13 were toddlers (1–3-years-old), 24 were school age (6–12-years-old), and 46 were preschool age (3–6-years-old). Most participants (N = 66; 77%) were male. Most experiments did not report participants' ethnicity (N = 49; 94%) or bodyweight (N = 40; 75%). Forty percent of all experiments (N = 21) described participants' skills in more (e.g., "Anna could communicate verbally, was able to make requests, and followed single-step and multiple-step instructions..." Knox, Rue, Wildenger, Lamb, & Luiselli, 2012, p. 409) or less detail (e.g., "He was ambulatory and communicated with gestures and cards"; Groff, Piazza, Zeleny, & Dempsey, 2011, p. 950). However, there is an increasing trend toward researchers describing participants' skill level (e.g., low-to-average cognitive and language abilities, followed a visual schedule, communicated with gestures and cards, engaged in conversation, followed complex instructions, self feeder, etc.). Twenty-seven (52%) experiments reported information about participants' medical conditions (i.e., presence or lack thereof; e.g., asthma, dysphagia, gastrostomy tube, GERD). Information regarding participants' diet prior to intervention was reported by 44 experiments (85%), but only 31 experiments (60%) specified foods or liquids the participants consumed prior to intervention. Most experiments (N = 30; 58%) did not report participants' feeding treatment history prior to intervention.

To derive meaning from data on feeding problem characteristics, we compiled a set of the most commonly recognized feeding problems in the literature and then calculated the percentage of experiments in which researchers described each characteristic feeding problem. We display the results of this analysis in Fig. 2.2. We

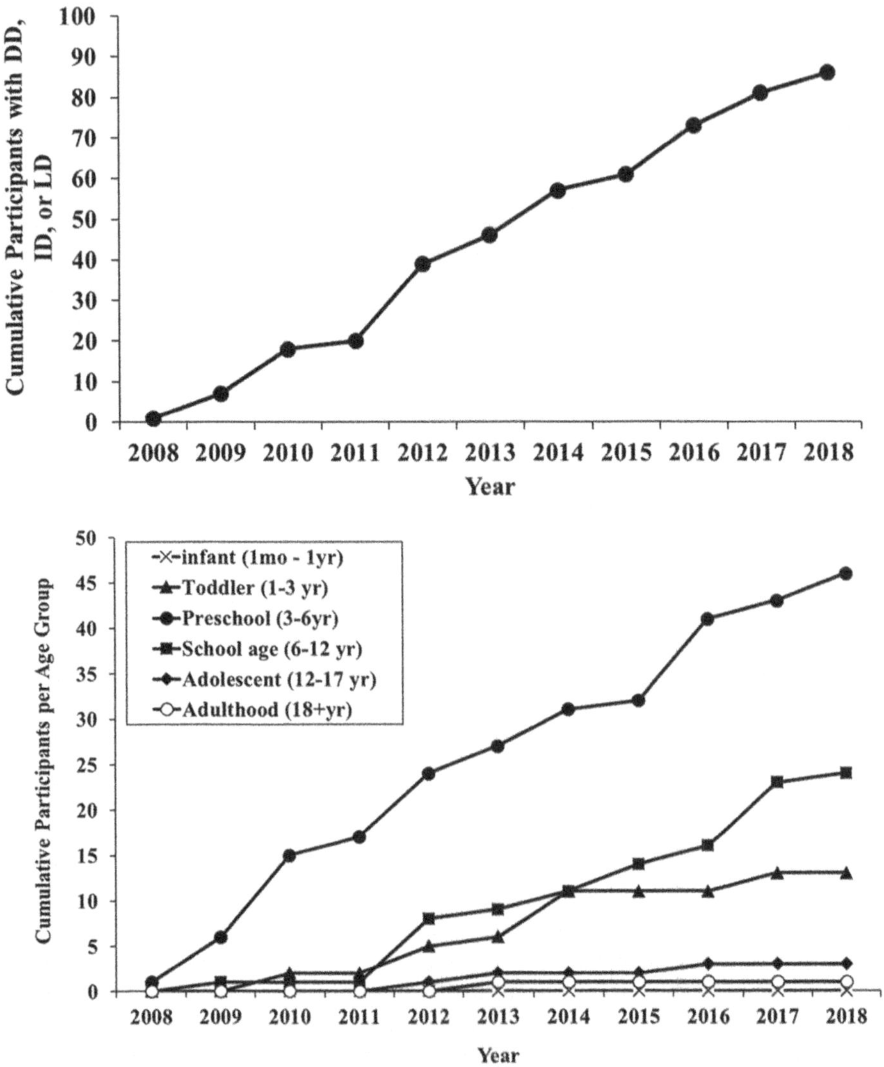

Fig. 2.1 The cumulative number of participants with developmental, intellectual, learning disabilities, or ASD (top), and the cumulative number of participants per age group (bottom)

identified at least 22 different feeding problems (excluding the classifications of FS, FR, and ARFID) and the five most frequently reported feeding problems, in order of most-to-least frequent, were IMB ($N = 48$; 92%), expulsion ($N = 27$; 52%), packing ($N = 17$; 33%), gagging ($N = 16$; 31%), and vomiting ($N = 15$; 29%). However, authors did not necessarily intervene on, measure, or otherwise assess all of the feeding problem characteristics reported. The five feeding problem characteristics that were most commonly measured for the purpose of conducting treatment evaluation, in order of most-to-least frequent, were IMB ($N = 22$; 42%), expulsion ($N = 12$; 23%), packing ($N = 8$; 15%), food volume ($N = 6$; 12%), and gagging ($N = 4$; 8%).

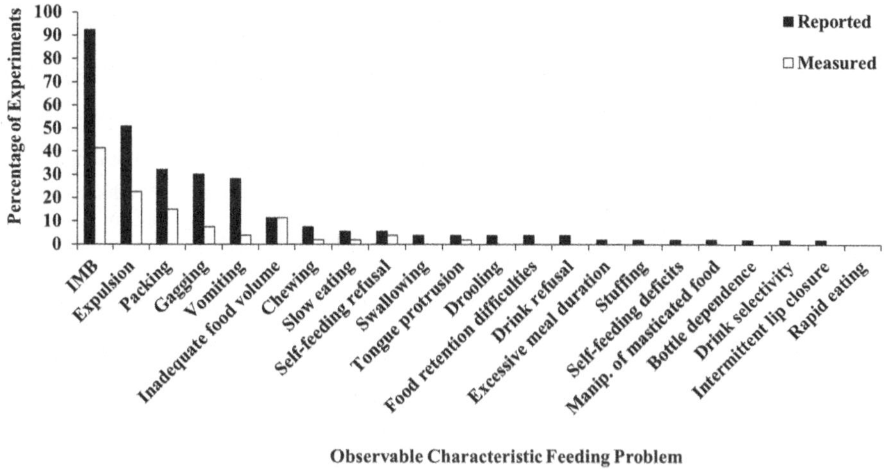

Fig. 2.2 The percentage of experiments (i.e., not participants or studies) in which researchers described each characteristic feeding problem

2.3.2 *Study Characteristics*

For the purpose of this chapter, we have limited our summary to the treatment components that were evaluated, and those study characteristics that directly impacted classification of evidential certainty.

Researchers evaluated at least 51 different treatment components, summarized in Table 2.1. Most experiments ($N = 51$; 98%) reported IOA. Of those experiments, mean IOA exceeded 90% for all dependent variables for 48 experiments (92%) and no experiments reported mean IOA below 80%. Most experiments assessed IOA based on 30% or more of sessions for all participants and conditions ($N = 34$; 65%). A minority of experiments ($N = 22$; 42%) reported treatment fidelity. For 22 of those experiments, researchers reported mean treatment fidelity of 90% or higher but researchers assessed treatment fidelity based on 30% or more of sessions for each condition and all participants for only 14 (61%) experiments.

Classification of evidential certainty indicated that 51 experiments (98%) used an experimental design (i.e., we determined that experiment 1 in Rivas et al., 2014 did not use an experimental design but we opted to include this experiment in our analysis because Experiment 2 did use an experimental design), 16 (31%) reported greater than 80% mean IOA and fidelity assessed based on at least 30% of sessions, 51 (98%) experiments provided operational definitions of dependent variables, 49 (94%) experiments provided sufficient details for replication of intervention procedures, and 38 (73%) experiments used a design that provided strong controls against alternative explanations for treatment outcomes. The average level of evidential certainty was 1.5 (i.e., between suggestive and preponderant). The evidential certainty was classified as suggestive for 36 (69%) experiments due largely to underreporting IOA and treatment fidelity, preponderant for five (9%) experiments, and conclusive for 11 (21%) experiments.

Table 2.1 Number of experiments that evaluated intervention components in isolation or as part of a treatment package, listed from most-to-least replications; for evidential certainty, *S* suggestive, *P* preponderant, *C* conclusive, numbers in parentheses indicate total number of experiments with that classification.

Intervention component	Experiments	Evidential certainty	FR/FS/ Both	Age range
DRA	30	S (18)/ P (4)/ C (8)	Both[a]	Toddler ➔ Adult
NRS	24	S (19)/ P (4)/ C (1)	Both	Toddler ➔ Adolescent
Representation	21	S (14)/ P (2)/ C (5)	Both	Toddler ➔ School age
Rules	10	S (6)/ P (2)/ C (2)	FS[a]	Toddler ➔ Adolescent
Demand fading	8	S (4)/ P (1)/ C (3)	FS	Toddler ➔ Adult
NCR	8	S (7)/ C (1)	Both	Toddler ➔ Preschool
Bite presentation (i.e., flipped spoon or upright spoon)	6	S (6)	Both	Toddler ➔ School age
Nonremoval of the cup	6	S (3)/ P (1)/ C (2)	Both	Toddler ➔ School age
Bite fading	5	S (3)/ P (1)/ C (1)	Both	Toddler ➔ School age
Antecedent choice	3	S (2)/ P (1)	Both	Preschool ➔ school age
High-probability instructional sequence	3	S (2)/ C (1)	FS	Preschool ➔ Adolescent
Nonremoval of the meal	3	S (2)/ C (1)	FS	Preschool ➔ School age
Positive practice	3	S (2)/ C (1)	Both	Toddler ➔ School age
Redistribution	3	S (2)/ C (1)	Both	Toddler ➔ Preschool
Apparatus fading	2	S (1)/ P (1)	FR	Toddler ➔ Preschool
Attention extinction	2	S (2)	Both	Preschool
Chaser	2	S (2)	Both	Preschool ➔ School age
Lag schedule of differential positive and negative reinforcement	2	C (2)	FS	Preschool
Modeling	2	S (1)/ C (1)	FS	School age

(continued)

Table 2.1 (continued)

Intervention component	Experiments	Evidential certainty	FR/FS/ Both	Age range
Reduction in response requirements (i.e., bite size and type manipulations)	2	S (1)/ C (1)	FS	Preschool ➔ school age
Stimulus fading	2	S (2)	FR	Preschool
Verbal or physical prompts	2	S (1)/ P (1)	FS[a]	School age ➔ adult
Visual schedule	2	S (2)	FS	Preschool ➔ adult
Avoidance procedure (extra bites of NPF contingent on refusal)	1	C	FS	Preschool
Backward chaining	1	C	FS	Preschool
Blending	1	S	FR	Preschool
Cup distance fading	1	S	FS	School age
Descriptive chew prompts	1	S	FR	Adolescent
DNRA	1	S	FS	School age
EE (hand-over-hand to self- feed)	1	C	FS	Preschool
Extinction of disruptive behavior	1	S	FS	Toddler ➔ preschool
Food type manipulation	1	S	FS	Toddler
LTM prompting	1	C	FS	Preschool
Modeling contingencies	1	C	FS	School age
Multiple bite instructions	1	P	[a]	School age
Mystery motivator	1	S	FS	Preschool
Nonremoval of the bottle	1	P	FR	Toddler
Nonremoval of the bite	1	C	FS	Preschool
Nonremoval of the fork	1	S	FS	Preschool
Nonremoval of the straw	1	S	Both	Preschool ➔ school age
Nonremoval of the strip	1	S	FR	Preschool
Nonremoval of the tube	1	S	FR	Preschool
Paced prompting	1	C	FS	Adolescent
Pre-session EO manipulation	1	C	FS	School age
Pre-session food or liquid deprivation	1	S	Both	Preschool ➔ school age
Reinforcer magnitude manipulation	1	P	FS	Preschool
Response blocking	1	C	FS	Preschool
Schedule thinning	1	P	FS	Preschool
Swallow facilitation	1	S	FR	Preschool
Texture fading	1	S	FS	Preschool
Volume fading	1	C	FR	School age

DNRA - Differential negative Reinforcement of Alternative Behavior
EE - environmental enrichment
LTM - least to most
EO - Establishing operation
S suggestive, *P* preponderant, *C* conclusive
Numbers in parentheses indicate total number of experiments with that classification
[a]Indicates one or more experiments that evaluated the intervention component for a feeding problem other than food refusal (FR) or food selectivity (FS)

2.3.3 Results Aggregated by Age Group

For each age group, we report participant and treatment characteristics of all experiments that contained participants from a target age group. Some experiments included participants from more than one age group.

2.3.3.1 Toddler

Most toddlers exhibited FS, and the most frequent feeding problem characteristics reported were IMB, packing, gagging, expulsion, and vomiting. Other characteristics included chewing problems, swallowing problems, inadequate food volume, self-feeding problems, food retention difficulties, and tongue protrusion. The most common dependent variables used to evaluate the effects of treatment were IMB, expulsion, packing, self-feeding, and food volume. The highest level of certainty provided by studies that included toddlers was preponderant (Alaimo, Seiverling, Anderson, & Sturmey, 2018; Najdowski et al., 2010) and the interventions in both studies were treatment packages. We classified two studies as preponderant, and the remaining studies as suggestive. In Alaimo et al.'s, 2018 study, consumption, IMB, and grams of the target food consumed were most improved coinciding with a treatment package consisting of apparatus fading, differential reinforcement of alternative behavior (DRA), and escape extinction (EE) using nonremoval of the spoon (NRS) with representation of expulsions. In Najdowski et al., bites swallowed and IMB were most improved coinciding with a treatment package consisting of DRA, NRS, and demand fading.

2.3.3.2 Preschool

Most preschool-age children exhibited FS, and the most frequent feeding problem characteristics reported were IMB, packing, gagging, expulsion, and vomiting. Other characteristics included inadequate volume, swallowing difficulties, slow eating, food retention, tongue protrusion, and chewing difficulties. The most common dependent variables used to evaluate treatment effects were IMB, packing, gagging, expulsion, and food volume. The highest level of evidential certainty provided by studies that included preschool-age children was conclusive (Hodges et al., 2018; Kozlowski, Taylor, Pichardo, & Girolami, 2016; Peterson, Piazza, & Volkert, 2016; Seiverling, Williams, Sturmey, & Hart, 2012; Silbaugh & Falcomata, 2017; Silbaugh, Wingate, & Falcomata, 2017; Wood, Wolery, & Kaiser, 2009). We classified seven studies as conclusive, two studies as preponderant, and the remaining studies as suggestive.

In Hodges et al. (2018), IMB and appropriate mealtime behavior were most improved coinciding with a treatment package consisting of DRA, demand fading,

EE with a three-step prompting hierarchy, and nonremoval of the bite and rules. In Kozlowski et al. (2016), acceptance and IMB were most improved coinciding with a treatment package consisting of DRA and nonremoval of the cup. In Peterson et al. (2016), acceptance, mouth clean, IMB, and grams consumed were most improved coinciding with a treatment package consisting of DRA, noncontingent reinforcement, and NRS with either: (a) representation of expulsions alone, (b) with redistribution, or, (c) with an avoidance procedure and backward chaining. In Seiverling et al. (2012), acceptance, disruptive behavior, and bites during probe meals were most improved coinciding with a treatment package consisting of bite fading, nonremoval of the meal, and DRA. In Silbaugh and Falcomata (2017), independent variant consumption and the number of foods consumed within sessions were most improved coinciding with a lag schedule of positive reinforcement with preferred items. In Silbaugh et al. (2017), independent variant consumption and the number of different foods consumed within session were most improved coinciding with a treatment package consisting of a lag schedule of differential negative reinforcement established with response blocking. In Wood et al. (2009), consumption, rejection, gagging, and escape were most improved coinciding with a treatment package of DRA and EE using hand-over-hand guidance to evoke self-feeding.

2.3.3.3 School Age

Most school-age children exhibited FS, and the most frequent feeding problem characteristics reported were IMB, packing, gagging, expulsion, and vomiting. Other characteristics included inadequate food volume, drink selectivity or refusal to drink or self-feed, and excessive mealtime duration. The most common dependent variables used to evaluate treatment effects were IMB, packing, gagging, and expulsion. The highest level of evidential certainty provided by studies that included school-age children was conclusive (Fu et al., 2015; Penrod, Gardella, & Fernand, 2012; Peterson, Volkert, & Milnes, 2017; Seiverling et al., 2012). We classified four studies as conclusive, all of which were treatment packages, two studies as preponderant, and the remaining studies as suggestive. In Fu et al., the percentage of bites consumed was most improved coinciding with a treatment package consisting of rules, modeling DRA, and modeling NRS plus DRA. In Penrod et al., the percentage of compliance with low-probability instructions and percentage of bites consumed was most improved coinciding with a treatment package consisting of demand fading combined with high-probability instructions, model prompts, and DRA. In Peterson et al., self-fed acceptance and IMB were most improved coinciding with a treatment package consisting of nonremoval of the cup with hand-over-hand physical guidance, representation of expulsions, practice trials, and volume fading. In Seiverling et al., bite and drink consumption, IMB, and total grams consumed were most improved coinciding with a treatment package consisting of NRS with representation and DRA.

2.3.3.4 Adolescent

Two studies included adolescents with FS, one with FR. The most frequent feeding problem characteristics reported were IMB, packing, and chewing difficulties. The highest level of evidential certainty provided by studies that included adolescents was conclusive (Knox et al., 2012). The remaining two studies were classified as suggestive. In Knox et al., the participant was a 16-year-old girl with a diagnosis of ASD who was underweight for her age. The most improvements in the percentage of lunch meal consumed coincided with a treatment package consisting of DRA, demand fading, and paced prompting.

2.3.3.5 Adulthood

Only one study evaluated a behavioral intervention in an adult (Barahona, DuBard, Luiselli, & Kesterson, 2013). The participant was an 18-year-old female with FS and a history of problem feeding behavior who exhibited an excessively slow meal pace. We classified the evidential certainty provided by the intervention as suggestive, and the most improvement in consumption coincided with a treatment package consisting of demand fading, a visual schedule, DRA, verbal prompts, and planned ignoring for IMB.

2.4 Discussion

In summary, most experiments were conducted with preschool-age children followed by school-age children and then toddlers. The prominent reported feeding problem characteristics across all three of these age groups were FS, IMB, packing, gagging, expulsion, and vomiting. Eleven experiments were classified as conclusive, including seven experiments with preschool children, four with school-age children, and one with an adolescent (note that one experiment [Seiverling et al., 2012] included participants across two different age groups). All experiments with conclusive evidential certainty evaluated a treatment package. Across the 11 experiments classified as conclusive, the treatment components most frequently demonstrated to improve feeding (i.e., consumption or other mealtime behavior) were: (a) DRA; (b) EE (nonremoval of the spoon, bite, cup, or meal; three-step prompting; hand-over-hand guidance); and, (c) fading procedures (demand, bite, or volume fading).

In the preschool-age group, DRA was used across all experiments classified as conclusive, and EE was used in the majority (5/7) of experiments in the form of three-step prompting with nonremoval of the bite, nonremoval of the cup, NRS, nonremoval of the meal, or hand-over-hand guidance. Fading procedures (bite and demand fading) were only used in two experiments.

In school-age children and adolescents (the majority of experiments) classified as conclusive utilized DRA (4 of 5 experiments) and fading procedures including bite, volume, and demand fading (4 of 5 experiments), whereas EE was used in only two experiments in the form of nonremoval of the cup with hand-over-hand physical guidance and nonremoval of the meal.

These results are consistent with findings of Silbaugh et al. (2016). In a synthesis of behavioral interventions for food selectivity specifically, Silbaugh et al. found that DRA, EE (including NRS), and fading procedures (stimulus and demand fading) were among the most frequently replicated treatment components. Thus, the authors suggested that these treatment components be utilized first, either simultaneously or sequentially, prior to considering other treatment components with fewer replications. In the current review, we attempted to elucidate the evidence-base for behavioral feeding interventions across age groups. Considering the experiments with conclusive evidence, our findings suggest that DRA is consistently used in treatment packages to address feeding problems irrespective of age group, whereas EE procedures are more frequently used with pre-school children and fading procedures are more frequently used with school-age children and adolescents.

2.5 Recommendations

Based on this systematic review and previous reviews, we make the following five practice recommendations.

Recommendation 1. We recommend that practitioners start with DRA and EE when working with preschool-age children.

Recommendation 2. We recommend practitioners start with DRA combined with a fading procedure such as bite or demand fading and only introduce EE if necessary when working with school-age children or adolescents.

Researchers demonstrated a variety of ways that EE-based procedures can be adapted to match participant characteristics thereby potentially increasing the likelihood that the intervention is relevant, consistent with client values and context, and efficiency and effectiveness are maximized. In the preschool-age group, of the five conclusive experiments that utilized EE, a traditional nonremoval of the bite, spoon, or cup procedure was used most frequently (3 of 5 experiments); one experiment utilized nonremoval of the meal and one study used hand-over-hand guidance. Of the two conclusive experiments that utilized EE in the school-age and adolescent age groups, nonremoval of the cup *with* hand-over-hand physical guidance and nonremoval of the meal were applied. Furthermore, of the conclusive experiments that utilized EE in the form of a nonremoval of the bite, cup, or spoon procedure, two out of four experiments included representation of expulsions.

Recommendation 3. We recommend that when using EE practitioners select procedural variations based on age, self-feeding skills, tolerance of physical prompts, and the intensity or presence of certain forms of IMB (i.e., *active* versus *passive refusal behaviors;* Penrod et al., 2012*). For example, for younger children who do not self-feed, NRS may be the most obvious choice. For an older child who* *self-feeds, engages in passive refusal behaviors (*e.g., *does not respond to bite presentations in the absence of IMB; Penrod* et al.*), and tolerates physical prompts, hand-over-hand physical guidance may be appropriate. Finally, for an older child who self-feeds, engages in active refusal behaviors (*i.e., *IMB), and does not tolerate physical prompting, nonremoval of the meal may be the best option.*

When implementing EE in the form of a nonremoval of the bite, cup, or spoon procedure, practitioners should also consider whether to include a representation component. Re-presentation of expulsions may facilitate acceptance and consumption both by minimizing escape and providing increased opportunity for the child to practice managing and retaining the bolus in their mouth (Piazza et al., 2015). Other variations of nonremoval procedures that practitioners should consider include the frequency and rate of bite or drink presentations, session duration, and the manner in which bites or drinks are deposited into the child's mouth (Fernand, Saksena, Penrod, & Fryling, 2017). Commonly, a fixed number of bites are presented on a fixed-time (FT) schedule (e.g., FT-30s; Allison et al., 2012) and sessions continue until all bites have been presented or a cut-off time has been reached (e.g., "The session continued until the child consumed all five bites or 10 min elapsed from the start of the session," p. 494, Peterson et al., 2016 or "The experimenter terminated the session when the participant consumed all eight bites or following the first consumed bite after 30 min had elapsed, whichever occurred first"; p. 93, Fernand, Penrod, Fu, Whelan, & Medved, 2016). Many studies that evaluated NRS specify that the feeder deposits the bite when the child opens their mouth (e.g., Fernand et al., 2016; Peterson et al., 2016) but do not necessarily specify any limiting conditions that would preclude the feeder from inserting the bite (e.g., "Bite placement occurred if he opened his mouth at any time with the exception of gags, coughs, yawns, and emesis, following which the bite was placed only after those responses ceased"; p. 8, Taylor, 2018).

*Recommendation 4. We recommend, based on our clinical experience, that practitioners implementing NRS procedures only deposit a bite when the child independently opens their mouth to accept the bite in the absence of IMB and their head is in a neutral position (90° angle) or in a position recommended by a speech and language pathologist or occupational therapist based on any physical conditions that may compromise the child's safety during feeding (*e.g., *dysphagia). Although this may limit the opportunities for acceptance, this practice ensures optimal safety during oral feeding (*Arvedson, 2008*).*

Recommendation 5. We recommend, regardless of the procedural variation of EE selected, that EE be combined with a reinforcement- and/or antecedent-based intervention to mitigate potential side effects that may be associated with EE procedures.

This recommendation is supported by our observation that NRS was never used in isolation except to demonstrate its effects separate from other components of a treatment package; furthermore, in spite of EE-based procedures (namely NRS) being one of the most frequently replicated treatment components (see Table 2.1), relatively few studies with conclusive evidential certainty included EE-based procedures. When selecting reinforcement- and/or antecedent-based interventions to use in combination with an EE-based procedure, we recommend that practitioners consider utilizing other treatment components based on the frequency with which they have been replicated in the literature (see Table 2.1) and intensify progress monitoring when evaluating components with few replications or lower evidential certainty. In the current review, the most frequently replicated reinforcement- and antecedent-based intervention components were DRA, rules, demand fading, noncontingent reinforcement, and manipulation of bite presentation (e.g., flipped spoon), in addition to representation, all of which may enhance the effectiveness of EE procedures commonly included in treatment packages to address feeding problems.

2.6 Conclusions

Feeding problems are especially prevalent among individuals with IDD and ASD and can occur and vary across one's lifespan. Thus, the purpose of this chapter was to explore behavioral feeding interventions across various age groups for this population. We conducted a comprehensive review of the literature over the last 10 years with the aim of providing practitioners with an overview of the best available evidence and recommendations for practice. Interventions including DRA, EE, and fading procedures were found to have the most empirical support, though the evidence-base is largely restricted to individuals up to 12 years of age.

Based on results of the current review, in general we recommend that practitioners: (a) first consider intervention components that have been most frequently replicated in the literature, and, (b) implement reinforcement- and/or antecedent-based interventions when using EE procedures to address feeding problems in children. Though many of the intervention components evaluated in the behavioral feeding literature would likely benefit adolescents and adults, before specific recommendations can be prescribed, more research with these age groups is needed. We recommend that researchers introduce intervention components sequentially starting with those that are least intrusive when designing interventions for adolescents or adults, and we hope this chapter will encourage and inform such research.

References

Addison, L. R., Piazza, C. C., Patel, M. R., Bachmeyer, M. H., Rivas, K. M., Milnes, S. M., & Oddo, J. (2012). A comparison of sensory integrative and behavioral therapies as treatment for pediatric feeding disorders. *Journal of Applied Behavior Analysis, 45*(3), 455–471. https://doi.org/10.1901/jaba.2012.45-455

Alaimo, C., Seiverling, L., Anderson, K., & Sturmey, P. (2018). A comparison of two multicomponent treatment packages for food refusal. *Behavioral Interventions, 33*(1), 93–101. https://doi.org/10.1002/bin.1503

Allison, J., Wilder, D. A., Chong, I., Lugo, A., Pike, J., & Rudy, N. (2012). A comparison of differential reinforcement and noncontingent reinforcement to treat food selectivity in a child with autism. *Journal of Applied Behavior Analysis, 45*(3), 613–617. https://doi.org/10.1901/jaba.2012.45-613

American Psychiatric Association, DSM 5 Task Force. (2013). *DSM 5 – Diagnostic and statistical manual of mental disorders* (5th ed.). Arlington VA: American Psychiatric Publishing. https://doi.org/10.1176/appi.books.9780890425596.x00DiagnosticClassification

Arvedson, J. C. (2008). Assessment of pediatric dysphagia and feeding disorders: Clinical and instrumental approaches. *Developmental Disabilities Research Reviews, 14*, 118–127. https://doi.org/10.1002/ddrr.17

Bachmeyer, M. H. (2009). Treatment of selective and inadequate food intake in children: A review and practical guide. *Behavior Analysis in Practice, 2*, 43–50. https://doi.org/10.1007/bf03391736

Bachmeyer, M. H., Gulotta, C. S., & Piazza, C. C. (2013). Liquid to baby food fading in the treatment of food refusal. *Behavioral Interventions, 28*(4), 281–298. https://doi.org/10.1002/bin.1367

Bachmeyer, M. H., Piazza, C. C., Fredrick, L. D., Reed, G. K., Rivas, K. D., & Kadey, H. J. (2009). Functional analysis and treatment of multiply controlled inappropriate mealtime behavior. *Journal of Applied Behavior Analysis, 42*(3), 641–658. https://doi.org/10.1901/jaba.2009.42-641

Badalyan, V., & Schwartz, R. H. (2012). Mealtime feeding behaviors and gastrointestinal dysfunction in children with classic autism compared with normal sibling controls. *Open Journal of Pediatrics, 2*, 150–160. https://doi.org/10.4236/ojped.2012.22025

Ball, S. L., Panter, S. G., Redley, M., Proctor, C.-A., Bryne, K., Clare, I. C. H., & Holland, A. J. (2012). The extent and nature of need for mealtime support among adults with intellectual disabilities. *Journal of Intellectual Disability Research, 56*, 382–401. https://doi.org/10.1111/j.1365-2788.2011.01488.x

Bandini, L. G., Curtin, C., Phillips, S., Anderson, S. E., Maslin, M., & Must, A. (2017). Changes in food selectivity in children with autism spectrum disorder. *Journal of Autism and Developmental Disorders, 47*, 439–446. https://doi.org/10.1007/s10803-016-2963-6

Barahona, C., DuBard, M., Luiselli, J. K., & Kesterson, J. (2013). School-based feeding intervention to increase variety and quantity of foods consumed by an adolescent with autism. *Clinical Practice in Pediatric Psychology, 1*(4), 361–368. https://doi.org/10.1037/cpp0000035

Berlin, K. S., Davies, W. H., Lobato, D. J., & Silverman, A. H. (2009). A biopsychosocial model of normative and problematic pediatric feeding. *Children's Health Care, 38*, 263–282. https://doi.org/10.1080/02739610903235984

Bijou, S. W. (1993). *Behavior analysis of child development*. Reno, NV: Context Press.

Birch, L. L. (1999). Development of food preferences. *Annual Review of Nutrition, 19*, 41–62. https://doi.org/10.1146/annurev.nutr.19.1.41

Borrero, C. S. W., Schlereth, J. G., Rubio, E. K., & Taylor, T. (2013). A comparison of two physical guidance procedures in the treatment of pediatric food refusal. *Behavioral Interventions, 28*(4), 261–280. https://doi.org/10.1002/bin.1373

Bui, L. T. D., Moore, D. W., & Anderson, A. (2013). Using escape extinction and reinforcement to increase eating in a young child with autism. *Behaviour Change, 30*(1), 48–55. https://doi.org/10.1017/bec.2013.5

Clawson, E. P., & Elliott, C. A. (2014). Integrating evidence-based treatment of pediatric feeding disorders into clinical practice: Challenges to implementation. *Clinical Practice in Pediatric Psychology, 2*, 312 321. https://doi.org/10.1037/cpp0000076

Curtiss, S. L., & Ebata, A. T. (2019). The nature of family meals: A new vision of families of children with Autism. *Journal of Autism and Developmental Disorders, 49*(2), 441–452. https://doi.org/10.1007/s10803-018-3720-9

Ewry, D. M., & Fryling, M. J. (2016). Evaluating the high-probability instructional sequence to increase the acceptance of foods with an adolescent with autism. *Behavior Analysis in Practice, 9*(4), 380–383. https://doi.org/10.1007/s40617-015-0098-4

Farmer, C., Swineford, L., Swedo, S. E., & Thurm, A. (2018). Classifying and characterizing the development of adaptive behavior in a naturalistic longitudinal study of young children with autism. *Journal of Neurodevelopmental Disorders, 10*(1), 1–9. https://doi.org/10.1186/s11689-017-9222-9

Fernand, J. K., Penrod, B., Fu, S. B., Whelan, C. M., & Medved, S. (2016). The effects of choice between nonpreferred foods on the food consumption of individuals with food selectivity. *Behavioral Interventions, 31*(1), 87–101. https://doi.org/10.1002/bin.1423

Fernand J. K., Saksena K., Penrod, B., Fryling M .J. (2017). Feeding disorders. In: J. L. Matson (ed.) *Handbook of childhood psychopathology and developmental disabilities treatment*. New York, NY: Springer. https://doi.org/10.1007/978-3-319-71210-9_21

Fiese, B. H., Tomcho, T. J., Douglas, M., Josephs, K., Poltrock, S., & Baker, T. (2002). A review of 50 years of research on naturally occurring family routines and rituals: Cause for celebration? *Journal of Family Psychology, 16*, 381–390. https://doi.org/10.1037//0893-3200.16.4.381

Fu, S. B., Penrod, B., Fernand, J. K., Whelan, C. M., Griffith, K., & Medved, S. (2015). The effects of modeling contingencies in the treatment of food selectivity in children with autism. *Behavior Modification, 39*(6), 771–784. https://doi.org/10.1177/0145445515592639

Gal, E., Hardal-Nasser, R., & Engel-Yeger, B. (2011). The relationship between the severity of eating problems and intellectual developmental deficit level. *Research in Developmental Disabilities, 32*, 1464–1469. https://doi.org/10.1016/j.ridd.2010.12.003

Gale, C. M., Eikeseth, S., & Rudrud, E. (2011). Functional assessment and behavioral intervention for eating difficulties in children with autism: A study conducted in the natural environment using parents and ABA tutors as therapists. *Journal of Autism and Developmental Disorders, 41*(10), 1383–1396. https://doi.org/10.1007/s10803-010-1167-8

Gentry, J. A., & Luiselli, J. K. (2008). Treating a child's selective eating through parent implemented feeding intervention in the home setting. *Journal of Developmental and Physical Disabilities, 20*(1), 63–70. https://doi.org/10.1007/s10882-007-9080-6

Goday, P. S., Huh, S. Y., Silverman, A., Lukens, C. T., Dodrill, P., Cohen, S. S., … Phalen, J. A. (2019). Pediatric feeding disorder-consensus definition and conceptual framework. *Journal of Pediatric Gastroenterology and Nutrition, 68*, 124–129. https://doi.org/10.1097/MPG.0000000000002188

Groff, R. A., Piazza, C. C., Zeleny, J. R., & Dempsey, J. R. (2011). Spoon-to-cup fading as treatment for cup drinking in a child with intestinal failure. *Journal of Applied Behavior Analysis, 44*(4), 949–954. https://doi.org/10.1901/jaba.2011.44-949

Hodges, A., Davis, T., Crandall, M., Phipps, L., & Weston, R. (2017). Using shaping to increase foods consumed by children with autism. *Journal of Autism and Developmental Disorders, 47*(8), 2471–2479. https://doi.org/10.1007/s10803-017-3160-y

Hodges, A., Gerow, S., Davis, T. N., Radhakrishnan, S., Feind, A., O'Guinn, N., & Prawira, C. (2018). An initial evaluation of trial-based functional analyses of inappropriate mealtime behavior. *Journal of Developmental and Physical Disabilities, 30*(3), 391–408. https://doi.org/10.1007/s10882-018-9592-2

Jenkins, S. R., LeBlanc, L. A., & Lambert, G. P. (2017). Treating food approval-seeking behavior: One bite at a time. *Behavior Analysis in Practice, 10*(4), 411–416. https://doi.org/10.1007/s40617-016-0170-8

Kadey, H. J., Roane, H. S., Diaz, J. C., & McCarthy, C. M. (2013). Using a Nuk® brush to increase acceptance of solids and liquids for two children diagnosed with autism. *Research in Autism Spectrum Disorders, 7*(11), 1461–1480. https://doi.org/10.1016/j.rasd.2013.07.017

Kedesdy, J. H., & Budd, K. S. (1998). *Childhood feeding disorders: Biobehavioral assessment and intervention*. Baltimore, MD: Paul H. Brooks Publishing. https://doi.org/10.1002/bin.82

Kerzner, B., Milano, K., MacLean, W. C., Berall, G., Stuart, S. S., & Chatoor, I. (2015). A practical approach to classifying and managing feeding difficulties. *Pediatrics, 135*, 344–353. https://doi.org/10.1542/peds.2014-1630

Knox, M., Rue, H. C., Wildenger, L., Lamb, K., & Luiselli, J. K. (2012). Intervention for food selectivity in a specialized school setting: Teacher implemented prompting, reinforcement, and demand fading for an adolescent student with autism. *Education and Treatment of Children, 35*(3), 407–418. https://doi.org/10.1353/etc.2012.0016

Koegel, R. L., Bharoocha, A. A., Ribnick, C. B., Ribnick, R. C., Bucio, M. O., Fredeen, R. M., & Koegel, L. K. (2012). Using individualized reinforcers and hierarchical exposure to increase food flexibility in children with autism spectrum disorders. *Journal of Autism and Developmental Disorders, 42*(8), 1574–1581. https://doi.org/10.1007/s10803-011-1392-9

Kozlowski, A. M., Taylor, T., Pichardo, D., & Girolami, P. A. (2016). The impact of emerging liquid preference in the treatment of liquid refusal. *Journal of Developmental and Physical Disabilities, 28*(3), 443–460. https://doi.org/10.1007/s10882-016-9482-4

Ledford, J. R., & Gast, D. L. (2006). Feeding problems in children with autism spectrum disorders. *Focus on Autism and Other Developmental Disorders, 21*, 153–166. https://doi.org/10.1177/10883576060210030401

Levin, D. S., Volkert, V. M., & Piazza, C. C. (2014). A multi-component treatment to reduce packing in children with feeding and autism spectrum disorders. *Behavior Modification, 38*(6), 940–963. https://doi.org/10.1177/0145445514550683

Mansell, J., Ashman, B., Macdonald, S., & Beadle-Brown, J. (2002). Residential care in the community for adults with intellectual disability: Needs, characteristics and services. *Journal of Intellectual Disability Research, 46*, 625–633. https://doi.org/10.1046/j.1365-2788.2002.00440.x

Marshall, J., Ware, R., Ziviani, J., Hill, R. J., & Dodrill, P. (2014). Efficacy of interventions to improve feeding difficulties in children with autism spectrum disorders: A systematic review and meta-analysis. *Child: Care, Health, and Development, 41*, 278–302. https://doi.org/10.1111/cch.12157

Matson, J. L., Fodstad, J. C., & Boisjoli, J. A. (2008). Cutoff scores, norms, patterns of feeding problems for the screening tool of feeding problems (STEP) for adults with intellectual disabilities. *Research in Developmental Disabilities, 29*, 363–372. https://doi.org/10.1016/j.ridd.2007.06.001

Matson, J. L., & Fodstad, J. C. (2009). The treatment of food selectivity and other feeding problems in children with autism spectrum disorders. *Research in Autism Spectrum Disorders, 3*, 455–461. https://doi.org/10.1016/j.rasd.2008.09.005

Meier, A. E., Fryling, M. J., & Wallace, M. D. (2012). Using high-probability foods to increase the acceptance of low-probability foods. *Journal of Applied Behavior Analysis, 45*(1), 149–153. https://doi.org/10.1901/jaba.2012.45-149

Najdowski, A. C., Tarbox, J., & Wilke, A. E. (2012). Utilizing antecedent manipulations and reinforcement in the treatment of food selectivity by texture. *Education and Treatment of Children, 35*(1), 101–110. https://doi.org/10.1353/etc.2012.0004

Najdowski, A. C., Wallace, M. D., Reagon, K., Penrod, B., Higbee, T. S., & Tarbox, J. (2010). Utilizing a home-based parent training approach in the treatment of food selectivity. *Behavioral Interventions, 25*(2), 89–107. https://doi.org/10.1002/bin.298

Penrod, B., Gardella, L., & Fernand, J. (2012). An evaluation of a progressive high-probability instructional sequence combined with low-probability demand fading in the treatment of food selectivity. *Journal of Applied Behavior Analysis, 45*(3), 527–537. https://doi.org/10.1901/jaba.2012.45-527

Penrod, B., Wallace, M. D., Reagon, K., Betz, A., & Higbee, T. S. (2010). A component analysis of a parent-conducted multi-component treatment for food selectivity. *Behavioral Interventions, 25*(3), 207–228. https://doi.org/10.1002/bin.307

Peterson, K., & Ibañez, V. (2018). Food selectivity and autism spectrum disorder: Guidelines for assessment and treatment. *Teaching Exceptional Children, 50*, 322–332. https://doi.org/10.1177/0040059918763562

Peterson, K. M., Piazza, C. C., & Volkert, V. M. (2016). A comparison of a modified sequential oral sensory approach to an applied behavior-analytic approach in the treatment of food selectivity in children with autism spectrum disorder. *Journal of Applied Behavior Analysis, 49*(3), 485–511. https://doi.org/10.1002/jaba.332

Peterson, K. M., Volkert, V. M., & Milnes, S. M. (2017). Evaluation of practice trials to increase self-drinking in a child with a feeding disorder. *Behavior Analysis in Practice, 10*(2), 167–171. https://doi.org/10.1007/s40617-016-0147-7

Piazza, C. C., Fisher, W. W., Brown, K. A., Shore, B. A., Patel, M. R., Katz, R. M., … Blakely-Smith, A. (2003). Functional analysis of inappropriate mealtime behaviors. *Journal of Applied Behavior Analysis, 36*, 187–204. https://doi.org/10.1901/jaba.2003.36-187

Piazza, C. C., Milnes, S. M., & Shalev, R. A. (2015). A behavior-analytic approach to the assessment and treatment of pediatric feeding disorders. In H. S. Roane, J. L. Ringdahl, & T. S. Falcomata (Eds.), *Clinical and organizational applications of applied behavior analysis* (pp. 69–94). https://doi.org/10.1016/B978-0-12-420249-8.00004-6

Pizzo, B., Williams, K. E., Paul, C., & Riegel, K. (2009). Jump start exit criterion: Exploring a new model of service delivery for the treatment of childhood feeding problems. *Behavioral Interventions, 24*(3), 195–203. https://doi.org/10.1002/bin.285

Rivas, K. M., Piazza, C. C., Roane, H. S., Volkert, V. M., Stewart, V., Kadey, H. J., & Groff, R. A. (2014). Analysis of self-feeding in children with feeding disorders. *Journal of Applied Behavior Analysis, 47*(4), 710–722. https://doi.org/10.1002/jaba.170

Rommel, N., De Meyer, A. M., Feenstra, L., & Veereman-Wauters, G. (2003). The complexity of feeding problems in 700 infants and young children presenting to a tertiary care institution. *Journal of Pediatric Gastroenterology and Nutrition, 37*, 75–84. https://doi.org/10.1097/00005176-200307000-00014

Rudolph, C. D., & Link, D. T. (2002). Feeding disorders in infants and children. *Pediatric Gastroenterology and Nutrition, 49*, 97–112. https://doi.org/10.1016/S0031-3955(03)00110-X

Sanders, M. R., Patel, R. K., Le Grice, B., & Shepherd, R. W. (1993). Children with persistent feeding difficulties: An observational analysis of the feeding interaction of problem and non-problem eaters. *Health Psychology, 12*, 64–73. https://doi.org/10.1037/0278-6133.12.1.64

Sasaki, A. M., & Fryling, M. J. (2014). Cup distance fading to decrease inappropriate behavior in a child with autism. *Journal of Developmental and Physical Disabilities, 26*(5), 507–512. https://doi.org/10.1007/s10882-013-9355-z

Seiverling, L., Anderson, K., Rogan, C., Alaimo, C., Argott, P., & Panora, J. (2018). A comparison of a behavioral feeding intervention with and without pre-meal sensory integration therapy. *Journal of Autism and Developmental Disorders, 48*(10), 3344–3353. https://doi.org/10.1007/s10803-018-3604-z

Seiverling, L., Williams, K., Sturmey, P., & Hart, S. (2012). Effects of behavioral skills training on parental treatment of children's food selectivity. *Journal of Applied Behavior Analysis, 45*(1), 197–203. https://doi.org/10.1901/jaba.2012.45-197

Seubert, C., Fryling, M. J., Wallace, M. D., Jiminez, A. R., & Meier, A. E. (2014). Antecedent interventions for pediatric feeding problems. *Journal of Applied Behavior Analysis, 47*, 449–453. https://doi.org/10.1002/jaba.117

Sharp, W. G., Harker, S., & Jaquess, D. L. (2010). Comparison of bite-presentation methods in the treatment of food refusal. *Journal of Applied Behavior Analysis, 43*(4), 739–743. https://doi.org/10.1901/jaba.2010.43-739

Sharp, W. G., Jaquess, D. L., Morton, J. F., & Herzinger, C. V. (2010). Pediatric feeding disorders: A quantitative synthesis of treatment outcomes. *Clinical Child and Family Psychology Review, 13*, 348–365. https://doi.org/10.1007/s10567-010-0079-7

Sharp, W. G., Odom, A., & Jaquess, D. L. (2012). Comparison of upright and flipped spoon presentations to guide treatment of food refusal. *Journal of Applied Behavior Analysis, 45*(1), 83–96. https://doi.org/10.1901/jaba.2012.45-83
Sharp, W. G., Trumbull, A., & Lesack, R. (2015). Blending to treat expulsion in a child with food refusal. *Behavioral Interventions, 30*(3), 247–255. https://doi.org/10.1002/bin.1413
Silbaugh, B. C., & Falcomata, T. S. (2017). Translational evaluation of a lag schedule and variability in food consumed by a boy with autism and food selectivity. *Developmental Neurorehabilitation, 20*(5), 309–312. https://doi.org/10.3109/17518423.2016.1146364
Silbaugh, B. C., Penrod, B., Whelan, C. M., Hernandez, D. A., Wingate, H. V., Falcomata, T. S., & Lang, R. (2016). A systematic synthesis of behavioral interventions for food selectivity of children with Autism Spectrum Disorders. *Review Journal of Autism and Developmental Disorders, 3*(4), 345–357. https://doi.org/10.1007/s40489-016-0087-8
Silbaugh, B. C., Swinnea, S., & Penrod, B. (2017). Synthesis of applied behavior analytic interventions for packing in pediatric feeding disorders. *Behavior Modification, 42*, 249–272. https://doi.org/10.1177/0145445517724541
Silbaugh, B. C., Wingate, H. V., & Falcomata, T. S. (2017). Effects of lag schedules and response blocking on variant food consumption by a girl with autism. *Behavioral Interventions, 32*(1), 21–34. https://doi.org/10.1002/bin.1453
Silverman, A. H. (2010). Interdisciplinary care for feeding problems in children. *Nutrition in Clinical Practice, 25*, 160–165. https://doi.org/10.1177/0884533610361609
Sira, B. K., & Fryling, M. J. (2012). Using peer modeling and differential reinforcement in the treatment of food selectivity. *Education and Treatment of Children, 35*(1), 91–100. https://doi.org/10.1353/etc.2012.0003
Skinner, B. F. (1945). The operational analysis of psychological terms. *Psychological Review, 52*, 270–277. https://doi.org/10.1037/h00
Stubbs, K. H., Volkert, V. M., Rubio, E. K., & Ottinger, E. (2018). A comparison of flipped-spoon presentation and redistribution to decrease packing in children with feeding disorders. *Learning and Motivation, 62*, 103–111. https://doi.org/10.1016/j.lmot.2017.03.007
Tarbox, J., Schiff, A., & Najdowski, A. C. (2010). Parent-implemented procedural modification of escape extinction in the treatment of food selectivity in a young child with autism. *Education and Treatment of Children, 33*(2), 223–234. https://doi.org/10.1353/etc.0.0089
Taylor, T. (2018). Intensive paediatric feeding treatment and the use of a side deposit for a clinical case within the home setting in Australia. *European Journal of Behavior Analysis, 19*(2), 208–227. https://doi.org/10.1080/15021149.2018.1472852
Taylor, C. M., Wernimont, S. M., Northstone, K., & Emmett, P. M. (2015). Picky/fussy eating in children: Review of definitions, assessment, prevalence and dietary intakes. *Appetite, 95*, 349–359. https://doi.org/10.1016/j.appet.2015.07.026
Troughton, K. E., & Hill, A. E. (2001). Relation between objectively measured feeding competence and nutrition in children with cerebral palsy. *Developmental Medicine & Child Neurology, 43*, 187–190. https://doi.org/10.1111/j.1469-8749.2001.tb00185.x
Valdimarsdóttir, H., Halldórsdóttir, L. Y., & Sigurådóttir, Z. G. (2010). Increasing the variety of foods consumed by a picky eater: Generalization of effects across caregivers and settings. *Journal of Applied Behavior Analysis, 43*(1), 101–105. https://doi.org/10.1901/jaba.2010.43-101
Vaz, P. C. M., Piazza, C. C., Stewart, V., Volkert, V. M., Groff, R. A., & Patel, M. R. (2012). Using a chaser to decrease packing in children with feeding disorders. *Journal of Applied Behavior Analysis, 45*(1), 97–105. https://doi.org/10.1901/jaba.2012.45-97
Verschuur, R., Didden, R., Lang, R., Sigafoos, J., & Huskens, B. (2014). Pivotal response treatment for children with autism spectrum disorders: A systematic review. *Review Journal of Autism and Developmental Disorders, 1*, 34–61. https://doi.org/10.1007/s40489-013-0008-z
Volkert, V. M., Patel, M. R., & Peterson, K. M. (2016). Food refusal and selective eating. In J. Luiselli (Ed.), *Behavioral health promotion and intervention in intellectual and developmental disabilities. Evidence-based practices in behavioral health* (pp. 137–161). Cham, Switzerland: Springer. https://doi.org/10.1007/978-3-319-27297-9

Volkert, V. M., & Piazza, C. C. (2012). Pediatric feeding disorders. In M. Hersen & P. Sturmey (Eds.), *Handbook of evidence-based practice in clinical psychology, child and adolescent disorders* (pp. 323–338). Hoboken, NJ: John Wiley. https://doi.org/10.1002/9781118156391.ebcp001013

Volkert, V. M., Piazza, C. C., Vaz, P. C. M., & Frese, J. (2013). A pilot study to increase chewing in children with feeding disorders. *Behavior Modification, 37*(3), 391–408. https://doi.org/10.1177/0145445512474295

Volkert, V. M., Vaz, P. C. M., Piazza, C. C., Frese, J., & Barnett, L. (2011). Using a flipped spoon to decrease packing in children with feeding disorders. *Journal of Applied Behavior Analysis, 44*(3), 617–621. https://doi.org/10.1901/jaba.2011.44-617

Vollmer, T. R., & Iwata, B. A. (1991). Establishing operations and reinforcement effects. *Journal of Applied Behavior Analysis, 24*(2), 279–291. https://doi.org/10.1901/jaba.1991.24-279

Voulgarakis, H., & Forte, S. (2015). Escape extinction and negative reinforcement in the treatment of pediatric feeding disorders: A single case analysis. *Behavior Analysis in Practice, 8*(2), 212–214. https://doi.org/10.1007/s40617-015-0086-8

Wilkins, J. W., Piazza, C. C., Groff, R. A., Volkert, V. M., Kozisek, J. M., & Milnes, S. M. (2014). Utensil manipulation during initial treatment of pediatric feeding problems. *Journal of Applied Behavior Analysis, 47*(4), 694–709. https://doi.org/10.1002/jaba.169

Wood, B. K., Wolery, M., & Kaiser, A. P. (2009). Treatment of food selectivity in a young child with autism. *Focus on Autism and Other Developmental Disabilities, 24*(3), 169–177. https://doi.org/10.1177/1088357609338381

Chapter 3
Empirically Supported Strategies for Teaching Personal Hygiene Skills to People with Intellectual Disabilities

Laurie McLay, Jenna van Deurs, Rosina Gibbs, and Sarah Whitcombe-Dobbs

3.1 Personal Hygiene and Grooming Skills

The ability to perform the tasks necessary to maintain personal hygiene are important to an individual's health and well-being and are fundamental to enacting an individual's rights to autonomy and dignity. Appropriate personal hygiene can improve an individual's ability to access employment and education, and it facilitates a higher quality of life via increased independence and health (Kraemer, McIntyre, & Blacher, 2003; Miller & Chan, 2008). Contemporary conceptualizations of intellectual disability place an emphasis on what assistance is needed to support a person's daily functioning and participation in society. To this end, practitioners must be able to: (1) accurately assess people's current skills, (2) identify the key components of tasks that are essential to daily hygiene and grooming, and (3) design and implement a plan for teaching the missing component skills. These are core aspects of supporting individuals' learning and skill acquisition.

The ability of an individual to care for their own personal hygiene needs is central to promoting independent living in community settings. Being able to perform personal care tasks reduces reliance on caregivers and, for many individuals, is the difference between supported and independent housing. Daily personal care tasks (e.g., dressing and toileting) hold significant influence over access to living arrangements, support services, and independence. Access to independent living arrangements can be particularly salient to adolescents and young adults as they seek to move away from the family home, and the ability to perform daily living skills is a common focus for families during this transition (Landmark, Ju, & Zhang, 2010). For some individual's access to more independent living situations is vital to inclusion and connection in their communities as it allows access to employment, increased opportunity for social relationships, and a more varied and stimulating

L. McLay (✉) · J. van Deurs · R. Gibbs · S. Whitcombe-Dobbs
School of Health Sciences, University of Canterbury, Christchurch, New Zealand

R. Lang, P. Sturmey (eds.), *Adaptive Behavior Strategies for Individuals with Intellectual and Developmental Disabilities*, Autism and Child Psychopathology Series, https://doi.org/10.1007/978-3-030-66441-1_3

living environment. Failure to teach these key skills reduces agency and increases dependence on others (Lancioni, O'Reilly, & Campodonico, 2002).

The reliable and effective performance of personal hygiene activities has benefits to both personal and public health outcomes. Routines such as handwashing, teeth brushing, and bathing can reduce an individual's exposure to infection, illness, and health complications such as tooth decay. Personal responsibility for daily care may also increase an individual's awareness of his or her own physical health. For example, bathing can lead to the identification of changes that may indicate a need for medical care like skin infections or other ailments. Hygiene practices can also reduce the spread of infectious diseases and illness within the wider community, particularly within educational and employment settings. This is particularly salient for individuals with intellectual disabilities who experience higher rates of chronic illnesses that are exacerbated by infection.

Individuals with intellectual and developmental disabilities are also more vulnerable to physical and sexual abuse, and risk of abuse may increase in the presence of caregivers during intimate personal care (Basile, Breiding, & Smith, 2016; Byrne, 2018). Encouraging independent hygiene skills could be a protective factor in preventing abuse. It is advised that whenever an It is advised that whenever an individual can undertake their own personal care, they should be encouraged to do so care, they should be encouraged to do so care (Carnaby & Cambridge, 2006). Supporting individual responsibility for purposeful care and cleaning can provide opportunities for people to learn about the functionality of their bodies and promote familiarity with and confidence in their body, which may also be a protective factor for abuse.

The importance of personal hygiene extends beyond physical health to social access and inclusion. Maintaining a clean and well-groomed appearance means meeting expectations of societal norms. These normative behaviors are generally learned through modeling in typically developing children; however, individuals with intellectual disabilities may need to be explicitly taught these expectations. Fitting in with norms around body odor, body hair, and good hygiene can increase social acceptance and reduce stigma particularly in employment settings (Cramm, Finkenflügel, Kuijsten, & Van Exel, 2009; Garff & Storey, 1998; Graffam, Shinkfield, Smith, & Polzin, 2002). The independent performance of these skills can subsequently improve self-esteem, peer relationships, community access, and opportunities for employment (Garff & Storey, 1998).

Finally, teaching personal hygiene skills reduces the burden of care on caregivers, who are often parents or family members. Supporting or being responsible for personal hygiene tasks places significant pressure on parents' and carers' time and energy (Tadema & Vlaskamp, 2009). As individuals age, some tasks can become physically difficult due to a restricted range of movement (e.g., dressing). Caregivers' emotional and physical capacity to continue supporting these tasks can also be compromised as they themselves age (Haley & Perkins, 2004; Taggart, Truesdale-Kennedy, Ryan, & McConkey, 2012). Increasing independence in personal hygiene routines can reduce the caregiver burden associated with the time-consuming task of providing hygiene and grooming care (Martin, Rusch, & Heal, 1982).

3.1.1 *Challenges in Acquisition of Personal Hygiene Skills*

People with intellectual disabilities face a number of challenges with regard to hygiene and grooming. Some of these are associated with the intellectual disability, including gross and fine motor difficulties as well as cognitive difficulties affecting non-verbal reasoning, attentional control, memory, planning, and sequencing (Danielsson et al., 2012). Cognitive deficits, in particular, affect the acquisition of hygiene skills as individuals tend to have difficulty learning and retaining the sequences of behaviors necessary to complete self-care skills. Sensory issues (e.g., extreme responses to tactile stimulation), difficulties with receptive and expressive communication (e.g., communicating the need to use the restroom) and challenging behaviors (e.g., non-compliance) are also more common among people with intellectual and developmental disabilities and deleteriously affect the learning process (Baranek, Foster, & Berkson, 1997; DeLeon et al., 2008; Ellis, Ala'i-Rosales, Glenn, Rosales-Ruiz, & Greenspoon, 2006; Matson, Neal & Kozlowski, 2012).

3.2 Assessment and Treatment Formulation

3.2.1 *Selecting Developmentally Appropriate Target Hygiene Skills*

In order to select appropriate intervention targets, it is often necessary to consider the developmentally appropriate sequence of skill acquisition. The majority of self-care skills are typically acquired between 2 and 6 years of age. Table 3.1 illustrates the age range in which most typically developing children have acquired specific hygiene and self-care skills. The information presented was consolidated from several sources (e.g., Dosman, Andrews, & Goulden, 2012; Frank & Esbensen, 2015; O'Connor Leppert, 2011; Scharf, Scharf, & Stroustrup, 2016; Schum et al., 2002).

In order to design effective individualized treatments for self-care skills, it is often necessary to assess the individual's foundational developmental skills (O'Connor Leppert, 2011). For example, assessment of pre-requisite skills such as gross and fine motor strength may be helpful in identifying challenges related to holding and using a toothbrush. Assessment of receptive language (e.g., ability to follow instructions), expressive language (e.g., ability to communicate need to use the toilet), cognitive ability, as well as possible sensory issues (e.g., aversion to the sound of brushing teeth) is also important to consider. The assessment of these underlying domains and skills also informs the order in which skills are taught by allowing focus on developmentally appropriate skills in the appropriate developmental sequence (Allen & Marotz, 2000; Frank & Esbensen, 2015). If specific higher-order skills are not yet attained, then it follows that intervention planning should be designed to teach the necessary pre-requisite skills. For example, Matson, DiLorenzo, and Esveldt-Dawson (1981) were required to provide body orientation

Table 3.1 Developmental norms for the acquisition of self-care skills

Age	Dressing skills	Toileting skills	Hygiene-related skills
12 mo	Removes hat		
15 mo	Attempts to use hair brush functionally	Fusses for diaper to be changed	
22 mo	Unfastens zip Partially puts shoes on		
24 mo	Takes off clothes without buttons, e.g., shoes, socks Pulls off pants Helps dress		
28 mo	Pulls pants up with assistance	Indicates toilet needs	
30 mo			Washes hands with assistance Brushes teeth with assistance
33 mo	Puts on coat unassisted		
36 mo	Puts on shoes without laces Unbuttons large buttons	Urinates independently Urinary continence during the day	
48 mo	Puts shoes on correct feet	Uses toilet independently for bowel movement Wipes after bowel movement	Washes face independently Washes and dries hands independently
52 mo	Buttons pants		
54 mo	Buttons shirts		
60 mo	Dresses independently		Dries hands thoroughly Brushes teeth independently Bathes independently
72 mo	Ties shoes Combs hair		

training to participants before they received intervention for independent showering that required responses to verbal cues relating to body parts. Similarly, before utilizing a modeling procedure to teach self-care tasks to children with Autism Spectrum Disorders (ASD), Charlop-Christy, Le, and Freeman (2000) first established that participants were able to maintain attention to a video for at least 30 minutes.

In addition to considering pre-requisite skills, standardized assessment tools can be used to determine age-appropriate self-care targets. Several standardized instruments are available to assess a range of developmental domains yielding standard scores and equivalent age-ranges; for example, the *Vineland Adaptive Behavior Scales, Second Edition* (VABS-II; Sparrow, Balla, & Cicchetti, 2005, 2006, 2008) *Scales of Independent Behavior-Revised* (SIB-R; Bruininks, Woodcock, Weatherman, & Hill, 1996), the *Ages and Stages Questionnaire* (ASQ-3; Squires, Twombley, Bricker, & Potter, 2009), the *Bayley Scales of Infant and Toddler Development, Third Edition* (Bayley-III; Bayley, 2006), and the *Peabody*

Developmental Motor Scales, Second Edition (PDMS-2; Folio & Fewell, 2000). (See Chap. 1, *Adaptive Behavior and Functional Life Skills Across the Lifespan: Conceptual and Measurement Issues,* by Tasse for a full discussion of this issue.)

In addition to standardized instruments, naturalistic observations are important components of a comprehensive assessment. Direct observation provides insight as to how an individual genuinely interacts with their environment. To gain an accurate accounting of an individual's functional capabilities, their behavior should be observed multiple times across multiple settings.

Finally, individuals with developmental disabilities often require training in a range of hygiene-related tasks. Therefore, in addition to following an appropriate developmental sequence, another important consideration of treatment design is which hygiene-related task to focus on first. According to Brown, Nietupski and Hamre-Nietupski's (1976) "criterion of ultimate functioning," a hierarchy of important therapeutic tasks can be generated based on whether the individual will be able to function independently in adulthood without learning a particular skill. For example, toilet training may be a more critical treatment target than nail clipping.

3.2.2 Task Analysis of the target skill

Many interventions for personal hygiene and grooming skills begin with a task analysis. Task analysis is an approach that involves breaking a complex, multi-faceted task into discrete, sequential, component steps (Klett & Turan, 2012). When completed, a task analysis should include all of the components necessary to complete the overall task (e.g., all of the components in a handwashing sequence). The steps identified in a task analysis form part of a behavior chain. Teaching each step of a behavior chain one step at a time is a useful way of teaching complex, multi-component activities. The steps involved in conducting a task analysis are summarized briefly below and Table 3.2 provides an example.

Table 3.2 Example of handwashing task analysis

Step	Instruction
1.	Turn water on
2.	Place hands under water and wet
3.	Put soap on hands
4.	Rub hands together until the soap makes bubbles
5.	Rub soap on both sides of hands
6.	Rub soap between fingers
7.	Place hands under water
8.	Rinse soap off
9.	Turn water off
10.	Get towel
11.	Dry hands for 10 seconds

1. Identify the skill to be targeted, e.g., brushing teeth or washing hands.
2. Identify the individual's current skill level and the pre-requisite skills that the individual needs in order to complete the task. The pre-requisite skills may need to be taught before teaching subsequent steps in the task analysis.
3. Identify the materials needed to teach the task. This may include assistive technologies that can support the person to demonstrate pre-requisite skills and/or perform the task.
4. Break the skill down into component parts so that, by completing these small steps, the individual will be able to complete the key task. This is often achieved by the interventionist and/or clinician completing the task themselves and documenting each step or observing another person and recording the steps. Each step recorded should be a discrete skill that can be taught.
5. Confirm that each step is accurately identified and recorded (i.e., ask a second person to complete these steps as they have been written).
6. Determine how the skills will be taught, including the evidence-based teaching procedures to be used and how to present the steps in the task analysis to the learner.
7. Implementation of the Teaching Strategies and Monitoring of Progress

3.3 Empirically Supported Intervention Approaches

The majority of research into interventions for personal hygiene and self-care is based on the principles of applied behavior analysis (ABA). Such interventions incorporate the principles of reinforcement, prompting, shaping, and chaining.

3.3.1 Chaining Procedures

The steps that are identified in a task analysis are often taught using chaining procedures. The term "behavior chain" is used to refer to a specific sequence of discrete responses that are associated with specific stimulus conditions. When these steps are linked together in sequence, they result in achievement of a key outcome (Cooper, Heron, & Heward, 2007). Each of the steps in the chain provides the discriminative stimulus for the next response, and performance of the behavior generates reinforcement for the previous response. For example, when washing hands, turning on the tap results in water running, which acts as reinforcement for the initial action of turning on the tap, and as a response prompt for the next action, picking up the soap.

There are several types of chaining procedures, but the most common of these are forward, backward, and total-task chaining procedures. Forward chaining begins by teaching the first step that is required to complete the task, and then prompting remaining steps in the sequence. For example, when teaching a child to brush their teeth, the child may first be taught to independently pick up their toothbrush and then be prompted to complete all remaining steps, such as adding toothpaste and so on. Each step of the task analysis is taught sequentially such that, when the first step is mastered, the second step in the chain is targeted. By contrast, backward chaining involves prompting all but the final step in the sequence/chain. For example, the child would be prompted to complete all steps in the tooth-brushing sequence, except the final step of putting the toothbrush back in the holder. In both forward and backward chaining, after a step is mastered, the next step or the previous step in the sequence is targeted, respectively. Total-task chaining involves teaching every step in the sequence during each instructional session as opposed to focusing on one step at a time. This may include the necessary prompting to complete all steps. For example, the child would be asked to complete the tooth-brushing sequence with prompting provided as necessary throughout the sequence. Chaining procedures have a number of advantages, including access to naturalistic contingencies of reinforcement that follow all steps in the behavior chain (Cooper et al., 2007). There is robust body of evidence to support the use of chaining procedures to teach personal hygiene skills, including management of menstruation (Richman, Reiss, Bauman, & Bailey, 1984; Veazey, Valentino, Low, McElroy, & LeBlanc, 2015), toileting skills (Drysdale, Lee, Anderson, & Moore, 2015), tooth-brushing (Horner & Keilitz, 1975), morning self-care routines (Jarman, Iwata, & Lorentzson, 1983), and dressing (Azrin, Schaeffer, & Wesolowski, 1976; Sisson, Kilwein, & Van Hasselt, 1988).

3.3.2 Prompting

Prompting strategies are instructional tools used to bridge the gap between the natural discriminative stimulus and the target behavior and are necessary when using chaining procedures to teach each step in a task analysis. Prompts increase the likelihood that an individual will respond correctly and access reinforcement. There are a number of prompting strategies that may be effective, including physical prompting (e.g., hand over hand guidance to turn on the tap), modeling prompts (e.g., somebody demonstrates the skill being performed), positional prompts (e.g., placing an item in a location so that success is ensured); gestural prompts (e.g., pointing to an item); visual prompts (e.g., pictures, written words, symbols); and verbal prompts (e.g., verbal cues). Prompts are conceptualized in a hierarchy according to level of intrusiveness and helpfulness. Prompts should be selected by considering the minimum amount of support a person needs to complete the target skill, while being as minimally invasive as possible. Careful consideration should be made to fade prompting over time so that the person receives less help and moves toward increased independence. For example, using a graduated guidance procedure, full manual guidance may be provided initially, then faded to light touch, then intermittent guidance, and then no assistance (Sisson et al., 1988). Prompts can also be directive when specific instructions or guidance are provided (e.g., "Turn on the tap"), or non-directive when information is provided in a suggestive manner (e.g., "I wonder what temperature the water will be?").

3.3.3 Modeling Procedures

Modeling procedures are another instructional strategy that involve the demonstration of a specific skill or component of a skill and can serve as a type of prompt for correct performance. Models may also show reinforcement contingencies operating for a target behavior. Various approaches to modeling have been reported as effective in the literature. These include in-vivo (live) modeling, video modeling (VM; in which the child watches a familiar or unfamiliar person demonstrating a task), video self-modeling (VSM; in which the person learning the target skill is depicted performing that task), and video point-of-view modeling (POV; in which the observer views the performance of the task, as if it were through the eyes of the model). After observing the model, the person is given the opportunity to perform the modeled task. Modeling procedures have been demonstrated to be effective in teaching a variety of daily-living, social, academic, and play skills to people with intellectual and developmental disabilities (Bidwell & Rehfeldt, 2004; Buffington, Krantz, McClannahan, & Poulson, 1998; Burton, Anderson, Prater, & Dyches, 2013; Coyle & Cole, 2004; D'Ateno, Mangiapanello, & Taylor, 2003; Gena, Couloura, & Kymissis, 2005; Hong et al., 2016; Van Laarhoven & Van Laarhoven-Myers, 2006; McLay, Carnett, van der Meer, & Lang, 2015; Mechling & Hunnicutt, 2011; Simó-Pinatella & Mumbardó-Adam, 2018; Taylor, 2003; Taylor, Levin, & Jasper, 1999; Walsh, Holloway, & Lydon, 2018; Wilson, 2013). Modeling has also been shown to facilitate the generalization and maintenance of treatment effects (Charlop-Christy et al., 2000; Haring, Kennedy, Adams, & Pitts-Conway, 1987). In order for modeling to be effective, people must: (a) attend to the behavior that is modeled; (b) retain the observed behavior and the conditions in which the behavior was demonstrated; (c) be capable of imitating the observed behavior; and, (d) be sufficiently motivated to perform the behavior that was modeled (i.e., sufficiently powerful reinforcer).

3.3.4 Activity-Based Intervention Approaches

Activity-based Intervention (ABI) provides a framework to integrate the principles of ABA into interactions or activities that are child-centered, transactional, and that encourage authentic engagement in daily activities (Pretti-Frontczak & Bricker, 2004). Within an ABI model, instruction and training is embedded in child-initiated or planned activities that are individualized through functional assessment, with the participation of the child and family. ABI involves the process of teaching functional skills within everyday contexts and daily activities, with naturally occurring antecedents and consequences (Bricker & Cripe, 1992). For example, teaching a child to put on their jacket occurs at a time when they want to go outside to play. The emphasis of ABI on functional and generative skills that promote independence aligns it as a promising instructional strategy for teaching personal care and hygiene skills. The majority of research has focused on the effectiveness of ABI as an early intervention approach. These studies indicate that ABI can promote skill acquisition and improvements across developmental domains (Apache, 2005; Bailey & Bricker, 1985; Bakkaloğlu, 2008; Bricker & Sheehan, 1981; Dada, Granlund, & Alant, 2007).

Embedded or naturalistic instructional strategies in general seem effective for teaching children with disabilities a variety of skills (Daugherty, Grisham-Brown, & Hemmeter, 2001; Fox & Hanline, 1993; Grisham-Brown, Schuster, Hemmeter, & Collins, 2000; Kurt & Tekin-İftar, 2008; McBride & Schwartz, 2003), including dressing (Sewell, Collins, Hemmeter, & Schuster, 1998). Although naturalistic-based instruction is thought to overcome some of the limitations of discrete trial teaching in terms of fluency, maintenance, and generalization (Alberto & Troutman, 2013), the frequency of learning opportunities is dependent on the person's daily routine, thus potentially impacting the rate of skill acquisition.

3.3.5 Visual Supports

Visual supports refer to visual prompts, visual activity schedules, and other types of visual aids. Visual prompts provide people with pictorial or symbolic representations of a task or of the steps necessary to complete that task. These aids can take the forms of photographs, drawings, generic images, or symbols. In the context of personal hygiene and self-care, they may take the forms of visual picture schedules showing the skill sequence, individual cue cards, or pictures and words that represent contingencies of reinforcement (e.g., first ____, then ____). Visual picture schedules may also be arranged in a story format wherein the reinforcement contingencies for completing the task are made salient in the pictures and narrative. These types of visual aids are thought to help people to understand and recall the expectations, steps, task requirements, and contingencies in place to support the completion of complex behavior chains (Gray, 1992, 2015; Hadwin, 2006; Lorimer, Simpson, Myles, & Ganz, 2002; Scattone, Wilczynski, Edwards, & Rabian, 2002; Soenksen & Alper, 2006).

3.4 Teaching Specific Hygiene Skills

3.4.1 Dressing Skills

Choosing appropriate clothes and getting dressed is a key part of the daily routine. Being able to dress independently reduces reliance on others and may reduce risk of some forms of abuse. Typically, children learn to dress themselves independently through a process of trial and error and by practicing during naturally occurring opportunities. This process may be complicated by the cognitive, motor, and behavioral difficulties commonly associated with intellectual disabilities. There is evidence to support the use of ABI strategies along with incidental approaches, to teach dressing skills to preschool-aged children with developmental delays (Kellegrew, 1998; McGee, Morrier, & Daly, 1999; Sewell et al., 1998). These approaches typically involve teaching dressing skills throughout the day, at times when dressing is an expected part of the routine. There is also evidence to support the use of a variety of prompting procedures to teach people with intellectual disabilities, including those with vision impairment. For example, simultaneous prompting with physical guidance, graduated guidance, and verbal prompting have all been used to support the acquisition of dressing skills (McKelvey, Sisson, Van Hasselt, & Hersen, 1992; Reese & Snell, 1991; Sisson et al., 1988). Evidence also supports the use of auditory (delivered via tape recording) and vibratory (delivered via a small wrist-worn device) prompting among adults with severe sensorimotor impairments and intellectual disability (Lancioni et al., 2007), a group often neglected within empirical studies. Chaining procedures, including forward, backward, and total task chaining are also commonly used to teach dressing skills to those with intellectual disabilities and have strong empirical support (Azrin et al., 1976; Batu, 2008; Lee, Muccio, & Osborne, 2009; Nida & Tjakrawiralaksana, 2018; Rayner, 2011; Richard III & Noell, 2019; Wibowo & Tedjasaputra, 2019).

To supplement the use of these empirically supported instructional strategies, physical adaptations to clothing and positioning can be useful. For example, using oversized clothing, presenting clothing in an accessible way, and ensuring that the individual is positioned according to their physical needs (e.g., seated to put socks on) may also assist in skill acquisition (Hughes, Schuster, & Michael Nelson, 1993; Reese & Snell, 1991; Sisson et al., 1988).

3.4.2 Oral Hygiene Skills

Many people with intellectual disabilities have poor oral hygiene as a consequence of inadequate oral care routines and/or infrequent dental visits. The Centre for Disease Control (CDC) has indicated that as many as 42% of children between 2 and 11 years of age have had a cavity in their baby teeth, and 21% of children between 6 and 11 years of age have had cavity in their permanent teeth (Dye et al., 2007). This issue extends to people with intellectual disabilities where dental problems, including gingivitis, plaque, oral injury, tooth decay, and cavities occur at higher rates than among the general population (DeMattei, Cuvo, & Maurizio, 2007; Klein & Nowak, 1999; Ward, Cooper, Hughes-McCormack, Macpherson, & Kinnear, 2019). Effective oral hygiene practices are fundamental in reducing the risk of developing cavities and periodontal disease (United States Department of Health and Human Services, 2000).

Problems with establishing appropriate oral hygiene practices are common in people with intellectual disabilities (Lewis, 2009). These problems are often the result of challenging behavior, including non-compliance with oral hygiene routines (Brickhouse, Farrington, Best, & Ellsworth, 2013; DeMattei et al., 2007; Farmer &

Aman, 2011; Lai, Milano, Roberts, & Hooper, 2012), fear of dental procedures, sensory sensitivity, poor dietary habits, avoidance of social contact, motor skills deficits, and poor comprehension, all of which can present major barriers to dental care (DeMattei et al., 2007; Graudins, Rehfeldt, DeMattei, Baker, & Scaglia, 2012; Marshall, Sheller, Williams, Mancl, & Cowan, 2007). Unfortunately, these problems can lead to the escalation of management strategies to those that are more invasive, such as sedation or restraint (Adair, Schafer, Rockman, & Waller, 2004).

A large body of evidence supports the use behavioral interventions to establish and maintain tooth-brushing skills. This includes video modeling, visual schedules, shaping, distraction, escape extinction, prompting, and differential reinforcement for the practice of cooperative behaviors (Allen & Stokes, 1989; Altabet, 2002; Conyers et al., 2004; Kemp, 2005; Piazza, Contrucci, Hanley, & Fisher, 1997; Pilebro & Bäckman, 2005; Popple et al., 2016; Rayner, 2010). Typically, behaviors that have been taught in analog settings have also generalized to in vivo settings (Cuvo, Godard, Huckfeldt, & DeMattei, 2010; Luscre & Center, 1996). According to Kemp (2005), the critical components of treatment packages include contingent positive reinforcement, differential reinforcement, and escape extinction.

Few studies have examined the pervasive problem of establishing children's compliance with caregiver implemented tooth-brushing and/or dental examinations and procedures (Bishop et al., 2013; Cuvo et al., 2010; Gillis, Matson, Roth, & Sevlever, 2016). A common intervention strategy is the use of stimulus-fading techniques, in which people are gradually exposed to a toothbrush or related items, by increasing the proximity or duration of that exposure (Cooper et al., 2007; Miltenberger, 2008). This strategy is typically incorporated within a treatment package that includes differential or non-contingent reinforcement, escape extinction, and/or modeling, and is a well-established technique to support people with developmental disabilities to acquire independent tooth-brushing, and to undergo dental procedures (Bishop et al., 2013; Cuvo et al., 2010). Additional procedures that have received some empirical support include in vivo or analog systematic desensitization (Altabet, 2002; Conyers et al., 2004; Kohlenberg, Greenberg, Reymore, & Hass, 1972; Luscre & Center, 1996).

Limited research has been undertaken exploring the effects of dental staff training on compliance with dental procedures (Graudins et al., 2012; Luscre & Center, 1996). In one study, (Graudins et al., 2012) provided a behavioral skills training package to teach dental hygiene students and staff to implement behavior analytic techniques. This program aimed to decrease rates of non-compliance and increase staff members' ability to perform oral care assessments and cleaning with patients. The training consisted of a 45-minute presentation that focused on differential reinforcement and escape extinction procedures, how to use reinforcement (e.g., reinforcing compliance), and the use of prompting and visual supports. Following the presentation, participants watched a video model and role-played the steps in the training checklist before being provided with feedback. Finally, these strategies were rehearsed with children with ASD. Training resulted in an increase in the ability of staff to apply techniques during examinations and cleaning and was viewed favorably, suggesting that group-based staff training packages may be an effective way to improve oral care for people with disabilities.

3.4.3 Menstrual Care

Very few studies have investigated strategies that support people with intellectual disabilities to manage menstruation independently. Typically, menstrual concerns in people with intellectual disabilities have been treated medically, using surgical or pharmacological procedures that suppress or eliminate menstruation (Richman, Ponticas, Page, & Epps, 1986). This has raised a number of important legal and ethical issues. Educational or behavioral approaches may offer a viable alternative to medical intervention, but such approaches are also met with challenges, as there are a number of important privacy considerations. Nearly all females will experience menarche, and teaching independent management of menstruation can increase personal privacy, enhance independence and community access, and reduce the need for medical interventions (Demetral, Driessen, & Goff, 1983).

Pioneering research in this area was undertaken by (Richman et al., 1984) who used task analysis, forward chaining procedures, simulated training, and differential reinforcement to teach menstrual care skills to five women with intellectual disability. In this study, these skills generalized to naturally occurring menses and gains were maintained at 5 months follow-up. Subsequent research has replicated the positive effects of simulated training and related procedures (Epps, Stern, & Horner, 1990; Richman et al., 1986). In the majority of cases, simulation training has involved a doll that was used for changing stained underwear and stained pads, or self-teaching procedures. Training has also often included the use of negative examples, such as teaching people not to change their underwear in the absence of a stain (Epps et al., 1990). Epps et al. (1990) compared simulation training using a doll, with in-vivo training. This included task analysis, forward chaining, and multiple exemplar training. While results were favorable in both conditions, limited generalization occurred for the doll training procedure. In another study, (Veazey et al., 2015) used total task chaining and forward chaining procedures, combined with prompting and reinforcement, to successfully teach menstrual care to two, 9- and 11-year-old females with ASD.

In a final unique study, Klett and Turan (2012), used a parent-implemented program which included an embedded, visually represented task analysis to teach independent menstrual care routines to three adolescents with ASD. The Social Story had three key sections: "Growing up," "My period," and "How to take care of my period." Each page included corresponding questions which parents asked their children as they read the story. This intervention resulted in an increase in participants' reproductive knowledge, independence in care for their menses, and importantly, parents reported high levels of satisfaction with intervention outcomes.

3.4.4 Washing and Bathing Skills

Few studies have evaluated treatments for washing/bathing procedures in individuals with developmental and intellectual disabilities. This is in spite of obvious immediate and tangential benefits to an individual's independence, health, safety, and social relationships (Garff & Storey, 1998; Stokes, Cameron, Dorsey, & Fleming, 2004). Evidently, there is also a dearth of research that has been undertaken in this area in the last two to three decades, particularly with children and adolescents (Konuk Sener, Aydin, & Cangur, 2019).

The majority of research targeting washing/bathing in individuals with intellectual disabilities has used multi-component treatment packages that begin with a task analysis, and subsequently include some combination of psychoeducation, self-management, modeling, prompting, and reinforcement procedures (Barry, Apolloni, & Cooke, 1977; Jarman et al., 1983; Konuk Sener et al., 2019; Matson et al., 1981; Matson, Marchetti, & Adkins, 1980; Saloviita & Tuulkari, 2000). For example, Matson et al. (1980) used self-management procedures within a standard treatment package to teach showering skills to adults with intellectual disability, living within an institution. Participants were assigned to either a no-treatment control group, standard treatment group (task analysis, prompts, modeling, shaping, fading, chaining, and social reinforcement), or standard treatment + self-management group (self-evaluation, self-monitoring, and self-reinforcement). Participants within the standard treatment + self-management treatment group experienced the largest increase in self-care tasks, with improvement maintained at an 8-week follow-up. Participants within the standard treatment group experienced a slight, gradual improvement. As expected, no improvement was demonstrated by participants in the no-treatment group. Similarly, Matson et al. (1981) demonstrated that a standard treatment package (psychoeducation, modeling, self-monitoring, and reinforcement) taught within a group setting to adults with intellectual disability was superior to a no-treatment control condition, and gains were maintained at a 3-month follow-up. More recently, Konuk Sener et al. (2019) utilized a group parent and adolescent personal hygiene education program, including psychoeducation, video/in-vivo modeling, and group discussions to teach bathing practices to young people with mild intellectual disability. These findings suggest multi-component instruction shows promise for the efficient and effective delivery of skills education for people with intellectual disabilities.

3.4.4.1 Handwashing

Adherence to handwashing routines is crucial in maintaining physical health and preventing the spread of contagious diseases. According to the CDC, simple handwashing procedures could reduce diarrheal disease-associated deaths by up to 50% and significantly reduce respiratory infections (Rabie & Curtis, 2006). A relatively large body of research has investigated the effects of home- and school-based interventions for handwashing in people with intellectual disabilities (Lee & Lee, 2014; Lee, Leung, Tong, Chen, & Lee, 2015; Vessey, Sherwood, Warner, & Clark, 2007; Walmsley, Mahoney, Durgin, & Poling, 2012). In the majority of these studies, intervention commenced with a task analysis of the steps in the handwashing sequence, and subsequently consisted of multiple components. These included visual supports depicting the steps in the handwashing sequence and/or the duration of hand scrubbing (often paired with songs), modeling, reinforcement, and prompting procedures (Lee et al., 2015; Vessey et al., 2007; Walmsley et al., 2012).

More recently, intervention packages have included the use of commercially available or individualized video models of the handwashing sequence (Deochand, Hughes, & Fuqua, 2019; Lee & Lee, 2014; Rosenberg, Schwartz, & Davis, 2010). For example, Lee and Lee (2014) evaluated a *5-step* handwashing intervention program in schools for children with mild intellectual disability. The intervention included a demonstration of a *5-step* handwashing technique, reward system, video models and songs, posters, and checklists. Those in the intervention group showed significant improvement, in comparison to the control group where the usual protocol for handwashing instruction was followed. In another study, Choi, Wong, and Chung (2012) used an "edutainment" video game to teach handwashing to 29, 6–11-year-old children with mild intellectual disability. The video game modeled the handwashing steps, and correct responses resulted in access to a preferred game. The computer-assisted teaching station included a user interface that consisted of a faucet, soap dispenser, and towel dispenser. Animations were based on the WHO *Guidelines on Hand Hygiene in Health Care* (2006).

In many cases, handwashing intervention packages have also included the use of glow gel (i.e., plastic simulated germs that fluoresce when placed under ultra-violet light) to assess the quality of handwashing by comparing change before and after handwashing (Deochand et al., 2019; Lee, Anderson, & Moore, 2014). These advances in recent research require further replication but offer significant promise as interventions for handwashing.

3.4.5 Grooming Skills

Satisfactory grooming skills, including shaving, trimming nails, brushing hair, and dressing appropriately, are critical to establishing and maintaining social relationships, employment, physical health, and community inclusion (Dowdy, Tincani, Nipe, & Weiss, 2018; Ellis et al., 2006; Garff & Storey, 1998). Individuals with developmental and intellectual disabilities may actively avoid or have difficulty completing grooming tasks. Non-compliance during grooming tasks, such as getting a haircut, is frequently maintained by escape from aversive stimuli. Therefore, a treatment consisting of escape extinction is often indicated. However, this can be unsafe when the routine involves dangerous instruments, such as scissors, which heighten the risk of injury during extinction bursts (Dowdy et al., 2018).

The majority of existing research has focused on either improving the independent grooming skills of adolescents and adults (Barry et al., 1977; Garff & Storey, 1998; Saloviita & Tuulkari, 2000) or improving compliance with grooming procedures (Dowdy et al., 2018; Ellis et al., 2006; Long, Hagopian, DeLeon, Marhefka, & Resau, 2005; Piazza et al., 1997; Schumacher & Rapp, 2011). As with previous hygiene-related tasks, most grooming interventions consisted of multiple components that include task analysis, modeling, prompting, and reinforcement procedures (Barry et al., 1977; Garff & Storey, 1998; Saloviita & Tuulkari, 2000). For example, Garff and Storey (1998) used in-vivo modeling, and self-management procedures, including a task analysis checklist and self-reinforcement (i.e., participants purchased self-selected reinforcers) to improve the grooming behaviors (shaving, fresh breath, clean face) of three adults with developmental disabilities.

Studies that have focused on escape-maintained non-compliance with grooming procedures (e.g., cutting toenails, haircuts) have typically used differential reinforcement procedures or non-contingent access to competing stimuli in combination with escape extinction to increase compliance with these procedures (Long et al., 2005; Piazza et al., 1997). In more recent research, however, procedures have been implemented without the use of escape extinction and have demonstrated positive outcomes in teaching compliance with nail cutting (Dowdy et al., 2018) and haircutting (Schumacher & Rapp, 2011). For example, Dowdy et al. (2018), used differential reinforcement without escape extinction to address escape-maintained behavior (e.g., pulling hand away) during nail cutting routines with two non-verbal adolescents with ASD and intellectual disability. Participants earned an edible treat following each successful nail cut. The edible items were visible throughout the task and participants could consume them at any time once earned. Escape behavior resulted in the therapist withdrawing the task for 5 s before re-attempting to cut the target nail. The intervention was successful in enabling the participant's therapist to cut all of their nails, and these gains were maintained at a 1- and 2-month follow-up for one participant.

Similarly, Schumacher and Rapp (2011) successfully increased tolerance to haircuts with a 5-year-old male with autism without using escape extinction. A preferred edible item and a 30 s escape from the chair was provided to the child contingent on sitting for increased time periods during haircuts. Prior to treatment, the child remained seated during a haircut for 10.5 s, and by the end of treatment was able to remain seated for 5 minutes, allowing his caregiver sufficient time to cut his hair. Behavior change was maintained at follow-up, but generalization to other settings (e.g., hair salon) was not assessed.

One unique study was also identified that investigated the use of graduated exposure, modeling, and contingent social attention, to increase the tolerance of skincare products (e.g., moisturizer and sunscreen) in two children with autism (Ellis et al., 2006). While such studies are scarce, they have a number of important clinical implications that provide an impetus for further research in this area.

3.4.6 Toilet Training Skills

Toilet training is a complex process that depends on both developmental maturation and learning. Although toileting skills are typically acquired between 2 and 4 years of age, not all children acquire the necessary skills within this timeframe or using conventional techniques. To achieve independence, children must acquire daytime and nocturnal continence, recognition of the need to urinate/defecate, as well as the general skills of dressing, undressing, and washing hands—all skills that are performed within the context of toileting. This process can be complicated by the communication, behavior, and motor difficulties experienced by people with intellectual disability. Toileting difficulties can result in social stigma and reduce access to community settings, and inadequate hygiene can lead to physical ailments such as infection and skin irritation (Cicero & Pfadt, 2002; Lang, McLay, Carnett, Ledbetter-Cho, Sun, & Lancioni, 2017).

The seminal work in the toilet training domain was conducted by Azrin and Foxx (1971), who pioneered the Rapid Toilet Training (RTT) method. A 2009 review of the literature conducted by Kroeger and Sorensen-Burnworth identified 28 studies focused on teaching toileting skills to people with developmental disabilities and found that the most frequently recommended approaches were based upon the RTT approach. The RTT approach involves: (a) scheduling regular opportunities for toileting, (b) increasing fluid intake, (c) reinforcement for voiding on the toilet, (d) graduated guidance prompting, and (e) punishment procedures (e.g., overcorrection, verbal reprimands) contingent on voiding outside of the toilet (Rinald & Mirenda, 2012). While RTT has strong empirical support (Kroeger & Sorensen-Burnworth, 2009), it does not always address the collateral behaviors necessary to independently complete the full toileting sequence (e.g., flushing the toilet, washing hands, and dressing), and the use of punishment techniques is not always viewed favorably by parents.

Alternative strategies that have received some empirical support are predominantly based on intervention packages. These include the use of video modeling and video self-modeling, which is commonly paired with prompting and reinforcement procedures and regularly scheduled practice opportunities (Bainbridge & Smith Myles, 1999; Drysdale et al., 2015; Keen, Brannigan, & Cuskelly, 2007; Lee et al., 2014; Sutherland, Carnett, van der Meer, Waddington, Bravo, & McLay, 2018; McLay et al., 2015). There are also a limited number of studies that have investigated the use of environmental or stimulus modification procedures such as the modification or removal of diapers. For example, Luiselli (Luiselli, 1996) describe a process of teaching children to void in the toilet by first reinforcing the child for in-diaper urination while seated on the toilet, and then cutting increasingly large holes in the diaper, placing the child on the toilet while wearing the diaper to provide a discriminative stimulus for urination, and then reinforcing in-toilet voiding. Taylor, Cipani, and Clardy (1994) also manipulated the environment by removing undergarments prior to toilet sittings, and then gradually and systematically re-introduced these garments, as in-toilet urination was achieved. While there is a strong body of research investigating the effectiveness of toilet training strategies, very few have focused defecation procedures, or initiation of toileting. Thus, further research is required in this area.

3.4.7 Self-Care Routines

The majority of research has focused on self-care tasks in isolation, though a few studies exist that have taught multiple skills concurrently, as a part of daily routine activities. To fulfill the goal of achieving independence across everyday situations, people must complete a series of self-care tasks in succession. For example, a morning self-care routine may consist of toileting, washing your face, dressing, brushing your teeth, and brushing your hair. It is, therefore, logical to consider interventions that support the acquisition of whole-routine self-care skills. Varying combinations of teaching methods have empirical support for teaching self-care routines including psychoeducation, picture schedules, checklists, reinforcement, modeling, and prompting procedures (Barry et al., 1977; Doleys, Stacy, & Knowles, 1981; Jarman et al.,1983; Konuk Sener et al., 2019; Matson et al., 1980; Piazza et al., 1997; Thinesen & Bryan, 1981). Interestingly, the majority of these studies were implemented in residential care or hospital settings (Piazza et al., 1997; Thinesen & Bryan, 1981) and thus replication in the home, with parents and children as change agents, is required.

A small number of studies have demonstrated the effects of video modeling procedures to teach a sequence of hygiene-related tasks (Charlop-Christy et al., 2000; Thompson & Faibish, 1970). In one such study, Charlop-Christy et al. (2000) used video and in-vivo modeling procedures to teach a 7-year-old male with ASD to independently brush his teeth and wash his face. Three video model presentations led to the acquisition and generalization of the target behavior across different settings, stimuli, and people. Interestingly, seven in vivo tooth-brushing presentations were required before this skill was acquired and generalization did not occur. Similarly, Thompson and Faibish (1970) showed that a combined approach of both video model and demonstration was more effective than demonstration alone to teach hygiene skills (handwashing, face washing, showering, menstrual care) to 53 adolescents with intellectual disability (14–17 years of age). The combined approach appeared to better facilitate generalization in the school and home setting. Videos are highly engaging as they direct the viewer's focus to relevant stimuli and reduce reliance on social communication skills (such as eye contact with the model; Charlop-Christy et al., 2000). As such, video modeling may be a more effective method than in-vivo modeling alone for teaching hygiene self-care skills.

3.5 Recommendations for Further Research

Several areas require further research, including the application of behavior analytic techniques to other hygiene practices not covered here and further exploration of innovative teaching technologies. Despite evidence supporting toileting interventions for people with intellectual disabilities, there are few studies examining the independent management of defecation. Research was also particularly limited regarding the teaching of menstrual management to females with intellectual disability. Given the personal nature of these hygiene practices and the intensive level of support required for people who cannot manage independently, this should be a high priority for future research. Modern technologies, such as the aforementioned computer program used to teach handwashing, could be trialed in a variety of settings and situations and have potential to improve outcomes when other methods have been unsuccessful.

There are several limitations to the evidence described here for the teaching of specific grooming and hygiene practices. Many studies were conducted within residential and institutional settings and/or were implemented by trained therapists. Ideally, interventions can be implemented in homes by parents. However, many of the procedures described here require repeated practice opportunities and a consistency of implementation that may not be feasible for parents or carers to implement in less-structured environments such as homes and communities. Future research should focus on the effects of parent- or carer-implemented teaching procedures for grooming and hygiene-related skills. The research was also limited with regard to group training procedures, both for staff learning effective techniques and for teaching new skills to people with disabilities in small groups. Individual- vs. group-based programs could be trialed using the same procedures to determine the most efficient and effective methods to support people to learn new skills.

3.6 Conclusion

Independent management of personal grooming and hygiene contributes to the freedom, social inclusion, autonomy, and self-esteem of people with intellectual disabilities. Daily routines related to personal care are central to adaptive functioning in society, so every effort should be made to support people to attain the highest possible level of independence. The evidence clearly shows that the most effective way to improve outcomes in this area is through structured teaching approaches that include the thorough assessment of individual capacities, task analysis, and intervention planning and implementation that closely scaffolds new skills and behavior sequences. Effective teaching methods for these news skills include behavior chaining, prompting strategies, modeling, ABI, reinforcement, and visual supports. There is also an emerging body of research that has investigated the use of innovative technologies including video modeling and edutainment-based instruction that warrant further research. By increasing individuals' self-care skills, parent and careers' burdens are reduced. Most importantly, however, it increases people's ability to live with greater dignity and freedom within wider society.

References

Allen, K. E., & Marotz, L. R. (2000). *By the ages: Behavior and development of children pre-birth through eight*. Canada: Delmar Cengage Learning as publisher. New York, USA.

Allen, K. D., & Stokes, T. F. (1989). Pediatric behavioral dentistry. In M. Hersen, R. Eisler, & P. Miller (Eds.), *Progress in behavior modification* (pp. 60–90). Newbury Park, CA: Sage.

Adair, S., Schafer, T., Rockman, R., & Waller, J. (2004). Survey of behavior management teaching in predoctoral pediatric dentistry programs. *Pediatric Dentistry, 26*, 143–150.

Alberto, P., & Troutman, A. C. (2013). *Applied behavior analysis for teachers* (9th ed.). Boston: Pearson.

Altabet, S. C. (2002). Decreasing dental resistance among individuals with severe and profound mental retardation. *Journal of Developmental and Physical Disabilities, 14*, 297–305. https://doi.org/10.1023/A:1016032623478

Apache, R. R. G. (2005). Activity-based intervention in motor skill development. *Perceptual and Motor Skills, 100*, 1011–1020. https://doi.org/10.2466/pms.100.3c.1011-1020

Azrin, N. H., & Foxx, R. M. (1971). A rapid method of toilet training the institutionalized retarded. *Journal of Applied Behavior Analysis, 4*, 89–99. https://doi.org/10.1901/jaba.1971.4-89

Azrin, N. H., Schaeffer, R. M., & Wesolowski, M. D. (1976). A rapid method of teaching profoundly retarded persons to dress by a reinforcement – guidance method. *Mental Retardation, 14*, 29–33.

Bailey, E., & Bricker, D. (1985). Evaluation of a three-year early intervention demonstrations project. *Topics in Early Childhood Special Education, 5*, 52–56.

Bainbridge, N., & Smith Myles, B. (1999). The use of priming to introduce toilet training to a child with autism. *Focus on Autism and Other Developmental Disabilities, 14*, 106–109. https://doi.org/10.1177/108835769901400206

Bakkaloğlu, H. (2008). The effectiveness of activity-based intervention program on the transition skills of children with developmental disabilities aged between 3 and 6 years. *Educational Sciences: Theory and Practice, 8*, 393–406.

Baranek, G. T., Foster, L. G., & Berkson, G. (1997). Sensory defensiveness in persons with developmental disabilities. *The Occupational Therapy Journal of Research, 17*, 173–185. https://doi.org/10.1177/153944929701700302

Barry, K., Apolloni, T., & Cooke, T. P. (1977). Improving the personal hygiene of mildly retarded men in a community-based residential training program. *Corrective & Social Psychiatry & Journal of Behavior Technology, Methods & Therapy, 23*, 65–68.

Basile, K. C., Breiding, M. J., & Smith, S. G. (2016). Disability and risk of recent sexual violence in the United States. *American Journal of Public Health, 106*(5), 928–933. https://doi.org/10.2105/AJPH.2015.303004

Batu, S. (2008). Caregiver-delivered home-based instruction using simultaneous prompting for teaching home skills to individuals with developmental disabilities. *Education and Training in Developmental Disabilities, 43*, 541–555.

Bayley, N. (2006). *Bayley scales of infant and toddler development screening test* (3rd ed., p. Harcourt Assessment, Inc.). San Antonio, TX.

Bidwell, M. A., & Rehfeldt, R. A. (2004). Using video modeling to teach a domestic skill with an embedded social skill to adults with severe mental retardation. *Behavioral Interventions, 19*, 263–274. https://doi.org/10.1002/bin.165

Bishop, M. R., Kenzer, A. L., Coffman, C. M., Tarbox, C. M., Tarbox, J., & Lanagan, T. M. (2013). Using stimulus fading without escape extinction to increase compliance with toothbrushing in children with autism. *Research in Autism Spectrum Disorders, 7*, 680–686. https://doi.org/10.1016/j.rasd.2013.02.004

Bricker, D., & Cripe, J. J. W. (1992). *An activity-based approach to early intervention*. Baltimore, MD: Paul Brookes.

Bricker, D., & Sheehan, R. (1981). Effectiveness of an early intervention program as indexed by child change. *Journal of the Division for Early Childhood, 4*, 11–27.

Brickhouse, T., Farrington, F., Best, A., & Ellsworth, C. (2013). Barriers to dental care for children in Virginia with autism spectrum disorders. *Journal of Dentistry for Children, 76*, 188–193. https://doi.org/10.1007/s40368-013-0075-y

Brown, L., Nietupski, J., & Hamre Nietupski, S. (1976). The criterion of ultimate functioning and public school services for severely handicapped students. In M. A. Thomas (Ed.), *Hey, don't forget about me: Education's investment in the severely, profoundly and multiply handicapped* (pp. 2–15). Reston, VA: Council for Exceptional Children.

Bruininks, R., Woodcock, R., Weatherman, R., & Hill, B. (1996). *Scales of independent behaviour – Revised*. Itasca, IL: Riverside.

Buffington, D. M., Krantz, P. J., McClannahan, L. E., & Poulson, C. L. (1998). Procedures for teaching appropriate gestural communication skills to children with autism. *Journal of Autism and Developmental Disorders, 28*, 535–545. https://doi.org/10.1023/A:1026056229214

Burton, C. E., Anderson, D. H., Prater, M. A., & Dyches, T. T. (2013). Video self-modeling on an iPad to teach functional math skills to adolescents with autism and intellectual disability. *Focus on Autism and Other Developmental Disabilities, 28*, 67–77. https://doi.org/10.1177/1088357613478829

Byrne, G. (2018). Prevalence and psychological sequelae of sexual abuse among individuals with an intellectual disability: A review of the recent literature. *Journal of Intellectual Disabilities, 22*, 294–310. https://doi.org/10.1177/1744629517698844

Carnaby, S., & Cambridge, P. (2006). *Intimate and personal care with people with learning disabilities*. Philadelphia, PA: Jessica Kingsley Publishers.

Charlop-Christy, M. H., Le, L., & Freeman, K. A. (2000). A comparison of video modeling with in vivo modeling for teaching children with autism. *Journal of Autism and Developmental Disorders, 30*, 537–552. https://doi.org/10.1023/A:1005635326276

Choi, K.-S., Wong, P.-K., & Chung, W.-Y. (2012). Using computer-assisted method to teach children with intellectual disabilities handwashing skills. *Disability and Rehabilitation: Assistive Technology, 7*(6), 507–516. https://doi.org/10.3109/17483107.2011.652998

Cicero, F., & Pfadt, A. (2002). Investigation of a reinforcement-based toilet training procedure for children with autism. *Research in Developmental Disabilities, 23*, 319–331. https://doi.org/10.1016/S0891-4222(02)00136-1

Conyers, C., Miltenberger, R. G., Peterson, B., Gubin, A., Jurgens, M., Selders, A., & Barenz, R. (2004). An evaluation of in vivo desensitization and video modeling to increase compliance with dental procedures in persons with mental retardation. *Journal of Applied Behavior Analysis, 37*, 233–238. https://doi.org/10.1901/jaba.2004.37-233

Cooper, J. O., Heron, T. E., & Heward, W. L. (2007). *Applied behavior analysis* (2nd ed.). Upper Saddle River, NJ: Pearson.

Coyle, C., & Cole, P. (2004). A videotaped self-modelling and self-monitoring treatment program to decrease off-task behaviour in children with autism. *Journal of Intellectual & Developmental Disability, 29*, 3–16. https://doi.org/10.1080/08927020410001662642

Cramm, J. M., Finkenflügel, H., Kuijsten, R., & Van Exel, N. J. (2009). How employment support and social integration programmes are viewed by the intellectually disabled. *Journal of Intellectual Disability Research, 53*, 512–520. https://doi.org/10.1111/j.1365-2788.2009.01168.x

Cuvo, A. J., Godard, A., Huckfeldt, R. M., & DeMattei, R. R. (2010). Training children with autism spectrum disorders to be compliant with an oral assessment. *Research in Autism Spectrum Disorders, 4*, 681–696.

Dada, S., Granlund, M., & Alant, E. (2007). A discussion of individual variability, in activity-based interventions, using the niche concept. *Child: Care, Health and Development, 33*, 424–431. https://doi.org/10.1111/j.1365-2214.2006.00700.x

Danielsson, H., Henry, L., Messer, D., Rönnberg, J., Institutet for, h., Linköpings, u., … Filosofiska, f. (2012). Strengths and weaknesses in executive functioning in children with intellectual disability. *Research in Developmental Disabilities, 33*, 600–607. https://doi.org/10.1016/j.ridd.2011.11.004

D'Ateno, P., Mangiapanello, K., & Taylor, B. (2003). Using video modeling to teach complex play sequences to a preschooler with autism. *Journal of Positive Behavior Interventions, 5*, 5–11. https://doi.org/10.1177/10983007030050010801

Daugherty, S., Grisham-Brown, J., & Hemmeter, M. L. (2001). The effects of embedded skill instruction on the acquisition of target and nontarget skills in preschoolers with developmental delays. *Topics in Early Childhood Special Education, 21*, 213–221.

DeLeon, I. G., Hagopian, L. P., Rodriguez-Catter, V., Bowman, L. G., Long, E. S., & Boelter, E. W. (2008). Increasing wearing prescription glasses in individuals with mental retardation. *Journal of Applied Behavior Analysis, 41*, 137–142. https://doi.org/10.1901/jaba.2008.41-137

Demetral, G. D., Driessen, J., & Goff, G. A. (1983). A proactive training approach designed to assist developmentally disabled adolescents deal effectively with their menarche. *Sexuality and Disability, 6*, 38–46.

DeMattei, R., Cuvo, A., & Maurizio, S. (2007). Oral assessment of children with an Autism Spectrum Disorder. *American Dental Hygienists' Association, 81*, 65–65.

Deochand, N., Hughes, H., & Fuqua, R. (2019). Evaluating visual feedback on the handwashing behavior of students with emotional and developmental disabilities. *Behavior Analysis: Research and Practice*. https://doi.org/10.1037/bar0000154

Doleys, D. M., Stacy, D., & Knowles, S. (1981). Modification of grooming behavior in adult retarded: Token reinforcement in a community-based program. *Behavior Modification, 5*, 119–128. https://doi.org/10.1177/014544558151009

Dosman, C. F., Andrews, D., & Goulden, K. J. (2012). Evidence-based milestone ages as a framework for developmental surveillance. *Pediatrics & Child Health, 17*, 561–568.

Dowdy, A., Tincani, M., Nipe, T., & Weiss, M. J. (2018). Effects of reinforcement without extinction on increasing compliance with nail cutting: A systematic replication. *Journal of Applied Behavior Analysis, 51*, 924–930. https://doi.org/10.1002/jaba.484

Drysdale, B., Lee, C. Y. Q., Anderson, A., & Moore, D. W. (2015). Using video modeling incorporating animation to teach toileting to two children with autism spectrum disorder. *Journal of Developmental and Physical Disabilities, 27*, 149–165. https://doi.org/10.1007/s10882-014-9405-1

Dye, B. A., Tan, S., Smith, V., Lewis, B. G., Barker, L. K., Thornton-Evans, G., & Li, C. H. (2007). Trends in oral health status, United States, 1988-1994 and 1999-2004. *External Vital Health Statistic, 11*, 1–92.

Ellis, E. M., Ala'i-Rosales, S. S., Glenn, S. S., Rosales-Ruiz, J., & Greenspoon, J. (2006). The effects of graduated exposure, modeling, and contingent social attention on tolerance to skin care products with two children with autism. *Research in Developmental Disabilities, 27*, 585–598. https://doi.org/10.1016/j.ridd.2005.05.009

Epps, S., Stern, R. J., & Horner, R. H. (1990). Comparison of simulation training on self and using a doll for teaching generalized menstrual care to women with severe mental retardation. *Research in Developmental Disabilities, 11*, 37–66. https://doi.org/10.1016/0891-4222(90)90004-R

Farmer, C. A., & Aman, M. G. (2011). Aggressive behavior in a sample of children with autism spectrum disorders. *Research in Autism Spectrum Disorders, 5*, 317–323. https://doi.org/10.1016/j.rasd.2010.04.014

Folio, M. K., & Fewell, R. (2000). *Peabody developmental motor scales: Examiner's manual* (2nd ed.). Austin, TX: PRO-ED.

Fox, L., & Hanline, M. F. (1993). A preliminary evaluation of learning within developmentally appropriate early childhood settings. *Topics in Early Childhood Special Education, 13*, 308–327.

Frank, K., & Esbensen, A. J. (2015). Fine motor and self-care milestones for individuals with Down syndrome using a retrospective chart review: Down syndrome milestones. *Journal of Intellectual Disability Research, 59*, 719–729. https://doi.org/10.1111/jir.12176

Garff, J. T., & Storey, K. (1998). The use of self-management strategies for increasing the appropriate hygiene of persons with disabilities in supported employment settings. *Education and Training in Mental Retardation and Developmental Disabilities, 33*, 179–188.

Graudins, M. M., Rehfeldt, R. A., DeMattei, R., Baker, J. C., & Scaglia, F. (2012). Exploring the efficacy of behavioral skills training to teach basic behavior analytic techniques to oral care providers. *Research in Autism Spectrum Disorders, 6*, 978–987. https://doi.org/10.1016/j.rasd.2011.12.010

Gena, A., Couloura, S., & Kymissis, E. (2005). Modifying the affective behavior of preschoolers with autism using in-vivo or video modeling and reinforcement contingencies. *Journal of Autism and Developmental Disorders, 35*, 545–556. https://doi.org/10.1007/s10803-005-0014-9

Graffam, J., Shinkfield, A., Smith, K., & Polzin, U. (2002). Factors that influence employer decisions in hiring and retaining an employee with a disability. *Journal of Vocational Rehabilitation, 17*, 175–181.

Gray, C. (1992). *How to write social stories*. Jenison, MI: Jenison Public Schools.

Gray, C. (2015). *The new social story book, revised and expanded 15th anniversary edition*. Arlington TX: Future Horizons Incorporated.

Grisham-Brown, J. L., Schuster, J. W., Hemmeter, M. L., & Collins, B. C. (2000). Using embedded strategy to teach preschoolers with significant disabilities. *Journal of Behavior Education, 10*, 139–162.

Haley, W. E., & Perkins, E. A. (2004). Current status and future directions in family caregiving and aging people with intellectual disabilities. *Journal of Policy and Practice in Intellectual Disabilities, 1*, 24–30. https://doi.org/10.1111/j.1741-1130.2004.04004.x

Haring, T. G., Kennedy, C. H., Adams, M. J., & Pitts-Conway, V. (1987). Teaching generalization of purchasing skills across community settings to autistic youth using videotape modeling. *Journal of Applied Behavior Analysis, 20*, 89–96. https://doi.org/10.1901/jaba.1987.20-89

Hong, E. R., Ganz, J. B., Mason, R., Morin, K., Davis, J. L., Ninci, J., & Gilliland, W. D. (2016). The effects of video modeling in teaching functional living skills to persons with ASD: A meta-analysis of single-case studies. *Research in Developmental Disabilities, 57*, 158–169. https://doi.org/10.1016/j.ridd.2016.07.001

Horner, R. D., & Keilitz, I. (1975). Training mentally retarded adolescents to brush their teeth. *Journal of Applied Behavior Analysis, 8*, 301–309. https://doi.org/10.1901/jaba.1975.8-301

Hughes, M. W., Schuster, J. W., & Michael Nelson, C. (1993). The acquisition of independent dressing skills by students with multiple disabilities. *Journal of Developmental and Physical Disabilities, 5*, 233–252. https://doi.org/10.1007/BF01047066

Jarman, P. H., Iwata, B. A., & Lorentzson, A. M. (1983). Development of morning self-care routines in multiply handicapped persons. *Applied Research in Mental Retardation, 4*, 113–122. https://doi.org/10.1016/0270-3092(83)90004-8

Keen, D., Brannigan, K., & Cuskelly, M. (2007). Toilet training for children with autism: The effects of video modeling. *Journal of Developmental and Physical Disabilities, 19*, 291–303.

Kellegrew, D. H. (1998). Creating opportunities for occupation: An intervention to promote the self-care independence of young children with special needs. *American Journal of Occupational Therapy, 52*, 457–465. https://doi.org/10.5014/ajot.52.6.457

Kemp, F. (2005). Alternatives: A review of non-pharmacologic approaches to increasing the cooperation of patients with special needs to inherently unpleasant dental procedures. *The Behavior Analyst Today, 6*, 88–108. https://doi.org/10.1037/h0100060

Klein, U., & Nowak, A. J. (1999). Characteristics of patients with Autistic Disorder (AD) presenting for dental treatment: A survey and chart review. *Special Care in Dentistry, 19*, 200–207. https://doi.org/10.1111/j.1754-4505.1999.tb01386.x

Klett, L. S., & Turan, Y. (2012). Generalized effects of social stories with task analysis for teaching menstrual care to three young girls with autism. *Sexuality and Disability, 30*, 319–336. https://doi-org.ezproxy.canterbury.ac.nz/10.1007/s11195-011-9244-2

Kohlenberg, R. J., Greenberg, D., Reymore, L., & Hass, G. (1972). Behavior modification and the management of mentally retarded dental patients. *ASDC Journal of Dentistry for Children, 39*, 61–67.

Konuk Sener, D., Aydin, M., & Cangur, S. (2019). Evaluating the effects of a personal hygiene program on the knowledge, skills, and attitudes of intellectual disabilities teenagers and their parents. *Journal of Policy and Practice in Intellectual Disabilities, 16*, 160–170. https://doi.org/10.1111/jppi.12277

Kraemer, B., Mcintyre, L., & Blacher, J. (2003). Quality of life for young adults with mental retardation during transition. *Mental Retardation, 41*, 250–262. https://doi.org/10.1352/0047-6765(2003)41<250:QOLFYA>2.0.CO;2

Kroeger, K. A., & Sorensen-Burnworth, R. (2009). Toilet training individuals with autism and other developmental disabilities: A critical review. *Research in Autism Spectrum Disorders, 3*, 607–618.

Kurt, O., & Tekin-İftar, E. (2008). A comparison of constant time delay and simultaneous prompting within embedded instruction on teaching leisure skills to children with autism. *Topics in Early Childhood Special Education, 28*, 53–64.
Lai, B., Milano, M., Roberts, M. W., & Hooper, S. R. (2012). Unmet dental needs and barriers to dental care among children with autism spectrum disorders. *Journal of Autism and Developmental Disorders, 42*, 1294–1303. https://doi.org/10.1007/s10803-011-1362-2
Lancioni, G. E., O'Reilly, M. F., & Campodonico, F. (2002). Promoting fluency of performance of self-help tasks with a person with multiple disabilities. *Behavioral Interventions, 17*, 15–20. https://doi.org/10.1002/bin.101
Lancioni, G., O'Reilly, M., Singh, N., Sigafoos, J., Oliva, D., Campodonico, F., & Groeneweg, J. (2007). Helping three persons with multiple disabilities acquire independent dressing through assistive technology. *Journal of Visual Impairment and Blindness, 101*, 768–773. https://doi.org/10.1177/0145482X0710101207
Landmark, L. J., Ju, S., & Zhang, D. (2010). Substantiated best practices in transition: Fifteen plus years later. *Career Development for Exceptional Individuals, 33*, 165–176. https://doi.org/10.1177/0885728810376410
Lang, R., McLay, L., Carnett, A., Ledbetter-cho, K., Sun, X., & Lancioni, G. (2017). Complications and side effects associated with a lack of toilet training skills. In J. L. Matson (Ed.), *Clinical guide to toilet training children* (pp. 19–31). Cham: Springer
Lee, C. Y. Q., Anderson, A., & Moore, D. W. (2014). Using video modeling to toilet train a child with autism. *Journal of Developmental and Physical Disabilities, 26*, 123–134.
Lee, S. C., Muccio, B., & Osborne, N. L. (2009). The effect of chaining techniques on dressing skills of children with moderate mental retardation: A single-subject design study. *Journal of Occupational Therapy, Schools, & Early Intervention, 2*, 178–192. https://doi.org/10.1080/19411240903392590
Lee, R., & Lee, P. (2014). To evaluate the effects of a simplified hand washing improvement program in schoolchildren with mild intellectual disability: A pilot study. *Research in Developmental Disabilities, 35*, 3014–3025. https://doi.org/10.1016/j.ridd.2014.07.016
Lee, R., Leung, C., Tong, W., Chen, H., & Lee, P. (2015). Comparative efficacy of a simplified handwashing program for improvement in hand hygiene and reduction of school absenteeism among children with intellectual disability. *American Journal of Infection Control, 43*, 907–912. https://doi.org/10.1016/j.ajic.2015.03.023
Lewis, C. W. (2009). Dental care and children with special health care needs: A population-based perspective. *Academic Pediatrics, 9*, 420–426. https://doi.org/10.1016/j.acap.2009.09.005
Long, E. S., Hagopian, L. P., DeLeon, I. G., Marhefka, J. M., & Resau, D. (2005). Competing stimuli in the treatment of multiply controlled problem behavior during hygiene routines. *Research in Developmental Disabilities, 26*, 57–69. https://doi.org/10.1016/j.ridd.2003.01.001
Lorimer, P. A., Simpson, R. L., Myles, B. S., & Ganz, J. B. (2002). The use of social stories as a preventative behavioral intervention in a home setting with a child with autism. *Journal of Positive Behavioral Interventions, 4*, 53–60.
Luiselli, J. K. (1996). A transfer of stimulus control procedure applicable to toilet training programs for children with developmental disabilities. *Child and Family Behavior Therapy, 18*, 29–34. https://doi.org/10.1300/J019v18n02_04
Luscre, D. & Center, D. (1996). Procedures for reducing dental fear in children with autism. *Journal of Autism and Developmental Disorders, 26*, 547–556. https://doi.org/10.1007/BF02172275
Marshall, J., Sheller, B., Williams, B. J., Mancl, L., & Cowan, C. (2007). Cooperation predictors for dental patients with autism. *Pediatric Dentistry, 29*, 369–376.
Martin, J., Rusch, F., & Heal, L. (1982). Teaching community survival skills to mentally retarded adults: A review and analysis. *Journal of Special Education, 16*, 243–267. https://doi.org/10.1177/002246698201600303
Matson, J. L., DiLorenzo, T. M., & Esveldt-Dawson, K. (1981). Independence training as a method of enhancing self-help skills acquisition of the mentally retarded. *Behaviour, Research and Therapy, 19*, 399–405. https://doi.org/10.1016/0005-7967(81)90128-5

Matson, J. L., Neal, D., & Kozlowski, A. M. (2012). Treatments for the challenging behaviours of adults with intellectual disabilities. *Canadian Journal of Psychiatry, 57*, 587–592

Mattson, J.M.G., Roth, M., & Sevlever M. (2016) Personal Hygiene. In: Luiselli J. (eds) *Behavioral Health Promotion and Intervention in Intellectual and Developmental Disabilities. Evidence-Based Practices in Behavioral Health* (pp. 43–72). Springer

Matson, J. L., Marchetti, A., & Adkins, J. A. (1980). Comparison of operant- and independence-training procedures for mentally retarded adults. *American Journal of Mental Deficiency, 84*, 487–494.

McBride, B. J., & Schwartz, I. S. (2003). Effects of teaching early interventionists to use discrete trials during ongoing classroom activities. *Topics in Early Childhood Special Education, 23*, 5–17. https://doi.org/10.1177/027112140302300102

McGee, G. G., Morrier, M. J., & Daly, T. (1999). An incidental teaching approach to early intervention for toddlers with Autism. *Journal of the Association for Persons with Severe Handicaps, 24*, 133–146. https://doi.org/10.2511/rpsd.24.3.133

McKelvey, J. L., Sisson, L. A., van Hasselt, V. B., & Hersen, M. (1992). An approach to teaching self-dressing to a child with dual sensory impairment. *Teaching Exceptional Children, 25*, 12–15. https://doi.org/10.1177/004005999202500104

McLay, L., Carnett, A., van der Meer, L., & Lang, R. (2015). Using a video modeling-based intervention package to toilet train two children with autism. *Journal of Developmental and Physical Disability, 27*, 431–451. https://doi.org/10.1007/s10882-015-9426-4

Mechling, L., & Hunnicutt, J. (2011). Computer-based video self-modeling to teach receptive understanding of prepositions by students with intellectual disabilities. *Education and Training in Autism and Developmental Disabilities, 46*, 369–385.

Miller, S., & Chan, F. (2008). Predictors of life satisfaction in individuals with intellectual disability. *Journal of Intellectual Disability Research, 52*, 1039–1047. https://doi.org/10.1111/j.1365-2788.2008.01106.x

Miltenberger, R. G. (2008). *Behavior modification: Principles and procedures* (6th ed.). Belmont, CA: Thomson Wadsworth.

Nida, D., & Tjakrawiralaksana, M. (2018). Teaching self-dressing skill behavior in a child with moderate intellectual disability and low vision with backward chaining technique. Conference: *1st International Conference on Intervention and Applied Psychology* (ICIAP 2017). https://doi.org/10.2991/iciap-17.2018.14

O'Connor Leppert, M. L. (2011). Neurodevelopmental assessment and medical evaluation. In R. G. Voigt, M. M. Macias, & S. M. Myers (Eds.), *Developmental and behavioral paediatrics* (pp. 93–120). Elk Grove Village: IL: American Academy of Pediatrics.

Piazza, C. C., Contrucci, S. A., Hanley, G. P., & Fisher, W. W. (1997). Nondirective prompting and noncontingent reinforcement in the treatment of destructive behavior during hygiene routines. *Journal of Applied Behavior Analysis, 30*, 705–708. https://doi.org/10.1901/jaba.1997.30-705

Pilebro, C., & Bäckman, B. (2005). Teaching oral hygiene to children with autism. *International Journal of Paediatric Dentistry, 15*, 1–9. https://doi.org/10.1111/j.1365-263X.2005.00589.x

Popple, B., Wall, C., Flink, L., Powell, K., Discepolo, K., & Keck, D. … Shic, F. (2016). Brief report: Remotely delivered video modeling for improving oral hygiene in children with ASD: A pilot study. *Journal of Autism and Developmental Disorders, 46*, 2791–2796. https://doi.org/10.1007/s10803-016-2795-4

Pretti-Frontczak, K., & Bricker, D. D. (2004). *An activity-based approach to early intervention* (3rd ed.). Baltimore, MD: Brookes.

Rabie, T., & Curtis, V. (2006). Handwashing and risk of respiratory infections: a quantitative systematic review. *Tropical Medicine and International Health, 11*, 258–267.

Rayner, C. (2010). Video modelling to improve task completion in a child with autism. *Developmental Neurorehabilitation, 13*, 225–230. https://doi.org/10.3109/17518421003801489

Rayner, C. (2011). Teaching students with autism to tie a shoelace knot using video prompting and backward chaining. *Developmental Neurorehabilitation, 14*(6), 339–347. https://doi.org/10.3109/17518423.2011.606508

Reese, G., & Snell, M. (1991). Putting on and removing coats and jackets: The acquisition and maintenance of skills by children with severe multiple disabilities. *Education and Training in Mental Retardation, 26*, 398–410. Retrieved from www.jstor.org/stable/23878703

Richard, P. R., III, & Noell, G. H. (2019). Teaching children with autism to tie their shoes using video prompt-models and backward chaining. *Developmental Neurorehabilitation, 22*, 509–515. https://doi.org/10.1080/17518423.2018.1518349

Richman, G. S., Reiss, M. L., Bauman, K. E., & Bailey, J. S. (1984). Teaching menstrual care to mentally retarded women: Acquisition, generalization, and maintenance. *Journal of Applied Behavior Analysis, 17*, 441–451. https://doi.org/10.1901/jaba.1984.17-441

Richman, G. S., Ponticas, Y., Page, T. J., & Epps, S. (1986). Simulation procedures for teaching independent menstrual care to mentally retarded persons. *Applied Research in Mental Retardation, 7*, 21–35. https://doi.org/10.1016/0270-3092(86)90015-9

Rinald, K., & Mirenda, P. (2012). Effectiveness of a modified rapid toilet training workshop for parents of children with developmental disabilities. *Research in Developmental Disabilities, 33*, 933–943. https://doi.org/10.1016/j.ridd.2012.01.003

Rosenberg, N., Schwartz, I., & Davis, C. (2010). Evaluating the utility of commercial videotapes for teaching hand washing to children with autism. *Education and Treatment of Children, 33*, 443–455. https://doi.org/10.1353/etc.0.0098

Saloviita, T. J., & Tuulkari, M. (2000). Cognitive-behavioural treatment package for teaching grooming skills to a man with an intellectual disability. *Scandinavian Journal of Behaviour Therapy, 29*, 140–147. https://doi.org/10.1080/028457100300049773

Scattone, D., Wilczynski, S. M., Edwards, R. P., & Rabian, B. (2002). Decreasing disruptive behaviors of children with autism using social stories. *Journal of Autism Developmental Disorders, 32*, 535–543.

Scharf, R. J., Scharf, G. J., & Stroustrup, A. (2016). Developmental milestones. *Pediatrics in Review, 37*, 25–38.

Schum, T. R., Kolb, T. M., McAuliffe, T. L., Simms, M. D., Underhill, R. L., & Lewis, M. (2002). Sequential acquisition of toilet-training skills: A descriptive study of gender and age differences in normal children. *Pediatrics, 109*, 1–9.

Schumacher, B. I., & Rapp, J. T. (2011). Increasing compliance with haircuts in a child with autism. *Behavioral Interventions, 26*, 67–75. https://doi.org/10.1002/bin.321

Sewell, T. J., Collins, B. C., Hemmeter, M. L., & Schuster, J. W. (1998). Using simultaneous prompting within an activity-based format to teach dressing skills to preschoolers with developmental delays. *Journal of Early Intervention, 21*, 132–145. https://doi.org/10.1177/105381519802100206

Simó-Pinatella, D., & Mumbardó-Adam, C. (2018). Using an intervention package, which included video prompting and video modeling to teach students with disabilities to find a word in the dictionary. *Journal of Developmental and Physical Disabilities, 30*, 807–818. https://doi.org/10.1007/s10882-018-9621-1

Sisson, L. A., Kilwein, M. L., & Van Hasselt, V. B. (1988). A graduated guidance procedure for teaching self-dressing skills to multihandicapped children. *Research in Developmental Disabilities, 9*, 419–432. https://doi.org/10.1016/0891-4222(88)90035-2

Soenksen, D., & Alper, S. (2006). Teaching a young child to appropriately gain attention of peers using a social story intervention. *Focus on Autism Other Developmental Disabilities, 21*, 36–44.

Sparrow, S., Balla, D., & Cicchetti, D. (2005). *Vineland adaptive behaviour scales-II. Survey forms manual*. Bloomington, MN: Pearson.

Sparrow, S., Balla, D., & Cicchetti, D. (2006). *Vineland adaptive behaviour scales-II. Teacher rating form manual*. Bloomington, MN: Pearson.

Sparrow, S., Balla, D., & Cicchetti, D. (2008). *Vineland adaptive behaviour scales-II. Expanded interview form manual*. Bloomington, MN: Pearson.

Squires, J., Twombley, E., Bricker, D., & Potter, L. (2009). *Ages and stages questionnaires (ASQ): A parent-completed child monitoring system* (3rd ed.). Baltimore, MD: Brooke.

Stokes, J. V., Cameron, M. J., Dorsey, M. F., & Fleming, E. (2004). Task analysis, correspondence training, and general case instruction for teaching personal hygiene skills. *Behavioral Interventions, 19*, 121–135. https://doi.org/10.1002/bin.153

Sutherland, J., Carnett, A., van der Meer, L., Waddington, H., Bravo, A., & McLay, L. (2018). Intensive toilet training targeting defecation for a child with Autism Spectrum Disorder. *Research and Practice in Intellectual and Developmental Disabilities, 5*, 87–97. https://doi.org/10.1080/23297018.2017.1360153

Tadema, A., & Vlaskamp, C. (2009). The time and effort in taking care for children with profound intellectual and multiple disabilities: A study on care load and support. *British Journal of Learning Disabilities, 38*, 41–48. https://doi.org/10.1111/j.1468-3156.2009.00561.x

Taylor, B. A., Levin, L., & Jasper, S. (1999). Increasing play-related statements in children with autism toward their siblings: Effects of video modeling. *Journal of Developmental and Physical Disabilities, 11*, 253–264. https://doi.org/10.1023/A:1021800716392

Taylor, S., Cipani, E., & Clardy, A. (1994). A stimulus control technique for improving the efficacy of an established toilet training program. *Journal of Behavior Therapy and Experimental Psychiatry, 25*, 155–160. https://doi.org/10.1016/0005-7916(94)90010-8

Taggart, L., Truesdale-Kennedy, M., Ryan, A., & McConkey, R. (2012). Examining the support needs of ageing family carers in developing future plans for a relative with an intellectual disability. *Journal of Intellectual Disabilities, 16*, 217–234. https://doi.org/10.1177/1744629512456465

Thinesen, P. J., & Bryan, A. J. (1981). The use of sequential pictorial cues in the initiation and maintenance of grooming behaviors with mentally retarded adults. *Mental Retardation, 19*, 247–250.

Thompson, M. M., & Faibish, G. M. (1970). The use of filmstrips in teaching personal hygiene to the moderately retarded adolescent. *Education and Training of the Mentally Retarded, 5*, 113–118.

Toplis, R., & Hadwin, J. A. (2006). Using social stories to change problematic behavior in school. *Educational Psychology Practice, 22*, 53–67.

United States Department of Health and Human Services. (2000). *Healthy people 2010* (Conference ed.). Washington, DC: U.S. Department of Health and Human Services.

Van Laarhoven, T., & Van Laarhoven-Myers, T. (2006). Comparison of three video-based instructional procedures for teaching daily living skills to persons with developmental disabilities. *Education and Training in Developmental Disabilities, 41*, 365–381.

Veazey, S. E., Valentino, A. L., Low, A. I., McElroy, A. R., & LeBlanc, L. A. (2015). Teaching feminine hygiene skills to young females with Autism Spectrum Disorder and Intellectual Disability. *Behavior Analysis in Practice, 9*, 184–189. https://doi.org/10.1007/s40617-015-0065-0

Vessey, J., Sherwood, J., Warner, D., & Clark, D. (2007). Comparing hand washing to hand sanitizers in reducing elementary school students' absenteeism. *Pediatric Nursing, 33*, 368–372.

Walmsley, C., Mahoney, A., Durgin, A., & Poling, A. (2012). Fostering hand washing before lunch by students attending a special needs young adult program. *Research in Developmental Disabilities, 34*, 95–101. https://doi.org/10.1016/j.ridd.2012.08.002

Walsh, E., Holloway, J., & Lydon, H. (2018). An evaluation of a social skills intervention for adults with autism spectrum disorder and intellectual disabilities preparing for employment in Ireland: A pilot study. *Journal of Autism and Developmental Disorders, 48*, 1727–1741. https://doi.org/10.1007/s10803-017-3441-5

Ward, L. M., Cooper, S. A., Hughes-McCormack, L., Macpherson, L., & Kinnear, D. (2019). Oral health of adults with intellectual disabilities: A systematic review. *Journal of Intellectual Disability Research, 63*, 1359–1378. https://doi.org/10.1111/jir.12632

Wilson, K. P. (2013). Teaching social-communication skills to preschoolers with autism: Efficacy of video versus in vivo modeling in the classroom. *Journal of Autism and Developmental Disorders, 43*, 1819–1831. https://doi.org/10.1007/s10803-012-1731-5

World Health Organization. (2006). WHO guidelines on hand hygiene in health care (advanced draft) : global safety challenge 2005–2006: clean care is safer care. World Health Organization. Retrieved from: https://apps.who.int/iris/handle/10665/69323

Wibowo, S., & Tedjasaputra, M. (2019). The effectiveness of backward chaining in improving buttoning skills in a child with moderate intellectual disability and poor vision: Single-case design. Conference: *Proceedings of the 2nd International Conference on Intervention and Applied Psychology* (ICIAP 2018). https://doi.org/10.2991/iciap-18.2019.11

Chapter 4
Teaching Communication Skills to People with Intellectual and Developmental Disabilities

Jeff Sigafoos

4.1 Communication in Developmental and Intellectual Disabilities

Although communication is difficult to define (Littlejohn & Foss, 2011), it can be broadly conceptualized as a domain of adaptive behavior functioning that involves the exchange of information from one person to another. A more comprehensive definition of communication is that it refers to:

> any act by which one person gives to or receives from another person information about that person's needs, desires, perceptions, knowledge, or affective states. Communication may be intentional or unintentional, may involve conventional or unconventional signals, may take linguistic or nonlinguistic forms, and may occur through spoken or other modes. (National Joint Committee for the Communication Needs of Persons with Severe Disabilities, 1992, para. 10)

As indicated in the above definition, communication acts can occur in a variety of modes. Reichle and Karlan (1985) classified communicative acts into three distinct modalities, specifically: (a) vocal or spoken mode, (b) gesture mode, and (c) graphic mode. The vocal mode includes vocalizations and speech. Gesture-mode communication involves the use of body movements, facial expressions, and natural, informal, and/or formal gestures. Examples include pointing, shaking one's head to indicate "yes" or "no", and producing manual signs from an organized sign language system (e.g., American Sign Language; Kennedy, 2019). Finally, graphic mode communication requires some type of external aide, such as pointing to photographs and line drawings or selecting icons from the visual display of an electronic speech-generating device.

J. Sigafoos (✉)
School of Education, Victoria University of Wellington, Wellington, New Zealand
e-mail: jeff.sigafoos@vuw.ac.nz

R. Lang, P. Sturmey (eds.), *Adaptive Behavior Strategies for Individuals with Intellectual and Developmental Disabilities*, Autism and Child Psychopathology Series, https://doi.org/10.1007/978-3-030-66441-1_4

Communication via the vocal, gesture, or graphic modes are not mutually exclusive and often occur simultaneously, such as when a child vocalizes while also pointing to a desired toy (Esteve-Gibert & Prieto, 2014; Fenlon, Cooperrider, Keane, Brentari, & Goldin-Meadow, 2019). In addition, the information exchanged via any of these modes could involve sending and/or receiving messages related to a wide range of wants and needs. Information exchange can also involve messages about one's observations or perceptions as well as "highly complex thoughts, feelings, and ideas" (Reed, 2018, p. 4).

While communication is just one domain of adaptive behavior functioning, it would be safe to conclude that participation in nearly all aspects of daily life requires effective and socially appropriate communication skills. Communication is not only an important domain of adaptive behavior functioning, it is also a basic human need and a basic human right (United Nations, 2008). In short, the ability to effectively receive and exchange information is critically important for learning, development, and overall quality of life (Brady et al., 2016).

Unfortunately, many people with intellectual disability (ID) experience significant communication impairment (American Association on Intellectual and Developmental Disabilities, 2010). Their communication difficulties can range from delayed speech and language to a total lack of speech and language skills and subsequent reliance on prelinguistic communication forms (Brady & Halle, 2002). Pavelko (2018) pointed out that "All children with ID can be expected to exhibit some type of communication and/or linguistic deficit" (p. 223).

Because ID is a heterogeneous condition that varies along a continuum of severity (American Psychiatric Association, 2013), the associated communication and/or linguistic deficits can also vary widely across individuals. Some of this variation stems from differing etiologies and differing severity levels (Abbeduto, McDuffie, Thurman, & Kover, 2016), but the influence of environmental factors, such as poor language models and ineffective language learning environments, should not be discounted (Sigafoos, O'Reilly, & Green, 2007). Generally, persons with more severe to profound levels of ID and persons with certain types of genetic syndromes (e.g., Angelman syndrome and Rett syndrome) will fail to acquire any appreciable amount of speech (Pavelko, 2018; Sigafoos et al., 2007). Such individuals have been described as having a severe communication impairment or as having complex communication needs (Beukelman & Mirenda, 2013). In contrast, individuals with mild to moderate degrees of ID and people with other specific syndromes (e.g., Down syndrome) can generally be expected to develop speech, although acquisition is likely to be delayed and linguistic deficits (e.g., poor syntax) may persist (Pavelko, 2018; Sigafoos et al., 2007).

Communication impairment is also prevalent among individuals with other types of developmental disabilities (DD), for example, cerebral palsy (Påhlman, Gillberg, & Himmelmann, 2019) and autism spectrum disorder (ASD; Tager-Flusberg & Kasari, 2013). In fact, social communication deficits are defining characteristics of ASD (American Psychiatric Association, 2013). As with ID, the nature and severity of the associated communication impairments will vary across individuals in line with the heterogeneous nature of DD. For example, while most children with ASD acquire some degree of spoken language, the quantity of social communication produced is impoverished when compared to typically developing children (Bacon, Osuna, Courchesne, & Pierce, 2019). And, at the more severe end of the autism spectrum, about 30% of children with ASD fail to acquire any appreciable amount of speech. These children have been described as being minimally verbal (Tager-Flusberg & Kasari, 2013).

Unlike typically developing children who generally acquire speech and language incidentally (Crain, 2019), children with intellectual and developmental disabilities (IDD), particularly children with severe levels of intellectual impairment, may require more intensive, explicit, deliberate, and structured teaching programs in order to develop effective communication skills. As noted before, the lack of effective communication skills is a major hindrance to community participation, learning, social and emotional development, and overall quality of life (Brady et al., 2016). Consequently, communication intervention is a major treatment priority for many people with IDD. Communication intervention for people with IDD could be broadly conceptualized as the provision of systematic instruction to develop effective message exchange capabilities via one or more communication modalities.

4.1.1 Chapter Aim

Given the prevalence of communication impairment among people with IDD, it is not surprising that a significant amount of research has focused on teaching communication skills to such individuals. This research has led to a number of evidence-based intervention approaches. The primary aim of this chapter is to provide an overview of contemporary evidence-based approaches for teaching communication skills to people with IDD.

The literature on teaching communication skills to people with IDD is vast— far too vast to cover in a single chapter. Consequently, this chapter concentrates on three selected communication intervention approaches, specifically: (a) Applied Verbal Behavior, (b) Functional Communication Training, and (c) Naturalistic Developmental Behavioral Interventions. Each of these approaches is supported by a considerable amount of empirical evidence. In addition, these approaches reflect contemporary practice and have been widely used with people of differing ages and with differing degrees and types of IDD. Even with this relatively narrow focus, it would not be possible to consider all of the nuances of the many hundreds of relevant intervention studies related to each approach. Instead, this chapter aims to provide a general overview of each intervention approach. As part of this general overview, exemplary studies are reviewed to illustrate how various approaches have been applied for the purpose of teaching communication skills to people with IDD.

Appreciating contemporary intervention approaches for teaching communication skills to people with IDD depends to some extent on understanding how these approaches evolved. The next section provides a brief historical overview of research in the field of communication intervention for persons with IDD. The aim of this historical overview is to illustrate how prior research has contributed to the evolution of contemporary intervention approaches.

4.2 Historical Overview

The genesis of communication intervention for people with IDD dates back to at least the mid-nineteenth century. One of the most important contributions occurred when Jean-Étienne-Dominique Esquirol recognized that ID was distinct from mental illness (Esquirol, 1845). His accompanying description of ID highlighted the significance of communication impairment in the diagnosis and classification of ID. Some heroic intervention efforts were also reported in the 1800s (Itard, 1962/1894; Seguin, 1971/1866). Itard (1962/1894) for example, described his 5-year effort to establish speech in a mute, and probably developmentally disabled, child named Victor. Victor had been discovered living feral in the wilds of France and was assumed to be about 12-years old when he was found. He presented with significant deficits in adaptive behavior and cognitive functioning, presumably from lack of human interaction. Itard's rehabilitation of Victor included efforts to teach speech and more generally socialize the child in home and community living. Unfortunately, despite 5 years of effort, Victor showed little progress with respect to the acquisition of speech. He did, however, become more socially appropriate and reportedly learned to use a few gestures and word cards to express his desires.

Although the communication difficulties associated with IDD and the consequent need for communication intervention have long been recognized, it was not until the 1970s that the first research-based and replicable intervention programs emerged. Lovaas (1977), for example, published a program for developing vocal-mode language in children with ASD. The program's curriculum progressed from initial vocal imitation training to the teaching of increasingly complex receptive (e.g., selecting named objects) and then expressive language skills (naming objects and actions). The curriculum and accompanying teaching procedures were based on previous intervention research by Lovaas and colleagues (e.g., Lovaas, Berberich, Perloff, & Schaeffer, 1966; Lovaas, Koegel, Simmons, & Long, 1973). Lovaas et al. (1966), for example, showed successful acquisition of imitative speech by two children with autism using behavior analytic/operant conditioning procedures (e.g., shaping, discrimination training, and reinforcement). In a report on the long-term outcomes from a comprehensive behavioral intervention program, Lovaas et al. (1973) reported favorable outcomes in a range of adaptive domains, including appropriate and spontaneous speech. This report was significant for evaluating the effects of intensive behavioral intervention with a relatively large sample ($N = 20$) of children with ASD.

Guess, Sailor, and Baer (1974) also developed a language training program that was in many ways similar to the Lovaas (1977) program. For instance, both programs targeted a range of vocal-mode communication skills (receptive and expressive labeling) as well as more advanced linguistic targets. In addition, both programs used teaching procedures based on operant learning principles (e.g., reinforcement, stimulus control). And both programs emerged from a series of experimental studies aimed at evaluating the effects of operant conditioning procedures on the acquisition of various language structures/linguistic skills. Guess, Sailor, Rutherford, and Baer (1968), for example, demonstrated that operant procedures (e.g., reinforcement, discrimination training) were effective in teaching correct use of the plural morpheme to a girl with severe ID. Using similar teaching procedures, Baer and Guess (1971) taught three individuals with ID to discriminately apply size-related adjectives (e.g., big versus bigger, small versus smaller). This program was significant in demonstrating acquisition of complex language via a carefully sequenced progression of skills that were taught using behavior analytic procedures.

Bricker and Bricker (1970) and Stremel (1972) also published programs for teaching vocal-mode communication to children and adults with ID, respectively. Both programs made use of various operant/behavior analytic teaching procedures to achieve progressively more complex language ability, including speech imitation training, building receptive vocabulary, naming objects and sentence production, for example.

Overall, these pioneering programs, and the underlying intervention research on which they were based, represented significant advances. The intervention research from which these programs were derived has had a lasting and major impact on the field of communication intervention for persons with IDD (LeBlanc, Esch, Sidener, & Firth, 2006; Scheifelbusch & Lloyd, 1974). Intervention success with this population provided convincing evidence that people with IDD, even people with severe IDD, could learn a wide range of speech and language skills with systematic intervention; systematic intervention involving the application of behavioral analytic teaching procedures. The successful outcomes often reported from this research highlighted the relevance of applied behavior analysis to the communication/language domain. Clinicians also benefited in a very practical way because they now had access to numerous evidence-based programs to guide their intervention work.

However, this initial era of research also highlighted a number of intervention challenges. For example, acquisition of vocal-mode communication often proved elusive for minimally verbal participants (Tager-Flusberg & Kasari, 2013). In addition, newly acquired language skills often failed to occur outside of the specific language training environment (Cooke, Cooke, & Apolloni, 1976). Lack of spontaneity, as evidenced by the need for intrusive prompts to evoke communication, was another noted challenge (Halle, 1987). Ensuring functional use of acquired vocabulary also proved challenging (Goldstein & Hontz Hockenberger, 1991). Gaining a large receptive and expressive vocabulary, that is learning a large number of nouns and verbs for example, did not necessarily enable the child to use that acquired vocabulary for communicating important messages, such as expressing wants and needs.

4.3 Contemporary Intervention Approaches

In response to these challenges, new and more effective intervention approaches emerged with increasing attention given to generalization, spontaneity, and functional use of communication skills. Alternative communication modes (e.g., manual signing and picture-based communication systems) also came to be more widely adopted (Beukelman & Mirenda, 2013) and increasingly viewed as legitimate modes of communication for people with IDD. This section reviews three contemporary intervention approaches that reflect these advances and priorities, beginning with the Applied Verbal Behavior approach, followed by Functional Communication Training, and finally Naturalistic Developmental Behavioral Interventions.

4.3.1 Applied Verbal Behavior

Applied Verbal Behavior (AVB) is an approach for teaching communication skills to persons with IDD that: (a) makes explicit use of behavior analytic principles and procedures and (b) targets communication skills derived from Skinner's (1957) analysis of communication. In this analysis, Skinner interpreted communication as a form of operant behavior largely controlled by its social consequences.

With respect to the first characteristic, AVB interventions involve applying some combination of various operant/behavior analytic principles and procedures in a structured, systematic, and deliberate intervention. The specific procedures used in teaching include: (a) reinforcement; (b) stimulus control and transfer of stimulus control; (c) discrimination training; (d) prompting, fading, and chaining; and (e) generalization and maintenance programming (Ivy & Schreck, 2016). Thus the AVB approach, as indeed many other communication intervention programs for people with IDD, could be seen as the application of systematic instruction (Collins, 2012) to teach precisely defined communication skills.

The second, and perhaps the most unique, characteristic of the AVB approach is its embrace of Skinner's (1957) functional account of communication as verbal behavior. In Skinner's analysis, the term verbal behavior referred to any form of behavior that would be effective as a means of message exchange. Verbal behavior includes speech of course but also non-speech forms of communication, such as writing, gestures, manual signing, picture exchange, and selecting graphic symbols from the display of an electronic speech-generating device. Uniquely, Skinner (1957) classified communication skills (or verbal operants) in terms of their controlling antecedents and consequences rather than using traditional linguistic categories (e.g., nouns, verbs). The basic verbal operants were the mand, tact, intraverbal, and echoic. Training on these skills (or basic verbal operants) constitutes the core curriculum of the AVB approach.

4.3.1.1 Mand

The mand is a communication skill that relates to messages about wants and needs. Technically, a mand is evoked by deprivation or aversive stimulation and maintained by consequences that alleviate/reduce the impinging state of deprivation or aversive stimulation. For example, when thirsty (i.e., deprived of water), a child might produce the mand *Water, please*. Receiving a glass of water from the listener would be the functional reinforcer for this mand form. Requesting access to preferred or needed objects and rejecting non-preferred objects are two important subclasses of the mand relation (Sigafoos et al., 2004). Requesting is often selected as the initial intervention target in AVB programs because it enables the individual to gain reinforcement, exert control over the environment, and express wants and needs (Reichle, York, & Sigafoos, 1991). Reichle et al. (1991) outlined a paradigm for teaching a basic manding skill; specifically requesting access to preferred objects. In this paradigm, a highly preferred item (e.g., the child's favorite toy) is present, but not readily available, perhaps by being placed out of reach. This situation is intended to create a relatively mild state of deprivation, thus creating the need (or motivation) for the person to produce the targeted mand form. The mand form is individualized to suit the person's abilities and could consist of either saying, signing, or selecting graphic symbols to communicate a relevant message (e.g., *I want X*). A time delay procedure is then implemented in which the individual is given some reasonable amount of time (e.g., 10–20 s) to produce the targeted mand form. If the targeted mand form does not occur within this time interval, then the instructor would deliver a response prompt to evoke the desired mand form. For example, the instructor could model the correct response or physically assist the person to make the response. A key component of this type of mand training intervention is to ensure that correct responses are reinforced with access to the requested item. It is also critical to fade out the use of response prompts to promote spontaneous (i.e., unprompted) requesting (Gobbi, Cipani, Hudson, & Lapenta-Neudeck, 1986; Halle, 1987).

Although requesting preferred items is an important and highly functional communication skill, the ability to reject non-preferred objects could be seen as equally important. Indeed, escape and avoidance of aversive stimulation is a significant motivation for communication (Vicker, 2008). Consequently, people with IDD will likely benefit from mand training that is focused on teaching rejecting as well as requesting. Along these lines, Choi, O'Reilly, Sigafoos, and Lancioni (2010) successfully taught an integrated sequence of requesting and rejecting skills to four children with IDD. Children were specifically taught to request missing, but needed, items. They learned to do this using either a picture exchange communication mode or by selecting graphic symbols on a speech-generating device. During intervention, children were sometimes given an item that did not match the reference of their prior request. This presentation of a wrong item was intended to set the occasion for teaching the rejecting response. The results showed that all four children learned to request missing items and reject wrong items. These newly acquired skills generalized to untrained items and were maintained at a 4-week follow-up for three of the four participants.

In addition to requesting and rejecting, more advanced manding skills have also been successfully taught to people with IDD using variations on the basic mand training paradigm outlined above. Sundberg, Leob, Hale, and Eigenheer (2002), for example, created the need for children with ASD to ask questions (i.e., mand for information) by hiding a desired object and then instructing the children to *Find x.* To successfully comply with this instruction, the children first had to ask *Where?* [is the object]. The resulting information about the object's location was intended to function as reinforcement for asking *Where?* More recently, Carnett, Ingvarsson, Bravo, and Sigafoos (2020) demonstrated successful procedures for teaching three minimally verbal children with ASD to mand for information (*Where is x?*). A unique aspect of this study was that the children were taught to use speech-generating devices to ask this question. Instruction occurred within the context of toy/game play with motivation created by hiding missing parts. Children learned to mand for information using a least-to-most prompting procedure (gesture, vocal, and physical prompting).

Overall, there is considerable evidence to support the use of behavioral procedures (response prompting, time delay) and specific motivational arrangements (e.g., behavior chain interruption strategy, missing-item format, and wrong-item format) for teaching a range of vocal-mode, gesture-mode, and graphic-mode mands to people with IDD (see DeSouza, Akers, & Fisher, 2017; Shafer, 1995; Wallace, 2007 for reviews). DeSouza, for example, identified 91 studies that evaluated procedures for teaching various kinds of mands (requesting, rejecting, and manding for information) to children with ASD. Success has also been obtained with adolescents and adults and with a range of other IDD conditions (Gobbi et al., 1986; McCook, Cipani, Madigan, & LaCampagne, 1988; Nepo, Tincani, Axelrod, & Meszaros, 2017; Reichle & Brown, 1986; Reichle, Rogers, & Barrett, 1984; Sigafoos, Laurie, & Pennell, 1996; Tirapelle & Cipani, 1991; Ziomek & Rehfeldt, 2008).

4.3.1.2 Tact

The tact is a communication skill that relates to messages about environmental referents. Technically, tacts are evoked by nonverbal stimuli and maintained by generalized conditioned reinforcement (Skinner, 1957). An important aspect of the tact is that the communication form expressed by the person relates in some meaningful way to its nonverbal referent or stimulus. For example, the spoken response *Rain* could be classified as a tact if it was evoked by the sight or sound of rain falling (the nonverbal stimulus) and reinforced by a relevant listener reply. (e.g., *Yes, I see it is raining. Thank you for letting me know.*) Procedures to teach tacts related to naming objects (expressive labeling), describing actions, and commenting on aspects of the environment have historically been included as a major curriculum area in communication intervention programs for people with IDD (Bricker & Bricker, 1970;

Guess et al., 1974; Lovaas, 1977; Stremel, 1972). Sundberg (2015) noted that tacting is an important class of communication behavior for several reasons. First, the ability to tact (i.e., name/label) everyday objects and other environmental stimuli represents an important knowledge/vocabulary base, which can become potentially available for engaging in other communicative behavior, such as requesting and rejecting. In addition, successful functioning in home, school, vocational, and community settings requires knowing the names of objects and actions, for example. Being able to name or label a wide range of objects, concepts, and stimulus properties (e.g., big, small, hot, cold) is arguably one mark of an educated person. Furthermore, tacting represents an appropriate way to provide important information to others (e.g., *Your telephone is ringing*). Providing helpful information such as this might lead to increased positive social interactions. Commenting on the features of the environment, which is a type of tacting, might also be an effective means of initiating conversations.

A common arrangement for teaching tacts involves: (a) presenting an object or performing an action (e.g., showing the child a fork or clapping your hands), (b) providing a verbal cue (e.g., asking *What is this? or What am I doing?*), and (c) prompting correct responses as necessary. Unlike with mand training, correct tacting responses are reinforced with some unrelated consequence (e.g., a preferred edible, verbal acknowledgement, or praise). The important aspect of reinforcement in the tact relation is that the reinforcer should be unrelated to the form of the response. The use of generalized conditioned reinforcement versus response-specific reinforcement is one feature that distinguishes mand training from tact training (Reichle, Lindamood, & Sigafoos, 1986).

This general type of instructional arrangement has long been successfully used in teaching individuals with IDD to name or label objects, actions, and even abstract properties of objects, such as their color or shape (Bricker & Bricker, 1970; Guess et al., 1974; Lovaas, 1977; Stremel, 1972). Tacting behavior has been taught in the speech/vocal-mode (Guess et al., 1974; Lovaas, 1977), as well as with alternative modes of communication, such as manual signing (Partington, Sundberg, Newhouse, & Spengler, 1994), and picture-based communication systems (Murphy, Steele, Gilligan, Yeow, & Spare, 1977; Reichle et al., 1984).

An illustrative study on teaching tacting was published by Barbera and Kubina Jr. (2005). They evaluated variations of the general tact training paradigm outlined above for teaching object labels (e.g., feather, mitten, salad, and teapot) to a 7-year-old boy with mild ID and ASD. Intervention involved presenting a picture of each object and asking *What is it?* The prompting strategy used was rather novel, in that it included rapidly moving from a receptive language task (i.e., telling the child to point to a specified picture) and then modeling the correct spoken label for the child to imitate. Correct responses were followed by social praise. With this procedure, the child acquired 30 tact responses within 30 (5-min) teaching sessions. This is an important finding as it shows a procedure by which some children with mild ID and ASD could rapidly acquire a large number of tacting responses.

In another illustrative study, Kagohara et al. (2012) successfully taught two adolescents to tact pictures of various images. The participants were minimally verbal and had ASD. During teaching sessions, participants were shown photographs (e.g., a photograph of a river or dolphin) and asked *What do you see?* or *What is this?* A correct tacting response required the participants to select the colored line drawing (e.g., a line drawing of a river or a dolphin) corresponding to the photographic image they had just been shown. Importantly, the photographs and line drawings contained the same relevant detail (e.g., a depiction of a river or a dolphin), but the two respective images were not identical. A unique feature of the study was that the line drawings were presented on an iPad with speech-generating software. Thus, selecting line drawings produced relevant synthetic speech output (e.g., "*River*" or "*Dolphin*"). Using reinforcement, time-delay, and least-to-most prompting procedures, both participants initially acquired tacts for 12 different images, and they later learned an additional 18 tacts. Most of the acquired tacts were also maintained when assessed at a 4-week follow-up.

Another notable study on teaching tacts was reported by Conallen and Reed (2016). Their study included 10 primary-school-aged children with ASD. The study aimed to teach these children to tact emotional states (e.g., happy, sad, angry). Specifically, the children were taught to select from one of three emotion cards (showing either a happy, sad, or angry child) when presented with corresponding cartoon scenarios. For example, a cartoon of a child receiving a puppy was used to signify happiness. To teach these tacts, the instructor presented a cartoon scenario and also gave a verbal summary of the cartoon (e.g., *Mummy has brought home a puppy, how does he feel?*). Correct responses were followed by a [presumably reinforcing] social response from the trainer. (*Yes, that's right. The child is happy because his mummy brought him a puppy.*) To ensure responses would occur and to prevent errors, the children were pre-trained to match the emotion cards to their corresponding scenarios. With this procedure, correct tacting increased from less than 10% in baseline to 80% or better after intervention. Correct tacting was maintained at this high level after intervention, and generalization to untrained scenarios was noted. A second generalization test revealed that the children were also able to correctly identify scenarios that made them either happy, sad, or angry. This latter finding suggests that the intervention had in fact equipped the children to tact three of their own emotional states. A unique aspect of this study was the use of a graphic-mode response form (i.e., selecting emotion cards). It is noted that all 10 children had prior experience with the Picture Exchange Communication System (PECS; Bondy & Frost, 1998). (Parenthetically, PECS is a manualized intervention for teaching graphic-mode communication skills to people with IDD who are minimally verbal. With PECS, participants are first taught to exchange picture cards to mand preferred objects.) While, Conallen and Reed focused on teaching tacts, it is possible that this prior experience with PECS may have facilitated acquisition.

Overall, as with manding, there is considerable evidence to support the use of behavioral procedures for teaching tacting behavior to people with IDD. In their review of the AVB literature for children with ASD, DeSouza et al. (2017) identified 56 studies that included tact training. Within these studies, a range of behavior analytic teaching procedures were described, including different training configurations, for example, massed versus distributed teaching opportunities and different prompting and error correction strategies. The resulting data show that these procedures were all generally effective for teaching a range of tacting behavior.

4.3.1.3 Intraverbal

The intraverbal is a communication skill that relates to the prior verbal behavior of a communicative partner. Technically, an intraverbal response is evoked by verbal stimuli and maintained by generalized conditioned reinforcement (Skinner, 1957). The verbal stimulus and the verbal response are thematically related, but not identical. For example, the spoken response *lamb* could be classified as a intraverbal if it was evoked by the prior verbal stimulus *Mary had a little* _____ and reinforced by a relevant listener reply (e.g., *Yes, that's right. Mary did have a little lamb.)* Making topic relevant comments during conversation and answering questions are two familiar kinds of intraverbal behavior.

As with mands and tacts, the intraverbal is a key curriculum area of AVB programs and a range of behavior analytic principles and teaching tactics have been successfully applied in teaching intraverbals to people with IDD. Indeed, there appears to be a growing number of intervention studies targeting the intraverbal. DeSouza et al. (2017), for example, identified 40 studies in which behavior analytic interventions were used to establish intraverbal responses among children with ASD.

A precedent setting early example of intraverbal training was published in 1983 by Braam and Poling. Their study involved two adolescents and one young adult with severe ID and hearing impairment. Participants were taught to produce manual signs for items that exemplified different super-ordinate categories. For example, producing the intraverbal signs BOOK, BUS, CHILDREN, RULER, and TEACHER in response to the verbal stimulus given by the instruction: [items found at] SCHOOL. The teaching procedures varied somewhat across the three participants, but generally progressed as follows: First, the instructor would present the verbal stimulus (e.g., manual sign for a specific category, such as HOME or SCHOOL). Next, participants were given 10 s to produce one or more of the corresponding intraverbals (i.e., BOOK, RULER, etc.). Correct responses resulted in praise and tokens, which were later exchanged for preferred items. Incorrect or no responding resulted in the instructor turning away for 10 s (i.e., a local time-out procedure) and presenting the same category with a picture or word prompt (e.g., presenting a picture of a ruler). Presenting pictures could be seen as a type of tact prompt. Tact prompts were faded by using a 10-s time delay procedure. The combination of tact prompting and time delay was intended as a means of transferring stimulus control of the participants' manual signed responses from the tact prompt (i.e., from the pictures) to the prior verbal stimulus (i.e., the instructor's category sign). With these procedures, all three participants quickly learned to produce the targeted intraverbals without prompting. In addition, the acquired intraverbals were maintained at follow-up and participants also showed response generalization by producing novel intraverbal responses that had not been directly taught.

More recent work has provided additional evidence to support the use of similar procedures for teaching intraverbal behavior (see DeSouza et al., 2017 for relevant citations). Goldsmith, LeBlanc, and Sautter (2007), for example, provided intraverbal training to three children (4–7 years old) with ASD. Training occurred in the vocal mode with the children taught to respond to questions such as *What are some things you wear?* and *What are some colors?* Training involved asking one of the questions (e.g., *What are some fruits?*) and immediately also presenting a tact prompt (e.g., a picture of an apple). Preferred edibles and praise were used as reinforcing consequences for correct responses. If a correct response did not occur to the tact prompt, then an imitative (echoic) model (i.e., *Say apple*) was used. To transfer control from the prompts to the initial question (e.g., *What are some fruits?*), a 3-s time delay was introduced between the question and the prompt. With this training, all three children began to produce correct responses to the various questions being asked, indicating acquisition of intraverbal responding. However, maintenance and generalization to an untrained category were limited.

Success in teaching intraverbals to people with IDD using the general strategies outlined by Braam and Poling (1983) and Goldsmith et al. (2007) would seem to hinge on participants already having tacts or echoic/imitative response forms corresponding to the targeted intraverbal forms. The presence of such prerequisite skills would enable the instructor to teach intraverbals using tact or echoic prompts. Intervention would then involve transferring stimulus control from the tact or echoic prompt to intended verbal stimulus (e.g., the question or category name) by delaying its presentation or otherwise fading the prompt, such as reducing the amount or intensity of the prompt. The success of any such prompting may also depend on participants' prior experience with tact and/or echoic prompts (Roncati, Coelho Souza, & Miguel, 2019). An interesting, yet unresolved, issue is the ease with which intraverbal responses could be taught when the targeted vocabulary/response forms are not already present in the person's verbal repertoire as either tacts or echoics/imitative responses. One might be successful in teaching gesture-mode and graphic-mode intraverbals without needing tact or echoic prompts (e.g., by instead using physical guidance prompts), but prompting speech-mode intraverbals (and speech-mode mands and tacts for that matter) would seem to depend on the person already being able to at least respond to an echoic prompt.

4.3.1.4 Echoic

Echoic behavior involves imitating or repeating the prior communicative behavior of another person. Technically, the echoic is occasioned by a prior verbal stimulus and reinforced by generalized social reinforcement. The critical aspect of the echoic, which distinguishes it from the intraverbal, is that the form of the echoic response matches the form of the stimulus. Everyday examples of echoic behavior include saying *Hello* when similarly greeted by a friend (*Hello Robert*) and repeating a parent's instruction to *finish lunch* by replying with *Yes. I will finish my lunch*. Imitation of this type can occur in the vocal, gesture, and graphic modes. In the vocal mode, the person repeats verbatim the speech of another. In the gesture mode, the person repeats the communicative gestures/manual signs of another person. An example of graphic-mode echoic might be when a teacher points to a communicative symbol representing lunch time, and the child then points to that same symbol shortly afterward to indicate having received the teacher's intended message that it is now lunch time.

Echoic behavior, and the more general ability to imitate, is very useful for instructional purposes. Imitative ability has also been implicated in facilitating language development (Bloom, Hood, & Lightbown, 1974). Ledford and Wolery (2011) emphasized the general notion that imitation is an important means by which children learn new skills. Various communication skills (e.g., object labels and scripted answers to standard questions) can be learned via imitation. Good imitation skills often make it easier to teach new behaviors because the teacher can then model the correct response for the person to imitate.

However, echoic behavior is important for reasons beyond facilitating instruction and general language development. In fact, good echoic skills are important for effective message exchange and more generally for good conversation. Indeed, echoic behavior appears to be a common feature of social-communicative interactions, as when one person's initial message is partially repeated and then expanded upon by his or her communicative partner (Carnett, Raulston, & Charpentier, 2019).

Many people with IDD appear to have limited imitation skills, including an underdeveloped echoic repertoire (Greer & Ross, 2008). This situation indicates the need for intervention to develop this aspect of the person's communication repertoire. Historically, communication interventions for people with IDD typically included initial imitation training (Bricker & Bricker, 1970; Guess et al., 1974; Lovaas, 1977; Stremel, 1972). The classic procedure for teaching vocal-mode imitation was demonstrated by Lovaas et al. (1966). The procedure involved four phases. First, any vocalization produced by the individual was reinforced so as to increase the frequency of vocal behavior. Next, the instructor modeled a speech sound (e.g., *ma*, *ba*) and reinforced any vocalizations that occurred within a few seconds of the model. The aim here was to teach the child to respond contingently to the instructor's prior vocal stimulus. The third phase involved response shaping in which reinforcement was contingent upon the child's response being increasingly similar to the instructor's prior verbal model. In the final phase, response chaining was used to develop more complex imitative responses (*ba*, *ball*, *red ball*, *big red ball*, etc.).

Imitation training of communicative gestures and graphic mode responses (e.g., exchanging a picture card) can be taught with a more streamlined set of procedures. This is because, unlike vocal responses, motor responses can be prompted by using physical assistance. For example, the instructor could give an instruction (e.g., Sign drink) while also demonstrating the manual sign for DRINK. The child could then be physically assisted to produce this sign and reinforced for doing so. Over successive teaching opportunities, physical assistance would be faded using time delay and by reducing the amount of physical assistance provided, a procedure known as graduated guidance (Billingsley & Romer, 1983). Transfer of stimulus control is achieved when the child imitates the instructor's prior manual sign without requiring any additional prompts.

The standard echoic training paradigm generally involves: (a) presenting a model or verbal stimulus for the person to imitate and (b) delivering reinforcement for responses that closely follow the model in time and which also closely match the form of the prior verbal stimulus. Variations on this standard approach included (a) gradually shaping up imitative responses by reinforcing closer and closer approximations to the model and (b) directly prompting imitative responses and then fading out the prompts over successive opportunities. Overall, this standard (behavioral) approach to imitation training has been widely used and has generally proven to be a fairly successful method for teaching echoic behavior to persons with IDD (DeSouza et al., 2017; Mulhern et al., 2017; Stock, Schulze, & Mirenda, 2008).

To summarize, the AVB approach uses behavior analytic procedures to teach the specific classes of communication skills delineated by Skinner (1957); principally, mands, tacts, intraverbals, and echoic responses. Instructors can draw upon a large number of published AVB intervention studies to guide their teaching of these different classes of communication skills. Instruction can proceed in any mode appropriate for the individual (i.e., vocal, gesture, and/or graphic communication modalities). A good starting point for implementing AVB is the excellent recent review by DeSouza et al. (2017).

4.3.2 Functional Communication Training

Functional communication training (FCT) is primarily used in the treatment of problem behavior (Carr et al., 1994; Durand, 1990; Durand & Moskowitz, 2019; Reichle & Wacker, 2017). Problem behaviors, such as aggression, self-injury, and extreme tantrums, are prevalent among people with IDD (Simó-Pinatella, Mumbardó-Adam, Alomar-Kurz, Sugai, & Simonsen, 2019). Considerable evidence points toward a link between the nature and severity of communication impairment and frequency and severity of problem behavior among people with IDD (Curtis, Frey, Watson, Hampton, & Roberts, 2018; Matson, Wilkins, & Macken, 2009). Based on this link, Durand (1986) argued that some problem behavior could be interpreted as a form of communication. For individuals with IDD who have extremely limited speech and language development, problem behaviors might represent their only effective means of expressing basic wants, needs, and emotions. When problem behavior represents a form of communication, then such behaviors might be effectively reduced—or even completely replaced—by teaching the person to use more socially appropriate forms of communication (Durand & Moskowitz, 2019). This is the logic of FCT.

FCT is based on two concepts (a) functional equivalence and (b) response efficiency (Carr & Kemp, 1989; Horner & Day, 1991). Functional equivalence applies when topographically different responses nonetheless lead to (or would lead to) the same reinforcing outcome. For example, a person might successfully request assistance by saying *Can you help me please?* or by selecting a *HELP ME* symbol on a speech-generating device. In this example, the two responses are functionally equivalent because they would both result in the person receiving the requested help. A large amount of data from experimental assessment studies has shown that problem behavior (e.g., tantrums or self-injury) is often maintained by socially mediated reinforcers, primarily: (a) attention from a social partner, (b) escape from nonpreferred activities, and/or (c) access to preferred objects (Iwata et al., 1994). These types of problem behavior could thus be seen as functionally equivalent to the communication skills of: (a) recruiting attention, (b) rejecting nonpreferred activities, and (c) requesting preferred objects, respectively. Such problematic forms of behavior might therefore be reduced or replaced by teaching the person to use socially appropriate communication skills to gain attention, reject, and request, respectively.

The second fundamental concept underpinning FCT, i.e., response efficiency, means that any new communication skill will only replace an existing problem behavior if the former is made more efficient than the latter (Horner & Day, 1991). Response efficiency encompasses two main features. First, a response is more efficient when it produces more frequent, immediate, and consistent reinforcement. To achieve this, each and every instance of appropriate communication should be reinforced—at least during the initial stages of FCT—and problem behavior should no longer be reinforced. In addition, the targeted communication skills should be easy for the person to perform, both in terms of physical effort and cognitive demand. A child who screams to get attention is unlikely to shift to using appropriate speech if listeners expect complex sentences from the child. Better to begin by teaching the child to produce a single word (e.g., *Hi*) as the initial alternative to screaming.

4.3.2.1 Implementing FCT

FCT involves first identifying the function or purpose of the problem behavior and then teaching a functionally equivalent, and more socially appropriate, form of communicative behavior. Identifying the function or purpose of problem behavior is accomplished by undertaking a functional assessment. Functional assessment aims to identify the antecedents that set the occasion for problem behavior and the consequences that reinforce and maintain the behavior. Within an applied behavior analytic framework, behavior is explained when its controlling antecedents and consequences have been identified. Thus, a functional assessment could be seen as an attempt to explain problem behavior. It seeks to determine why a specific problem behavior is occurring, what function(s) it serves, and what reinforcing outcomes it produces for the person.

Several procedures have been developed to assess the function or purpose of problem behavior in people with IDD. These include the use of questionnaires, interview protocols, naturalistic observations, and structured observations. Matson (2012) provided a comprehensive survey of these varying assessment tactics and their associated pros and cons.

The gold standard protocol for identifying the function of problem behavior in people with IDD is the functional-experimental analysis methodology developed by Iwata, Dorsey, Slifer, Bauman, and Richman (1982). In a functional-experimental analysis, the assessor records the frequency of a person's problem behavior under a number of different conditions or contingencies. Commonly used assessment conditions include (a) attention, (b) task, and (c) tangible scenarios.

In the attention condition, the person and an assessor are situated in the same space and the assessor attends to the person contingent upon each instance of the person's problem behavior. High rates of problem behavior in this condition suggest the behavior is functioning as a means of recruiting attention. Logically, a functionally equivalent replacement would involve use of a more appropriate communicative skill for gaining attention. For example, the person might be taught to activate an attention signal switch (Sobsey & Reichle, 1989).

In the task condition, in contrast, the person is prompted to work on a demanding task, which is then interrupted in response to each instance of problem behavior. High rates of problem behavior in this condition suggest that problem behavior is functioning as a means of escaping from nonpreferred activities. A logical target for FCT would be to teach more appropriate means of escaping from task demands. The person might be taught to request a break from the task or ask for help in completing the task. Both of these skills might work to reduce the aversiveness of the task and thus reduce the use of escape-motivated problem behavior (Reichle & McComas, 2004).

To assess for a possible tangible function, preferred items are present but made accessible to the person only following instances of problem behavior. High rates of problem behavior in this condition suggest that problem behavior is functioning as a mand for tangible/preferred objects. A logical replacement strategy here would be to teach more socially appropriate mand forms. For example, the person could be taught to use speech, manual signs, or assistive devices (e.g., a speech-generating device) to request preferred objects (Durand, 1993).

As highlighted in the above scenarios, FCT interventions often focus on teaching different kinds of mands, such as vocal-mode, gesture-mode, or graphic-mode requests for: (a) attention, (b) breaks, (c) assistance, and (d) preferred objects and activities. In recognition of this, DeSouza et al. (2017) classified FCT as "a special case of mand training" (p. 236). When seen in this light, FCT is conceptually related to the more general AVB approach.

In terms of teaching the functionally equivalent communication alternative, FCT uses well-established behavior-analytic procedures which are generally of the same type used in the AVB approach and in the pioneering programs from the 1970s (Bricker & Bricker, 1970; Guess et al., 1974; Lovaas, 1977; Stremel, 1972). In a review of FCT studies using gesture- and graphic-mode alternatives, Walker, Lyon, Loman, and Sennott (2018) documented the range of behavior-analytic principles and procedures that were employed in different FCT studies. These included: (a) creating the need or motivation for communication (e.g., using the behavior chain interruption strategy or missing-item format), (b) applying various prompting and prompt fading strategies (e.g., least-to-most and most-to-least prompt hierarchies, time delay, and graduated guidance), and (c) programming reinforcement for the replacement skills and extinction for problem behavior. An important aspect of FCT is that instruction to teach alternative communication skills should occur under the same antecedent conditions that set the occasion for problem behavior. That is, intervention to teach functionally equivalent communication needs to be properly contextualized (Walker et al., 2018).

Contextualizing intervention may help to promote generalization and maintenance and ensure that the targeted communication skills will in fact come to serve as a functionally equivalent replacement for problem behavior.

In their classic study, Carr and Durand (1985) successfully used FCT to replace disruptive behavior in four children with IDD. A prior functional assessment indicated that some of the participating children engaged in disruption when attention from the teacher was infrequent. In contrast, the disruptive behavior of the other children was most frequent when they were working on difficult academic tasks. In the former case, the children were taught to recruit praise/attention, whereas the other children were taught to request assistance with the difficult task. Instruction occurred in the vocal mode. Children were taught to emit socially appropriate sentences when the instructor asked a priming question (i.e., *Do you have any questions*). The priming question was intended to set the occasion for the children to either recruit attention and praise (*Am I doing good work?*) or to request help by indicating a lack of understanding (e.g., *I don't understand*). If the children did not respond to the priming question, then an echoic prompt was provided (e.g., *Say am I doing good work*). The use of echoic prompts was eliminated after the children could reliably imitate the target phrase when given the verbal cue. With these procedures, the children learned to recruit attention or solicit help, respectively. Acquisition of these alternative communication skills was associated with collateral decreases in disruptive behavior. The success of this intervention was attributed to the teaching of vocal mands (i.e., requests for attention or requests for help) that enabled the children to obtain the same reinforcing outcomes that had previously followed disruptive behavior.

A decade later, Sigafoos and Meikle (1996) aimed to reduce problem behavior that served multiple communicative functions by teaching multiple communicative replacements. The study involved two 8-year-old boys with ASD. Results of an initial functional assessment suggested that the boys' problem behaviors (e.g., aggression, self-injury, and property destruction) served multiple functions, specifically to request attention and to request access to preferred tangibles, such as foods, beverages, and/or toys. The boys were therefore taught two communicative alternatives; one to recruit attention and one to request preferred objects. To recruit attention, one boy was taught to use a gesture (i.e., lightly tapping the teacher's hand) and the other boy was taught to say the teacher's name. To request preferred objects, one boy was taught to point to graphic symbols (i.e., line drawings representing *FOOD*, *DRINK*, and *TOYS*) and the other boy was taught to use single words. Under conditions that had previously evoked problem behavior (i.e., the teacher being present, but not attending to the child and preferred items being visible, but out of reach), the children were initially prompted to immediately produce the relevant communicative alternative. For the child being taught gesture-mode and graphic mode responses, prompting consisted of using physical assistance/graduated guidance. For the child being taught in the vocal mode, echoic prompts (*Say want drink.* or *Say want toy.*) were used. Over successive teaching opportunities, prompts were faded by waiting longer and longer before prompting (i.e., time delay prompting). With these procedures, both children showed increased use of the targeted communication alternatives and collateral decreases in problem behavior. This finding suggested that the newly taught communication skills served as effective alternatives to the children's problem behavior.

In a more recent FCT study, Muharib, Correa, Wood, and Haughney (2019) explored whether use of a high-tech speech-generating device could be taught as an alternative to problem behavior. Participants were a 6-year-old girl and a 5-year-old boy. Both children had ASD and were minimally verbal. Their problem behaviors included crying, grabbing, and head banging. The initial functional assessment involved recording the antecedents and consequences surrounding instances of problem behavior. The results of this A-B-C analysis suggested that both children used problem behavior to gain access to preferred objects, such as toys and books. The FCT intervention focused on teaching the children to request access to these preferred objects by selecting icons from the screen of the iPad®-based speech-generating device. Teaching involved briefly interrupting the child's use of a preferred object, waiting 10 s for an independent response, and then prompting an iPad-based request if one had not occurred independently within 10 s of the interruption. Prompts were faded using a least-to-most hierarchy. The hierarchy consisted of first giving a verbal cue. (e.g., *If you want your toy back, touch the picture.*) If this failed to evoke a correct response, the teacher then gave a variant of this verbal cue (*If you want your toy back, touch here*), while also pointing to the correct icon on the iPad® screen. If the combined use of a verbal and gesture prompt was ineffective, the teacher resorted to physically guiding the child's finger to tap the correct symbol. Correct responses produced relevant synthesized speech output (e.g., "*I want book.*") and immediate access to the requested object. The latter outcome represented natural reinforcement for making an iPad®-based requesting response. In addition, while delivering the requested object, the teacher also made relevant verbal comments (e.g., *Alright, it's your turn now. I liked that you touched the book picture*). It is also important to note that if problem behavior occurred during the 10-s interruption, this did not result in access to the preferred object. Instead this meant that the child was prompted to use the iPad®. The results of this intervention were positive in that both children learned to use the iPad® to make requests. Importantly, when iPad®-based requesting was acquired, problem behavior decreased. These results suggest that iPad®-based requesting had effectively replaced or displaced the children's problem behavior. The study represents an important development in the application of FCT given the increasing popularity of iPad®-based speech-generating devices for people with IDD and severe communication impairment (Ok, 2018; Rispoli, Franco, van der Meer, Lang, & Hoher Camargo, 2010).

In summary, the compelling logic of FCT is matched by an equally compelling (and extensive) evidence base. Since 1985, a plethora of studies have accumulated to support the effectiveness and efficacy of FCT in the treatment of problem behavior among people with IDD. Numerous reviews of FCT (Gerow et al., 2018; Gerow, Davis, Radhakrishnan, Gregori, & Rivera, 2018; Mancil, 2006; Mirenda, 1997; Neely, Garcia, Bankston, & Green, 2018; Walker et al., 2018) have confirmed its general effectiveness. These reviews indicate the wide applicability of FCT. FCT has been successfully used in helping children, adolescents, and adults with varying types and degrees of IDD. It has also been successfully applied in the treatment of a wide range of problem behaviors (e.g., aggression, self-injury, tantrums, stereotypy, and property destruction). Furthermore, a wide range of communication skills—from the vocal-mode, gesture-mode and graphic-mode—have been successfully taught to replace problem behavior. In addition, problem behaviors serving a range of different [communicative] functions (e.g., requesting, rejecting/protesting, recruiting attention) have been replaced using FCT. In conclusion, FCT can be a highly effective approach for developing socially appropriate communicative alternatives to problem behavior among people with IDD. It is indicated for use when problem behaviors have social-communicative functions as determined by a prior functional assessment.

4.3.3 Naturalistic Developmental Behavioral Intervention

Naturalistic Developmental Behavioral Interventions (NBDIs) represent a class of approaches that share a number of distinct characteristics. In an important consensus paper, Schreibman et al. (2015) delineated five key characteristics of NDBIs. These are: (a) implementation in natural settings, (b) shared control between child and therapist, (c) natural reinforcement, (d) use of behavior analytic/systematic instructional strategies, and (e) a focus on teaching developmentally appropriate skills. Further explanation of each of these characteristics may help to clarify the unique aspects of the NDBI approach.

First, a NDBI is meant to be implemented in natural, real-world settings and within everyday routines and social interactions. Thus, intervention should ideally occur in the settings and during the activities in which the targeted communication skills are ultimately expected to occur. For example, in an NDBI approach, instruction to teach mands related to gaining access to toys and turn taking might occur during play periods at both home and school. In contrast, instruction to teach mands related to food and drink would occur at the person's regular mealtimes. As another example, certain types of intraverbals (e.g., answering questions) might be taught during story time in both the home and preschool setting. The use of natural environments as the instructional setting stands in contrast to the use of pull-out models and clinical settings, which characterized many of the pioneering communication intervention programs. This difference in implementation setting might partially explain the often-noted lack of generalization in the communication intervention literature (Cooke et al., 1976; Drasgow, Halle, & Sigafoos, 1999; Stokes & Baer, 1977).

Second, NDBIs tend to mix child-initiated opportunities with therapist-directed instruction. Sometimes the therapist might deliberately create a teaching opportunity by picking up the child's preferred toy and asking a specific question (e.g., *What color is the car?*). On other occasions, however, the therapist might wait for the child to initiate a communicative interaction and then reinforce the child's intended meaning. This latter scenario represents an approach in which the therapist aims to capture and capitalize on the child's motivation to communicate, which provides optimal conditions for teaching new communication skills. The distribution of therapist-directed versus child-initiated opportunities is likely to change over time, and become more child-directed as the child's rate of initiation and range of communication skills increases. In NDBIs, therapists adjust the degree of directedness to match the child's changing developmental level. Also in NDBIs, various natural communication partners (e.g., parents, teachers, peers) could be enlisted as therapists, which would again likely help in promoting generalization.

Third, NDBIs emphasize the use of natural consequences rather than contrived reinforcers (Skinner, 1982). A young child who vocalizes while also pointing to a cookie, for example, should receive the cookie because this is the natural reinforcer for the child's behavior. In contrast, a child who correctly named a cookie when shown one and asked *What is this?* should receive a natural social consequence (e.g., *Yes, that's right. It is a cookie. Well done*!). The deliberate avoidance of contrived reinforcement is consistent with AVB and FCT. In all three approaches, ensuring a [functional] match between a person's communication responses and the resulting consequences is what helps to define the function or message underlying different types of communication skills (Carnett et al., 2019; Skinner, 1957).

Fourth, the nitty-gritty instructional tactics used in NDBIs are derived from behavior analytic principles. The specific teaching procedures are similar to those applied in many early communication intervention programs (Bricker & Bricker, 1970; Guess et al., 1974; Lovaas, 1977; Stremel, 1972). In line with contemporary descriptions of systematic instructional practices (Collins, 2012), NDBIs infuse instruction into the give and take of everyday social interactions. In addition, a NDBI protocol usually allows for considerable flexibility and individualization. This looser approach to training is also a possible facilitator of generalization (Campbell & Stremel-Campbell, 1982; Stokes & Baer, 1977).

Fifth, NDBIs target skills that match the child's developmental level. This could mean targeting prelinguistic vocalizations and basic gestures (e.g., reaching and pointing) in a young minimally verbal child or targeting peer-to-peer conversational skills in an older child. For some children, depending on their entry-level abilities, various prerequisite or cognitive skills (e.g., imitation, joint attention, and reciprocal turn taking) might be initial intervention targets.

In a classic study, Koegel, O'Dell, and Koegel (1987) evaluated a "natural language teaching paradigm" for increasing vocal-mode communication in two, 4 -to 5-year-old children with ASD. Intervention occurred during social/play interactions between the therapist and child. Intervention made use of the children's preferred toys, which were varied and rotated to prevent satiation. During interactions, the therapist responded to the child's communicative attempts by providing natural reinforcement. For example, initially reinforcing word approximations (e.g., *ba*), but also attempting to shape that approximation in a target word (e.g., *Ball*). Vocal imitation (*Say x.*) and responding to tact questions (e.g., *What is this*?) were also targeted. With this intervention, both children showed increases in correct imitation of speech and spontaneous (unprompted) use of words. Acquired responses also generalized to a different setting. An important aspect of this study is that both children had previously failed to show progress under a more structured, therapist-directed intervention program. This suggested that, at least for these two children, the NDBI approach was superior to a more structured and therapist-directed intervention.

4.3.3.1 Pivotal Response Treatment (PRT)

PRT is another research-based NDBI for enhancing communication and other adaptive behavior skills (Koegel, Ashbaugh, & Koegel, 2016; Koegel & Koegel, 2006; Schreibman et al., 2015; Vernon et al., 2019; Verschuur, Didden, Lang, Sigafoos, & Huskens, 2014). It represents a refinement of the natural language teaching paradigm. PRT has been widely applied as an intervention for children with ASD and there is sufficient research evidence to support its use in teaching communication and social skills, and also improving children's academic achievement (Koegel & Koegel, 2006; Verschuur et al., 2014). The architects of PRT (Koegel et al., 2016) explained that PRT emphasizes enhancement of children's motivation to learn. The critical need for motivation enhancement, particularly for children with ASD, is based in part on the phenomenon of learned helplessness (Koegel & Egel, 1979; Seligman, 1972). Koegel et al. (2016) argued that children with ASD may learn to be helpless due to various instructional experiences, such as inappropriate demands, unstimulating learning environments, and repeated failure. In a PRT intervention, reducing learned helplessness and increasing the child's motivation to learn are viewed as pivotal to achieving successful intervention outcomes. Other pivotal skills or abilities that are targeted in a PRT intervention include (a) initiation of communication and social bids, (b) self-management skills, and (c) responding to multiple cues, which is a type of stimulus generalization. To these ends, PRT involves reinforcing attempts and approximations as well as incorporating children's preferences. Children are also given opportunities to make choices regarding the reinforcers, materials, and types of learning tasks that are employed during intervention (Koegel et al., 2016). To maintain interest, learning tasks are varied. To ensure a high success rate—and a consequently dense reinforcement schedule—previously mastered tasks are interspersed with new learning tasks. As well, PRT incorporates other common elements of NDBIs, such as using natural reinforcement, providing instruction in natural settings, and adopting a more child-centric flow to intervention sessions rather than adopting a solely therapist-directed approach.

In a classic PRT study, Koegel, Camarata, Váldez-Menchaca, and Koegel, (1998) focused on the pivotal skill of asking questions. The study involved three children with IDD who ranged from 3- to 5-years of age. Children participated in 30-min sessions in which specific PRT techniques (e.g., incorporating child choice, task variation, natural reinforcement, and mixing previously learned skills with new tasks). Additional systematic instructional procedures were also applied to teach the targeted communication skills, specifically response prompting, time delay, and fading out visual cues to promote spontaneous question asking. With these procedures, all three children showed acquisition of spontaneous (i.e., unprompted) question asking. Children also showed an increase in correctly tacting objects. Impressively, these gains generalized to new settings and communication partners.

The positive results reported by Koegel et al. (1998) have been replicated in numerous other studies. Verschuur et al. (2014) identified 43 studies that evaluated the effects of PRT with a total of 420 children, primarily young (preschool-aged) children with ASD. In the main, these studies reported positive outcomes across a range of pivotal skill areas, including: (a) functional verbal utterances, (b) expressive and receptive language, (c) responding to others, and (d) maintaining social interactions. While the literature on PRT is relatively large and has demonstrated consistently positive outcomes, Verschuur et al. noted that about half of the studies had methodological limitations that reduce the certainty of evidence. Still, there is sufficient evidence to support the value of PRT for teaching communication skills, as well as a range of other skills, to children with IDD.

In another version of a NDBI, Waddington, van der Meer, Sigafoos, and Ogilvie (2019) evaluated an intervention based on the Early Start Denver Model (ESDM; Rogers & Dawson, 2010). The ESDM is a manualized early intervention program for young children with ASD. Intervention is delivered during play-based sessions. During sessions, the therapist configures interactions to capture the child's attention, establish joint attention, and make use of the child's preferences, such as by following the child's lead. Additional therapeutic techniques include adopting a highly responsive/positive affect and using well-established instructional procedures, such as time delay, expanding on the child's utterances, response prompting, and natural reinforcement. Intervention objectives can be individualized, but for young children these often include aiming to increase engagement, imitation, and spontaneous/functional utterances. Waddington et al. evaluated the effects of a relatively low intensity version of the ESDM (i.e., two or three, 60-min sessions per week for 10 weeks). Sessions were conducted in the home by trained therapists, and generalization to parent-implemented sessions was assessed. The results were generally positive, in that all four children showed increased engagement and communication, specifically either functional communicative utterances and/or intentional vocalizations. Imitation also increased, but to a lesser extent. Importantly, generalization to parent-led sessions was noted. These results are significant in showing benefits from a relatively low-intensity NDBI.

The NDBI approach has been packaged and applied in varying configurations. These include the natural language paradigm, PRT, and the ESDM (Schreibman et al., 2015). A considerable amount of research has evaluated these and other NDBI configurations (Schreibman et al., 2015; Verschuur et al., 2014). The overall results of this research suggest that a well-designed and carefully implemented NDBI is likely to produce improvements in children's communicative, social, play, and other adaptive skills. Given these positive results and its applicability to natural settings, it is not surprising that the NDBI approach appears to be growing in popularity, especially as an early intervention approach for young children with ASD (Schreibman et al., 2015). NDBIs could be seen as an evolution or refinement of the pioneering programs from the 1970s. In this refinement, operant conditioning/ behavior analytic principles and procedures have been shown to be effective even when applied in a looser or more naturalistic and child-centered approach.

4.4 Summary and Conclusions

Effective communication skills are essential for participation in nearly all aspects of life. Unfortunately, IDD is associated with communication impairments that can hinder participation, learning, and the ability to basic express wants, needs, and emotions. Without communication people with IDD may be unable to become fully involved in meaningful social interactions. The close association between IDD and communication impairments means that many, if not most, people with IDD should receive intervention to enhance their communication skills. Fortunately, effective, research-based approaches for teaching communication skills to people with IDD are available.

Pioneering research from the 1960s demonstrated that people with IDD could learn a range of communication skills using teaching procedures derived from behavior analytic/operant conditioning principles. From this pioneering research, a number of communication training programs emerged. These early programs typically outlined intervention protocols that were intended for implementation in clinical settings under highly structured conditions. Although communication skills were successfully taught through such programs, ensuring generalization, and functional and spontaneous use of newly taught communication skills remained elusive.

Since those pioneering days, significant progress has been made in teaching communication skills to people with IDD. Previous challenges regarding limited functional use of communication skills, generalization, and spontaneity—while not completely purged from concern—have been more effectively addressed in contemporary intervention approaches. Contemporary approaches, such as AVB, FCT, and various NDBIs, give greater attention to communicative functions rather than formal linguist structures. Contemporary approaches also give credence to the full range of communication modalities, which is enabling for people with severe impairments who are, and who are likely to remain, minimally verbal. Contemporary approaches also tend to embrace more naturalistic intervention contexts. Evidence accumulating since the 1960s continues to support the relevance of behavior analytic/operant conditioning principles to the teaching of communication skills to people with IDD. The contemporary intervention approaches of AVB, FCT, and

NDBI reflect refinements that have emerged from research into the application of such principles. These refinements include: (a) directly teaching a range of different communicative functions (e.g., mands and tacts), (b) teaching in context (e.g., teaching in natural settings using natural antecedents and consequences), and (c) selecting communication modes that will enable the person to effectively participate in the exchange of information from one person to another.

Author Note The author reports no conflicts of interest and is solely responsible for the content and writing of this chapter.

References

Abbeduto, L., McDuffie, A., Thurman, A. J., & Kover, S. T. (2016). Language development in individuals with intellectual and developmental disabilities: From phenotypes to treatments. *International Review of Research in Developmental Disabilities, 50*, 71–118. https://doi.org/10.1016/bs.irrdd.2016.05.006

American Association on Intellectual and Developmental Disabilities. (2010). *Intellectual disability: Definition, classification, and systems of support* (11th ed.). Washington, DC: Author.

American Psychiatric Association. (2013). *Diagnostic and statistical manual of mental disorders* (5th ed.). Washington, DC: American Psychiatric Publishing.

Bacon, E. C., Osuna, S., Courchesne, E., & Pierce, K. (2019). Naturalistic language sampling to characterize the language abilities of 3-year-olds with autism spectrum disorder. *Autism, 23*, 699–712. https://doi.org/10.1177/1362361318766241

Baer, D. M., & Guess, D. (1971). Receptive training of adjectival inflections in mental retardates. *Journal of Applied Behavior Analysis, 4*, 129–139. https://doi.org/10.1901/jaba.1971.4-129

Barbera, M. L., & Kubina, R. M., Jr. (2005). Using transfer procedures to teach tacts to a child with autism. *The Analysis of Verbal Behavior, 21*, 155–161. https://doi.org/10.1007/BF03393017

Beukelman, D. R., & Mirenda, P. (2013). *Augmentative and alternative communication: Supporting children and adults with complex communication needs* (4th ed.). Baltimore, MD: Paul H. Brookes Publishing.

Billingsley, F. F., & Romer, L. T. (1983). Response prompting and the transfer of stimulus control: Methods, research, and a conceptual framework. *Journal of the Association for Persons with Severe Handicaps, 8*, 3–12. https://doi.org/10.1177/154079698300800201

Bloom, L., Hood, L., & Lightbown, P. (1974). Imitation in language development: If, when, and why. *Cognitive Psychology, 6*, 380–420. https://doi.org/10.1016/0010-0285(74)90018-8

Bondy, A., & Frost, L. A. (1998). The picture exchange communication system. *Seminars in Speech and Language, 19*, 373–388. https://doi.org/10.1055/s-2008-1064055

Brady, N. C., Bruce, S., Goldman, A., Erickson, K., Mineo, B., Ogletree, B. T., … Wilkinson, K. (2016). Communication services and supports for individuals with severe disabilities: Guidance for assessment and intervention. *American Journal on Intellectual and Developmental Disabilities, 121*, 121–138. https://doi.org/10.1352/1944-7558-121.2.121

Brady, N. C., & Halle, J. W. (2002). Breakdowns and repairs in conversations between beginning AAC users and their partners. In J. Reichle, D. R. Beukelman, & J. Light (Eds.), *Exemplary practices for beginning communicators* (pp. 323–351). Baltimore, MD: Paul H. Brookes Publishing.

Braam, S. J., & Poling, A. (1983). Development of intraverbal behavior in mentally retarded individuals through transfer of stimulus control procedures: Classification of verbal operants. *Applied Research in Mental Retardation, 4*, 279–302. https://doi.org/10.1016/0270-3092(83)90030-9

Bricker, W. A., & Bricker, D. D. (1970). A program of language training for the severely language handicapped child. *Exceptional Children, 37*, 101–111. https://doi.org/10.1177/001440297003700203

Campbell, C. R., & Stremel-Campbell, K. (1982). Programming "loose training" as a strategy to facilitate language generalization. *Journal of Applied Behavior Analysis, 15*, 295–301. https://doi.org/10.1901/jaba.1982.15-295

Carnett, A., Ingvarsson, E. T., Bravo, A., & Sigafoos, J. (2020). Teaching children with autism spectrum disorder to ask "where" questions using a speech-generating device. *Journal of Applied Behavior Analysis., 53*(3), 1383–1403. https://doi.org/10.1002/jaba.663

Carnett, A., Raulston, T. J., & Charpentier, J. (2019). The application of Skinner's analysis of verbal behavior for teaching communication skills to persons with developmental disabilities. *Current Developmental Disorder Reports, 6*, 131–137. https://doi.org/10.1007/s40474-019-00170-0

Carr, E. G., & Durand, V. M. (1985). Reducing behavior problems through functional communication training. *Journal of Applied Behavior Analysis, 18*, 111–126. https://doi.org/10.1901/jaba.1985.18-111

Carr, E. G., & Kemp, D. C. (1989). Functional equivalence of autistic leading and communicative pointing: Analysis and treatment. *Journal of Autism and Developmental Disorders, 19*, 561–578. https://doi.org/10.1007/BF02212858

Carr, E. G., Levin, L., McConnachie, G., Carlson, J., Kemp, D., & Smith, C. (1994). *Communication-based intervention for problem behavior: A user's guide for producing positive change*. Baltimore, MD: Paul H. Brookes Publishing.

Choi, H., O'Reilly, M. F., Sigafoos, J., & Lancioni, G. (2010). Teaching requesting and rejecting sequences to four children with developmental disabilities using augmentative and alternative communication. *Research in Developmental Disabilities, 31*, 560–567. https://doi.org/10.1016/j.ridd.2009.12.006

Cooke, S., Cooke, T. P., & Apolloni, T. (1976). Generalization of language training with the mentally retarded. *Journal of Special Education, 10*, 299–304. https://doi.org/10.1177/002246697601000311

Collins, B. C. (2012). *Systematic instruction for students with moderate and severe disabilities*. Baltimore, MD: Paul H. Brookes Publishing.

Conallen, K., & Reed, P. (2016). A teaching procedure to help children with autistic spectrum disorder to label emotions. *Research in Autism Spectrum Disorders, 23*, 63–72. https://doi.org/10.1016/j.rasd.2015.11006

Crain, S. (2019). Meaning in first language acquisition. In K. von Heusinger, C. Maienborn, & P. Portner (Eds.), *Semantics – Typology, diachrony, and processing* (pp. 237–273). Berlin, Germany: de Gruyter.

Curtis, P. R., Frey, J. R., Watson, C. D., Hampton, L. H., & Roberts, M. Y. (2018). Language disorders and problem behaviors: A meta-analysis. *Pediatrics, 142*, e20173551. https://doi.org/10.1542/peds.2017-3551

DeSouza, A. A., Akers, J. S., & Fisher, W. W. (2017). Empirical application of Skinner's verbal behaviour to interventions for children with autism: A review. *The Analysis of Verbal Behavior, 33*, 229–259. https://doi.org/10.1007/s40616-017-0093-7

Drasgow, E., Halle, J. W., & Sigafoos, J. (1999). Teaching communication to learners with severe disabilities: Motivation, response competition, and generalization. *Australasian Journal of Special and Inclusive Education, 23*, 47–63. https://doi.org/10.1017/S103001200024507

Durand, V. M. (1986). Self-injurious behavior as intentional communication. In K. D. Gadow (Ed.), *Advances in learning and behavioral disabilities* (Vol. 5, pp. 141–155). Greenwich, CN: JAI Press.

Durand, V. M. (1990). *Severe behavior problems: A functional communication training approach*. New York, NY: Guilford Press.

Durand, V. M. (1993). Functional communication training using assistive devices. Effects on challenging behavior and affect. *Augmentative and Alternative Communication, 9*, 168–176. https://doi.org/10.1080/07434619312331276571

Durand, V. M., & Moskowitz, L. J. (2019). The link between problem behavior and communication impairment in persons with developmental disabilities. *Current Developmental Disorders Reports, 6*, 138–144. https://doi.org/10.1007/s40474-019-00172-y

Esquirol, J-E. D. (1845). *Mental maladies: A treatise on insanity*. E. K. Hunt (trans.). Philadelphia, PA: Lea and Blanchard.

Esteve-Gibert, N., & Prieto, P. (2014). Infants temporally coordinate gesture-speech combinations before they produce their first words. *Speech Communication, 57*, 301–316. https://doi.org/10.1016/j.specom.2013.06.006

Fenlon, J., Cooperrider, K., Keane, J., Brentari, D., & Goldin-Meadow, S. (2019). Comparing sign language and gesture: Insights from pointing. *Glossa: A Journal of General Linguistics, 4*(2), 1–26. https://doi.org/10.5334/gigl.499

Gerow, S., Davis, T., Radhakrishnan, S., Gregori, E., & Rivera, G. (2018). Functional communication training: The strength of evidence across disabilities. *Exceptional Children, 85*, 86–103. https://doi.org/10.1177/0014402918793399

Gerow, S., Hagan-Burke, S., Rispoli, M., Gregori, E., Mason, R., & Ninci, J. (2018). A systematic review of parent-implemented functional communication training for children with ASD. *Behavior Modification, 42*, 335–363. https://doi.org/10.1177/0145445517740872

Gobbi, L., Cipani, E., Hudson, C., & Lapenta-Neudeck, R. (1986). Developing spontaneous requesting among children with severe mental retardation. *Mental Retardation, 24*, 357–363.

Goldsmith, T. R., LeBlanc, L. A., & Sautter, R. A. (2007). Teaching intraverbal behavior to children with autism. *Research in Autism Spectrum Disorder, 1*, 1–13. https://doi.org/10.1016/j.rasd.2006.07.001

Goldstein, H., & Hontz Hockenberger, E. (1991). Significant progress in child language intervention: An 11-year retrospective. *Research in Developmental Disabilities, 12*, 401–424. https://doi.org/10.1016/0891-4222(91)90035-Q

Greer, R. D., & Ross, D. E. (2008). *Verbal behavior analysis: Inducing and expanding new verbal capabilities in children with language delays*. New York, NY: Pearson.

Guess, D., Sailor, W., & Baer, D. M. (1974). To teach *language* to retarded children. In R. Scheifelbusch & L. Lloyd (Eds.), *Language perspectives: Acquisition, retardation, and intervention* (pp. 529–536). Baltimore, MD: University Park Press.

Guess, D., Sailor, W., Rutherford, G., & Baer, D. M. (1968). An experimental analysis of linguistic development: The productive use of the plural morpheme. *Journal of Applied Behavior Analysis, 1*, 297–306. https://doi.org/10.1901/jaba.1968.1-297

Halle, J. W. (1987). Teaching language in the natural environment: An analysis of spontaneity. *Journal of the Association for Persons with Severe Handicaps, 12*, 28–37. https://doi.org/10.1177/154079698701200105

Horner, R., & Day, H. M. (1991). The effects of response efficiency on functionally equivalent competing behaviors. *Journal of Applied Behavior Analysis, 24*, 719–732. https://doi.org/10.1901/jaba.1991.24-719

Itard, J.-M. G. (1962/1894). *The wild boy of Aveyron*. East Norwalk, CT, US: Appleton-Century-Crofts. [Reprint of the 1894 edition of *Rapports et Memories sur le Sauvage de L'Aveyron. Paris:* Courrie].

Ivy, J. W., & Schreck, K. A. (2016). The efficacy of ABA for individuals with autism across the lifespan. *Current Developmental Disorders Reports, 3*, 57–66. https://doi.org/10.1007/s40474-016-0070-1

Iwata, B. A., Pace, G. M., Dorsey, M. F., Zarcone, J. R., Vollmer, T. R., Smith, R. G., … Willis, K. D. (1994). The functions of self-injurious behavior: An experimental-epidemiological analysis. *Journal of Applied Behavior Analysis, 27*, 215–240. https://doi.org/10.1901/jaba.1994.27-215

Iwata, B. A., Dorsey, M. F., Slifer, K. J., Bauman, K. E., & Richman, G. S. (1982). Toward a functional analysis of self-injury. *Analysis and Intervention in Developmental Disabilities, 2*, 3–20. https://doi.org/10.1016/0270-4684(82)90003-9

Kagohara, D. M., van der Meer, L., Achmadi, D., Green, V. A., O'Reilly, M. F., Lancioni, G. E., … Sigafoos, J. (2012). Teaching picture naming to two adolescents with autism spectrum disorders using systematic instruction and speech-generating devices. *Research in Autism Spectrum Disorders, 6*, 1224–1233. https://doi.org/10.1016/j.rasd.201204001

Kennedy, A. (2019). *Integrating American Sign Language into the inclusive classroom*. Undergraduate Honors thesis, State University of New York, New Paltz. Retrieved on 22 August 2019 from http://hdl.handle.net/1951/70775

Koegel, L. K., Ashbaugh, K., & Koegel, R. L. (2016). Pivotal response treatment. In R. Lang, T. B. Hancock, & N. N. Singh (Eds.), *Early intervention for young children with autism spectrum disorder* (pp. 85–112). Cham, Switzerland: Springer.

Koegel, L. K., Camarata, S. M., Váldez-Menchaca, M., & Koegel, R. L. (1998). Setting generalization of question-asking by children with autism. *American Journal on Mental Retardation, 102*, 346–357. https://doi.org/10.1352/0895-8017(1998)102<0346:SGOQBC>2.0CO:2

Koegel, R. L., & Egel, A. L. (1979). Motivating autistic children. *Journal of Abnormal Psychology, 88*, 418–426. https://doi.org/10.1037/0021-843X.88.4.418

Koegel, R. L., & Koegel, L. K. (2006). *Pivotal response treatments for autism: Communication, social, and academic development*. Baltimore, MD: Paul H. Brookes Publishing.

Koegel, R. L., O'Dell, M. C., & Koegel, L. K. (1987). A natural language paradigm for nonverbal autistic children. *Journal of Autism and Developmental Disorders, 17*, 187–200. https://doi.org/10.1007/BF01495055

LeBlanc, L. A., Esch, J., Sidener, T. M., & Firth, A. M. (2006). Behavioral language interventions for children with autism: Comparing applied verbal behavior and naturalistic teaching approaches. *The Analysis of Verbal Behavior, 22*, 49–60. https://doi.org/10.1007/bf03393026

Ledford, J. R., & Wolery, M. (2011). Teaching imitation to young children with disabilities: A review of the literature. *Topics in Early Childhood Special Education, 30*, 245–255. https://doi.org/10.1177/0271121410363831

Littlejohn, S. W., & Foss, K. A. (2011). *Theories of human communication* (10th ed.). Long Grove, IL: Waveland Press.

Lovaas, O. I. (1977). *The autistic child: Language development through behavior modification*. Oxford, UK: Irvington.

Lovaas, O. I., Berberich, J. P., Perloff, B. F., & Schaeffer, B. (1966). Acquisition of imitative speech by schizophrenic children. *Science, 151*, 705–707. https://doi.org/10.1126/science.151.3711.705

Lovaas, O. I., Koegel, R. L., Simmons, J. Q., & Long, J. S. (1973). Some generalization and follow-up measures of autistic children in behavior therapy. *Journal of Applied Behavior Analysis, 6*, 131–165. https://doi.org/10.1901/jaba.1973.6-131

Mancil, G. R. (2006). Functional communication training: A review of the literature related to children with autism. *Education and Training in Developmental Disabilities, 41*, 213–224. Retrieved from: https://pdfs.semanticscholar.org/47e0/1262fc0a91ab5f4bb56c9a507ec8f69ff737.pdf

Matson, J. L. (Ed.). (2012). *Functional assessment for challenging behavior*. New York, NY: Springer.

Matson, J. L., Wilkins, J., & Macken, J. (2009). The relationship of challenging behaviors to severity and symptoms of autism spectrum disorders. *Journal of Mental Health Research in Intellectual Disabilities, 2*, 29–44. https://doi.org/10.1080/19315860802611415

McCook, B., Cipani, E., Madigan, K., & LaCampagne, J. (1988). Developing requesting behavior: Acquisition, fluency, and generality. *Mental Retardation, 26*, 137–143.

Mirenda, P. (1997). Supporting individuals with challenging behavior through functional communication training and AAC: Research review. *Augmentative and Alternative Communication, 13*, 207–225. https://doi.org/10.1080/07434619712331278048

Muharib, R., Correa, V. I., Wood, C. L., & Haughney, K. L. (2019). Effects of functional communication training using GoTalk™ Now iPad® application on challenging behavior of children

with autism spectrum disorder. *Journal of Special Education Technology, 34*, 71–79. https://doi.org/10.1177/0162643418783479
Mulhern, T., Lydon, S., Healy, O., Mollaghan, G., Ramey, D., & Leoni, M. (2017). A systematic review and evaluation of procedures for the induction of speech among persons with developmental disabilities. *Developmental Neurorehabilitation, 20*, 207–227. https://doi.org/10.3109/17518423.2016.1150360
Murphy, G. H., Steele, K., Gilligan, T., Yeow, J., & Spare, D. (1977). Teaching a picture language to a non-speaking retarded boy. *Behaviour, Research and Therapy, 15*, 198–201. https://doi.org/10.1016/0005-7967(77)90107-3
National Joint Committee for the Communication Needs of Persons with Severe Disabilities. (1992, March). Guidelines for meeting the communication needs of persons with severe disabilities. *American Speech and Hearing Association, 34* (Supplement #7), 1–8. Retrieved from: https://www.asha.org/policy/GL1992-00201/#sec1.3.1
Neely, L., Garcia, E., Bankston, B., & Green, A. (2018). Generalization and maintenance of functional communication training for individuals with developmental disabilities: A systematic and quality review. *Research in Developmental Disabilities, 79*, 116–129. https://doi.org/10.1016/j.ridd.2018.02.002
Nepo, K., Tincani, M., Axelrod, S., & Meszaros, L. (2017). iPod Touch® to increase functional communication of adults with autism spectrum disorder and significant intellectual disability. *Focus on Autism and Other Developmental Disabilities, 32*, 209–217. https://doi.org/10.1177/1088357615612752
Ok, M. W. (2018). Use of iPads as assistive technology for students with disabilities. *TechTrends, 62*, 95–102. https://doi.org/10.1007/s11528-017-0199-8
Påhlman, M., Gillberg, C., & Himmelmann, K. (2019). One-third of school-aged children with cerebral palsy have neuropsychiatric impairments in a population-based study. *Acta Paediatrica, Early View, 108*, 2048. https://doi.org/10.1111/apa.14844
Partington, J. W., Sundberg, M. L., Newhouse, L., & Spengler, S. M. (1994). Overcoming an autistic child's failure to acquire a tact repertoire. *Journal of Applied Behavior Analysis, 27*, 733–734. https://doi.org/10.1901/jaba.1994.27.733
Pavelko, S. L. (2018). Language and children with intellectual disabilities. In V. A. Reed (Ed.), *An introduction to children with language disorders* (pp. 215–234). Boston, MA: Pearson.
Reed, V. A. (Ed.). (2018). *An introduction to children with language disorders*. Boston, MA: Pearson.
Reichle, J., & Brown, L. (1986). Teaching the use of a multipage direct selection communication board to an adult with autism. *Journal of the Association for Persons with Severe Handicaps, 11*, 68–73. https://doi.org/10.1177/154079698601100109
Reichle, J., & Karlan, G. (1985). The selection of an augmentative system in communication intervention: A critique of decision rules. *Journal of the Association for Persons with Severe Handicaps, 10*, 146–156. https://doi.org/10.1177/154079698501000304
Reichle, J., Lindamood, L., & Sigafoos, J. (1986). The match between reinforcer class and response class: Its influence on communication intervention strategies. *Journal of the Association for Persons with Severe Handicaps, 11*, 131–135. https://doi.org/10.1177/154079698601100207
Reichle, J., & McComas, J. (2004). Conditional use of a request for assistance. *Disability and Rehabilitation, 26*, 1255–1262. https://doi.org/10.1080/09638280412331280262
Reichle, J., Rogers, N., & Barrett, C. (1984). Establishing pragmatic discriminations among the communicative functions of requesting, rejecting, and commenting in an adolescent. *Journal of the Association for Persons with Severe Handicaps, 9*, 31–36. https://doi.org/10.1177/154079698400900105
Reichle, J., & Wacker, D. P. (2017). *Functional communication training for problem behavior*. New York, NY: The Guilford Press.
Reichle, J., York, J., & Sigafoos, J. (1991). *Implementing augmentative and alternative communication: Strategies for learners with severe disabilities*. Baltimore, MD: Paul H. Brookes Publishing Co..

Rispoli, M. J., Franco, J. H., van der Meer, L., Lang, R., & Hoher Camargo, S. P. (2010). The use of speech generating devices in communication interventions for individuals with developmental disabilities: A review of the literature. *Developmental Neurorehabilitation, 13*, 276–293. https://doi.org/10.3109/17518421003636794

Rogers, S. J., & Dawson, G. (2010). *Early Start Denver Model for young children with autism: Promoting language, learning, and engagement*. Guilford Press.

Roncati, A. L., Coelho Souza, A., & Miguel, C. F. (2019). Exposure to a specific prompt topography predicts its relative efficiency when teaching intraverbal behavior to children with autism spectrum disorder. *Journal of Applied Behavior Analysis, 52*, 739–745. https://doi.org/10.1002/jaba.568

Scheifelbusch, R., & Lloyd, L. (Eds.). (1974). *Language perspectives: Acquisition, retardation, and intervention*. Baltimore, MD: University Park Press.

Schreibman, L., Dawson, G., Stahmer, A. C., Landa, R., Rogers, S. J., McGee, G. G., ... Halladay, A. (2015). Naturalistic developmental behavioral interventions: Empirically validated treatments for autism spectrum disorder. *Journal of Autism and Developmental Disorders, 45*, 2411–2428. https://doi.org/10.1007/s10803-015-2407-8

Seguin, E. (1971/1866). *Idiocy and its treatment by the physiological method*. New York, NY: A.M. Kelley.

Seligman, M. E. P. (1972). Learned helplessness. *Annual Review of Medicine, 23*, 407–412. https://doi.org/10.1146/annurev.me.23.020172.002203

Sigafoos, J., Drasgow, E., Reichle, J., O'Reilly, M., Green, V. A., & Tait, K. (2004). Teaching communicative rejecting to children with severe disabilities. *American Journal of Speech-Language Pathology, 13*, 31–42. https://doi.org/10.1044/1058-0360(2004/005)

Sigafoos, J., Laurie, S., & Pennell, D. (1996). Teaching children with Rett syndrome to request preferred objects using aided communication: Two preliminary studies. *Augmentative and Alternative Communication, 12*, 88–96. https://doi.org/10.1080/07434619612331277538

Sigafoos, J., & Meikle, B. (1996). Functional communication training for the treatment of challenging behavior in two boys with autism. *Behavior Modification, 20*, 60–84. https://doi.org/10.1177/01454455960201003

Sigafoos, J., O'Reilly, M., & Green, V. A. (2007). Communication difficulties and the promotion of communication skills. In A. Carr, G. O'Reilly, P. N. Walsh, & J. McEvoy (Eds.), *The handbook of intellectual disability and clinical psychology practice* (pp. 606–642). New York, NY: Routledge.

Simó-Pinatella, D., Mumbardó-Adam, C., Alomar-Kurz, E., Sugai, G., & Simonsen, B. (2019). Prevalence of challenging behaviors exhibited by children with disabilities: Mapping the literature. *Journal of Behavioral Education, 28*, 323–343. https://doi.org/10.1007/s10864-019-09326-9

Skinner, B. F. (1982). Contrived reinforcement. *The Behavior Analyst, 5*, 308. https://doi.org/10.1007/BF03393135

Skinner, B. F. (1957). *Verbal behavior*. Englewood Cliffs, NJ: Prentice-Hall.

Sobsey, D., & Reichle, J. (1989). Components of reinforcement for attention signal switch activation. *Mental Retardation and Learning Disabilities Bulletin, 17*, 46–60.

Stock, R. A., Schulze, K. A., & Mirenda, P. (2008). A comparison of stimulus-stimulus pairing, standard echoic training, and control procedures on the vocal behavior of children with autism. *The Analysis of Verbal Behavior, 24*, 123–133. https://doi.org/10.1007/BF033933061

Stremel, K. (1972). Language training: A program for retarded children. *Mental Retardation, 10*, 47–49.

Stokes, T. F., & Baer, D. M. (1977). An implicit technology of generalization. *Journal of Applied Behavior Analysis, 10*, 349–367. https://doi.org/10.1901/jaba.1977.10.349

Sundberg, M. L. (2015). The most important verbal operant. *VB News, 14*, 3–5. Retrieved from: https://www.researchgate.net/publication/289528593_Sundberg_M_L_2015_The_most_important_verbal_operant_VB_NEWS_14_3-5

Sundberg, M. L., Loeb, M., Hale, L., & Eigenheer, P. (2002). Contriving establishing operations to teach mands for information. *The Analysis of Verbal Behavior, 18*, 15–29. https://doi.org/10.1007/bf03392968

Tager-Flusberg, H., & Kasari, C. (2013). Minimally verbal school-aged children with autism spectrum disorder: The neglected end of the spectrum. *Autism Research, 6*, 468–478. https://doi.org/10.1002/aur.1329

Tirapelle, L., & Cipani, E. (1991). Developing functional requesting: Acquisition, durability, and generalization of effects. *Exceptional Children, 58*, 260–269. https://doi.org/10.1177/001440299105800308

United Nations (2008). Final report of the ad hoc committee on a comprehensive and integral international convention on the protection and promotion of the rights and dignity of persons with disabilities. Retrieved from: https://www.un.org/development/desa/disabilities/resources/ad-hoc-committee-on-a-comprehensive-and-integral-international-convention-on-the-protection-and-promotion-of-the-rights-and-dignity-of-persons-with-disabilities.html

Vernon, T. W., Holden, A. N., Barrett, A. C., Bradshaw, J., Ko, J. A., McGarry, E. S., … German, T. C. (2019). A pilot randomized clinical trial of an enhanced pivotal response treatment approach for young children with autism: The PRISM model. *Journal of Autism and Developmental Disorders, 49*, 2358–2373. https://doi.org/10.1007/s10803-019-03909-1

Verschuur, R., Didden, R., Lang, R., Sigafoos, J., & Huskens, B. (2014). Pivotal response treatment for children with autism spectrum disorders: A systematic review. *Review Journal of Autism and Developmental Disorders, 1*, 34–61. https://doi.org/10.1007/s40489-013-0008-z

Vicker, B. (2008). Communicative functions or purposes of communication. *The Reporter, 14*(1), 13–17. Retrieved from: https://www.iidc.indiana.edu/pages/Communicative-Functions-or-Purposes-of-Communication

Waddington, H., van der Meer, L., Sigafoos, J., & Ogilvie, E. (2019). Evaluation of a low-intensity version of the Early Start Denver Model with four preschool-aged children with autism spectrum disorder. *International Journal of Developmental Disabilities, 66*, 257. https://doi.org/10.1080/20473869.2019.1569360

Walker, V. L., Lyon, K. J., Loman, S. L., & Sennott, S. (2018). A systematic review of Functional Communication Training (FCT) interventions involving augmentative and alternative communication in school settings. *Augmentative and Alternative Communication, 34*, 118–129. https://doi.org/10.1080/07434618.2018.1461240

Wallace, M. D. (2007). A comprehensive analysis of mand training. *Journal of Speech and Language Pathology – Applied Behavior Analysis, 2*(3), 278–286. https://doi.org/10.1037/h0100225

Ziomek, M. M., & Rehfeldt, R. A. (2008). Investigating the acquisition, generalization, and emergence of untrained verbal operants for mands acquired using the Picture Exchange Communication System in adults with severe developmental disabilities. *Analysis of Verbal Behavior, 24*, 15–30. https://doi.org/10.1007/bf03393054

Chapter 5
Teaching Academic Skills to People with Intellectual and Developmental Disability

So Yeon Kim, Catharine Lory, Soo Jung Kim, Emily Gregori, and Mandy Rispoli

5.1 Academic Skills

Academic skills are an essential part of daily life for most successful individuals. Reading text messages, checking the weather on the Internet, reading a clock, comparing prices, and following a recipe all require academic skills. School is the primary place where school-age children obtain academic skills that are fundamental for living a high-quality life in the future. In the US, the majority of students with intellectual and developmental disabilities (IDD) are educated in public schools and spend at least some time in general education classrooms (U. S. Department of Education, National Center for Educational Statistics, 2019). However, inclusion refers to more than just classroom placement or curriculum. Successful inclusion requires teachers equipped with evidence-based practices (EBPs) to provide students with IDD with individualized instruction to support them in making meaningful educational progress.

Students with IDD have a variety of educational needs. Although some students may require relatively minor accommodations to work toward grade level academic standards (e.g., extended time, sitting in a front row), some students are expected to achieve alternative or functional skills that are not directly related to grade-level standards. As students with more significant educational needs age, the focus of instruction often shifts from teaching academic to functional academic skills.

S. Y. Kim · C. Lory · S. J. Kim · M. Rispoli (✉)
Department of Educational Studies, College of Education, Purdue University, West Lafayette, IN, USA
e-mail: mrispoli@purdue.edu

E. Gregori
Department of Special Education, College of Education, University of Illinois at Chicago, Chicago, IL, USA

R. Lang, P. Sturmey (eds.), *Adaptive Behavior Strategies for Individuals with Intellectual and Developmental Disabilities*, Autism and Child Psychopathology Series, https://doi.org/10.1007/978-3-030-66441-1_5

However, the age or disability of students should not preclude students from accessing grade-level academic standards.

There are two broad approaches to curriculum design. In a standards-based curriculum, a state or national agency, professional body or panel of experts identified a body of knowledge or skills that it deems to be understood or done. In a functional curriculum, skills are taught that are of value immediately or in the near future. Functional skills can include not only vocational and social skills but also the everyday application of reading and writing to tasks, such as reading and following a recipe to produce food to eat or texting a message to call for a taxi to go home. The merits of standards-based versus functional curriculum are often debated when educating students with IDD who have extensive support needs (Ayres, Lowrey, Douglas, & Sievers, 2011; Ayres, Lowrey, Douglas, & Sievers, 2012; Courtade, Spooner, Browder, & Jimenez, 2012). Functional curriculum focuses on the needs and preference of each student and aims at teaching practical skills that can lead to a more independent adult life (Ayres et al., 2011). Adopting a functional curriculum can have practical value in maximizing time for teaching functional skills that can be directly used in everyday life (e.g., consumer skills, self-help skills, community living skills) by developing an individualized curriculum for each individual student (Ayres, 2012). However, adopting only a functional curriculum brings up some concerns related to preventing or limiting students from accessing the general education curriculum (Courtade et al., 2012). Researchers have also acknowledged that a standard-based curriculum can allow students to increase overall independence (e.g., reading a mail, participating in government) and prepare them for adult jobs (e.g., jobs that require mathematics) without precluding instruction that is personally relevant (Courtade et al., 2012).

It is worth noting that one curriculum does not need to be a replacement for another and functional skills (e.g., eating with a spoon) are not prerequisites to academic learning (e.g., learning to read, solving math problems) (Courtade et al., 2012). Such educational decisions should be made by a collaborative team involving the family and school. When planning academic interventions for students with IDD, the team must decide *what to teach* (i.e., learning objectives) and *how to teach* (i.e., instructional methods). The purpose of this chapter is to describe teaching procedures appropriate for both standard-based and functional curriculum goals, including research-based practices to teach literacy, mathematics, and science to students with IDD.

5.2 Review of Literature

5.2.1 Selecting Academic Goals and Objectives

Teaching academic skills to students with IDD who have varying cognitive abilities and prerequisite skills to engage with grade-level standards may be challenging for many educators. Within the past decade, there has been an increased emphasis on supporting all students, including students with IDD, to achieve meaningful progress in academic subject areas (e.g., *Every Student Succeeds Act*, 2015; Individuals with Disabilities Education Improvement Act, 2004; No Child Left Behind, 2002). However, curriculum for students with IDD, especially when they have moderate to severe educational needs, has mostly focused on teaching functional skills (e.g., preparing meals) or prerequisite skills (e.g., calling letters) (Snyder, Knight, Ayres, & Mims, 2017). Table 5.1 describes the characteristics and educational needs of three students with IDD across age groups. Based on the scenarios in Table 5.1, the focus of academic instruction for Santiago in the inclusive kindergarten classroom and Kayla in the high school self-contained classroom may look different. For example, reading instruction for Santiago can be designed to teach him letter-sound knowledge to decode the sound of each consonant (e.g., dog = /d/ and /g/) like other students, but reading instruction for Kayla may focus on increasing the number of sight words she can read in her community (e.g., open, close, stop, cereals, milk, check-out). The focus of academic instruction is often adjusted from teaching grade-level academic skills to teaching functional academic skills (e.g., reading food labels, money concepts) as students get older.

Before changing *what* the student learns and teaching functional academic skills, educators should consider changing *how* the student learns to provide equal access to grade-level academic contents first. Instruction for students with IDD may target: (a) *grade-level skills* with or without supports, (b) *alternative skills* that are relevant to grade level standards, or (c) *functional skills* that are not directly related to grade-level standards but essential to supporting independent functioning in home, school, and community settings. When educators select academic goals and objectives for students with IDD, they should first consider instructional methods to support the students' achievement of grade-level academic skills.

Table 5.1 Student examples

Santiago is a 5-year-old boy recently identified as having an intellectual disability. He has two older brothers, and his family primarily speaks Spanish at home. He attends an inclusive kindergarten classroom at a local school. He has delayed spoken language development but can communicate with others using sentences including 2–3 words. His classroom teacher is concerned that he is unaware of letters and letter-sound relationship.
Alex is a fifth grader with ASD and receives special education services in a resource room. He uses full sentences for communication but often has difficulties having a back-and-forth conversation with peers. He follows his favorite baseball team and searches it online every day and enjoys talking about that. He can read paragraphs aloud but has difficulties comprehending what he read. During reading, he tends to focus on small details rather than understanding the big picture. He has difficulties finding main ideas, understanding characters' motivations and feelings, and answering inferential questions.
Kayla is a tenth grader with Down syndrome who has extensive educational needs. She receives a life-skills curriculum at school and mainly uses words and gestures to communicate with others. She has delayed motor development and poor muscle tone that makes it difficult to write using a pencil. She is able to differentiate picture symbols and read 15 to 20 sight words. She requires repeated instruction to learn something new, but she is enthusiastic about every classroom activity and very social. After she enrolled in high school, her parents have taken a hard look at what she wants to do when her secondary education is over.

After appropriate academic goals and objectives are selected for students, the educators need to select instructional methods to support the students to achieve those goals and objectives. A framework to help educators decide what to teach and how to teach is displayed in Fig. 5.1. Accommodations and modifications are two different ways of promoting equal access to instruction and assessment for students with disabilities. The major difference between accommodations and modifications is whether the learning expectations are changed. Accommodations are intended to support students with disabilities to achieve the primary grade-level goals by changing *how* the student learns and modifications are intended to change *what* the

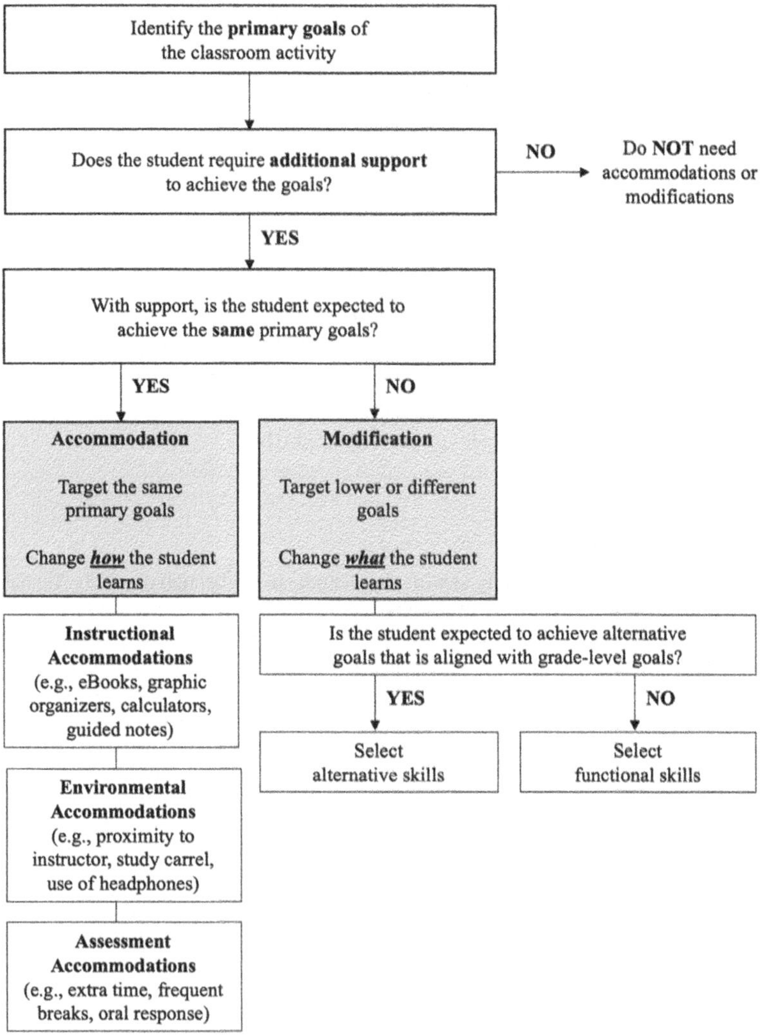

Fig. 5.1 A framework to decide academic goals and objectives

student learns by targeting alternate goals. For example, Alex's science teacher plans to teach the relationships between producers, consumers, decomposers, and predators within their ecosystem to the class. The teacher believes that Alex can achieve the same learning objectives with supports. To help Alex focus on important details, the teacher provides a graphic organizer and prompts him to visualize each organism's role within their ecosystem. The same worksheet is assigned to Alex at the end of the lesson, but he is allowed to use to his graphic organizer to answer the questions and received 20 extra minutes to complete the work. This is an example of accommodations as Alex is expected to achieve the same primary goals of the class activity with support (i.e., graphic organizer, extra time). Conversely, if Alex requires more intrusive supports than accommodations to achieve meaningful outcomes, the teacher may select different learning objectives for Alex (e.g., identifying producers, matching organisms with their food). This is an example of modifications.

5.2.2 Research-Based Practices

After appropriate academic goals and objectives are selected, educators need to consider how to support the students to achieve the goals and objectives effectively. Prominent organizations and research groups, such as the National Professional Development Center on Autism Spectrum Disorders, National Autism Center (NAC), and Autism Evidence-based Practice Review Group (Wong et al., 2013) have provided comprehensive reports on EBPs to teach individuals with autism spectrum disorder (ASD) across various outcome domains (e.g., social interaction, communication, behavior, academic). Although there is currently no comprehensive EBP report specifically for individuals with ID, existing literature does offer effective instructional strategies to guide teaching practices for this group of students. The terms 'evidence base' and 'research base' are often used interchangeably (Charlop, Lang, & Rispoli, 2018). EBP refers to practices that are well supported in the research base. EBPs value empirical evidence over anecdotal or indirect evidence, and EBPs are supported by multiple quality peer-reviewed studies. The purpose of this section is to aggregate and describe EBPs to teach academic skills to students with IDD based on comprehensive reports and literature reviews.

Before we describe EBPs to teach academic skills to students with IDD, it is necessary to clarify the terms *intervention component* and *intervention package*. The term intervention component refers to a single instructional strategy, and the term intervention package refers to a collection of intervention components (Charlop et al., 2018). For example, if a computer-assisted instruction (CAI) was designed to teach sight words using time-delay and least-to-most prompting, the CAI program can be considered as an intervention package and time delay and prompting can be considered as intervention components. In this chapter, both single intervention components and intervention packages were considered and listed in Table 5.2.

Table 5.2 Research-based practices to teach academic skills to individuals with IDD

	Literacy		Mathematics		Science	
Strategies	Academic	Functional	Academic	Functional	Academic	Functional
Systematic instruction						
Prompting	X	X	X	X	X	X
Time delay	X	X	X	X	X	X
Stimulus prompting/ fading		X	X	X		
Task analysis	X	X	X	X	X	X
Reinforcement	X	X	X	X	X	
Error correction	X	X	X	X	X	
Multiple exemplars		X				X
Visual support	X	X	X	X	X	
Video modeling		X	X	X		
Technology-assisted instruction	X	X	X	X	X	
Peer-mediated instruction	X	X	X		X	
Behavior skills training				X		
Explicit instruction	X	X	X	X	X	X

5.2.2.1 Systematic Instruction

Systematic instruction is based on the principles of applied behavior analysis (ABA) and has been identified as a particularly effective approach for teaching students with IDD (Browder, Ahlgrim-Delzell, Spooner, Mims, & Baker, 2009; Morse & Schuster, 2014; Spooner, Knight, Browder, Jimenez, & DiBiase, 2011). Components of systematic instruction include: (a) targeting meaningful skills, (b) defining target skills in observable and measurable terms, (c) using data to demonstrate the effectiveness of intervention on target outcomes, (d) using behavioral strategies to reinforce, prompt, and provide feedback, and (e) impacting outcomes that can be generalized across skills or settings (Spooner et al., 2011).

5.2.2.2 Prompting

Prompting is generally defined as any help given to a student that assists in using a specific skill (Cox, 2013). Physical, verbal, or gestural assistance is provided by an adult or peer immediately before or just as the student attempts to use the target skill. Prompts are generally classified as: (a) physical prompt (e.g., Tell a student to "Find the letter A" and physically guide the student to touch the letter A card); (b) modeling (e.g., Ask a student "What is this word?" and read the exact word aloud); (c) visual prompt (e.g., Ask a student "Where did Tommy go?" and the correct answer, a zoo, was highlighted in a sentence); (d) verbal prompt (e.g., Ask a student "What comes after Monday?" and state "Tu…"); and (e) gestural prompt (e.g., Ask a student "What did you just read about?" and point to the title of the book). A hierarchy of prompts can be pre-determined and delivered in a systematic procedure which allows educators to increase or decrease prompting systematically based on the student's response to instruction. Prompting procedures include simultaneous prompting, least-to-most prompting, most-to-least prompting, and physical guidance. Prompting is often used with other research-based practices, such as time-delay and reinforcement.

Simultaneous prompting Simultaneous prompting involves delivering a prompt (e.g., verbal prompt, gestural prompt) simultaneously with the instructional cue. Simultaneous prompting has been successfully used to teach discrete and chained skills to students with IDD (Pennington, Stenhoff, Gibson, & Ballou, 2012; Smith, Schuster, Collins, & Kleinert, 2011; Waugh, Fredrick, & Alberto, 2009). For example, Waugh et al. (2009) applied simultaneous prompting strategies to teach sounds and blending skills to students with moderate ID. During the intervention sessions for teaching sounds, a teacher presented a letter card and asked the student to touch the letter to obtain the student's attention. Then the teacher used simultaneous prompt with the instructional cue (i.e., This sound is [emitted sound]. What sound?). If the student did not imitate the word within 4 s, the teacher represented the instructional cue and simultaneous prompt.

Least-to-most prompting Least-to-most prompting delivers prompts only as needed to teach a discrete skill or a series of tasks (Browder, Wood, Thompson, & Ribuffo, 2014). In a least-to-most prompt system, an educator may provide a student with an opportunity to respond without providing a prompt first. If an error or no response occurs, the educator delivers the least intrusive form of prompt, followed by another opportunity to respond. This procedure is repeated until the student correctly responds or the most intrusive prompt (e.g., full physical) is delivered. Browder, Hudson, and Wood (2013) used a modified system of least intrusive prompting to assist middle school students with ID in answering reading comprehension questions. After the participants read a chapter, the interventionist asked a comprehension question and waited for 30 s. If the participants answered the question correctly, a descriptive verbal praise was given. If the participants answered the question incorrectly, the first prompt within a modified system of least intrusive prompting (i.e., restating the question and definition of WH words) was delivered. If the participants made another incorrect response, the second prompt (i.e., restating the question and definition, rereading appropriate text aloud, stating the correct answer) or third prompt (i.e., stating the correct answer and pointing to the correct response in the text) was delivered. In this way, prompts increased in helpfulness following errors until the student was able to respond correctly.

Most-to-least prompting Most-to-least prompting provides prompts in the hierarchy in the opposite sequence. When most-to-least intrusive prompting is applied, educators may begin with full physical prompt and then gradually reduce the intrusiveness of prompts until the student responds correctly to the natural cue (i.e., discriminative stimulus). Davenport and Johnston (2015) used most-to-least prompting in an inclusive early childhood setting to teach numeracy skills to students with disabilities. During intervention, a verbal task demand (e.g., "Point to the number 6") was paired with the full physical prompt (i.e., guiding the student's hand). The intrusiveness of prompt was reduced to partial physical prompt (i.e., gently nudging the participants elbow) and then faded further to a verbal prompt as correct responses increased.

Graduated guidance Graduated guidance involves following the student's movement closely with hands but not touching the student (Cooper, Heron, & Heward, 2007). Educators provide a controlling prompt to support the student to correctly perform the target skill and gradually remove the prompt as the student begins to use the skill (e.g., increasing distance of hands, changing location). Moment-to-moment decisions are required based on the student's performance during instruction, and the prompt is reinstated if the student regresses. Graduated guidance is typically used to teach chained skills that include physical components and multiple steps (e.g., getting dressed, using utensils). In terms of academics, van der Meer et al. (2015) evaluated effects of graduate guidance and differential reinforcement on correct picture and word matching of a student with ASD. Four pictures/words were presented on an iPad screen, and the students were prompted to select a matched picture/word by using graduated guidance.

5.2.2.3 Time Delay

Time delay is a systematic procedure that can be used to help fade prompts during instructional activities (Wong et al., 2013). Time delay has been demonstrated by rigorous experimental studies to be effective in teaching academic skills to students with IDD across different ages and severity of developmental disabilities (Collins, Hager, Creech- Galloway, 2011; Spooner et al., 2012). Critical features of time delay have been defined to include: (a) trials with 0 s delay of prompting, (b) opportunities for students to perform the target skill with 0 s delay prompting, (c) trials with delayed prompting with seconds as specific units of time, and (d) opportunities for students to perform the target skill with delayed prompting (Browder et al., 2009). Time delay can be further classified into constant time delay or progressive time delay. Both procedures start with 0-s time delay wherein the teacher presents the learning task and immediately prompts the learner to respond correctly. With constant time delay, subsequent trials involve increasing the amount of time between the presentation of the task and the prompt by a fixed number of seconds, such as 0 s, 3 s, 6 s, 9 s, and so on. With progressive time delay, subsequent trials involve increasing the delay of prompt by gradually increasing the number of seconds after each set of trials, such as 0 s, 3 s, 7 s, 12 s, and so on.

5.2.2.4 Stimulus Prompting and Fading

Stimulus prompting is a strategy to provide students with a cue to respond by embedding prompts into the instructional stimuli (Cooper et al., 2007). Stimulus prompts have been effectively used to teach functional academic skills, such as reading sight words (e.g., Hetzroni & Shalem, 2005). Target words may be color coded to provide more differentiation (e.g., blue is written in blue, red is written in red) or presented within pictures (e.g., letter A is written within a picture of an apple). However, one potential problem of using stimulus prompts is that students often associate the spoken word (e.g., "blue") with the additional cue (e.g., color of the word) instead of the written word (e.g., blue). In this case, the students may not read the word if the word is presented without the stimulus prompt. For this reason, stimulus prompting is generally used in conjunction with prompt fading procedures.

Stimulus fading involves exaggerating a dimension of a stimulus (e.g., color, size, position) to increase the likelihood of a correct response and the exaggerated dimension is gradually faded away (Cooper et al., 2007).

5.2.2.5 Task Analysis

Task analysis involves breaking down a complex task into smaller, more manageable steps or subskills. The steps can be sequenced as they are commonly performed or from easiest to most difficult (Cooper et al., 2007; Heward, Alber-Morgan, & Konrad, 2017). Ways to identify the steps of a task include: (a) observing students who are competent in performing the task, (b) performing the task yourself, and (c) consulting with an expert on the most efficient way to perform the task. Task analyses must be individualized according to each student's cognitive ability, motor skills, and current level of performance. For example, the steps of solving a word problem involving the area of quadrilaterals may be more specific for a student who requires some support to identify each type of quadrilateral versus a student who is fluent in identifying different types of quadrilaterals.

Although task analysis has been identified as an EBP across academic domains, including literacy, mathematics, and science, it is often used with other components of systematic instruction, such as prompting, error correction, and video modeling, etc. (Spooner et al., 2012). For example, Collins, Branson, Hall, and Rankin (2001) demonstrated that a combination of task analysis and least-to-most prompting can be effective for teaching the writing of personal letters to high school students with moderate intellectual disabilities (Collins et al., 2001).

5.2.2.6 Reinforcement

Reinforcement is a process of teaching new skills by strengthening specific behaviors (Cooper et al., 2007; Mayer, Sulzer-Azaroff, & Wallace, 2012). Reinforcement is a critical component of learning and can be categorized as positive or negative

(Cooper et al., 2007; Mayer et al., 2012). Positive reinforcement is defined as the provision of a stimulus (e.g., activity, game, tablet, food) following a behavior that increases the likelihood that the behavior will occur again in the future (Cooper et al., 2007; Mayer et al., 2012). For example, if Mrs. Martin gives Pedro a high five after he correctly responds to the question, "What is 2+2?," and he is more likely to answer correctly the next time Mrs. Martin asks the same question, then positive reinforcement has been implemented successfully.

Negative reinforcement is defined as the removal of an aversive or nonpreferred stimulus contingent on a target behavior (Cooper et al., 2007; Mayer et al., 2012) such that the target behavior occurs more often in the future. For example, Alex completes 10/10 problems on his math worksheet. His teacher, Mr. Nunez, allows Alex to take a 10 min break instead of completing the second assignment. The removal of additional work (i.e., negative reinforcement) increases the likelihood that Alex will complete all of his worksheet problems in the future.

The application of preferred stimuli (i.e., positive reinforcers) and the removal of nonpreferred stimuli (i.e., negative reinforcers) should be selected individually for each student. Failing to identify stimuli that are truly reinforcing will hinder the learners' performance. Reinforcers can be selected by interviewing the student about their preferences and interests or observing the student and recording their interactions with preferred/nonpreferred items or activities. It is important to note that reinforcers may change over time. Hence, it is imperative to re-assess preference periodically to ensure that appropriate stimuli are used. Identifying stimuli that are currently reinforcing for a student is often simple (e.g., ask the student), but for younger students or students with more significant needs, potential reinforcers may not be obvious. Various types of preference assessments (e.g., multiple stimuli without replacement, paired stimulus assessment, free operant observations) have been designed to identify one's preference hierarchy (Davis, Hodges, Weston, Hogan, & Padilla-Mainor, 2017). These assessments allow educators to determine most- and least-preferred stimuli, and the most preferred item can potentially serve as an effective reinforcer.

5.2.2.7 Error Correction

Error correction procedures involve systematically correcting the student's incorrect response by repeating a learning trial and having the student practice correct responses (Cooper et al., 2007). If the response is correct, a reinforcer is provided (e.g., verbal praise). If the response is incorrect, corrective feedback may be provided. Corrective feedback can involve a verbal cue (e.g., "No, that's not the letter A") or gestural cue (e.g., pointing to the letter A). Following corrective feedback, the learning trial is repeated to provide the student with another opportunity to respond independently (Leaf et al., 2016). A variety of error correction procedures can be used to facilitate skill acquisition, and the procedures are often used in conjunction with the other research-based practices, such as prompting, time delay, and reinforcement (Carroll, Joachim, St. Peter, & Robinson, 2015). A general error correction procedure is depicted in Fig. 5.2.

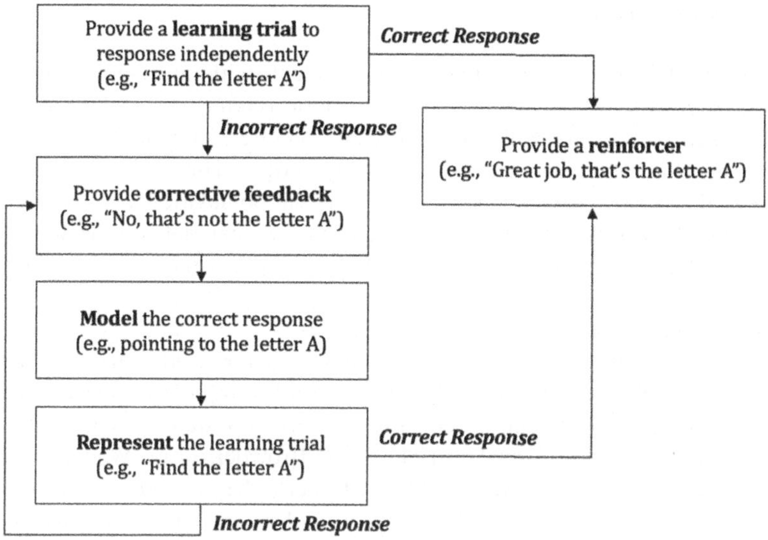

Fig. 5.2 Error correction procedures

In Waugh et al. (2009), simultaneous prompting and error correction procedures were used to teach sight words to students with ID. Once a sight word card is presented, the teacher provided an instructional cue with the simultaneous prompt (e.g., "What word? Cap"). If the student gave a correct response, the teacher provided a verbal praise (e.g., "Good reading"). If the student did not respond or responded incorrectly, the teacher provided error correction with a second opportunity for correct responding (e.g., "No this word is cap. What word?").

5.2.2.8 Multiple Exemplars

The use of multiple exemplars can be a component of systematic instruction to teach various skills, such as learning new words and naming objects (Fiorile & Greer, 2007), learning safety skills (Winterling, Gast, Wolery, & Farmer, 1992), and reading hazardous product labels and handling the products appropriately (Collins & Griffen, 1996). Collins and Griffen (1996) taught elementary-aged students with intellectual disabilities to read warning labels and respond appropriately to hazardous materials through a combination of constant time delay and multiple exemplars. The teacher utilized a wide range of examples across materials (e.g., liquid bleach, powdered insecticide, sprayed oven cleaner) and settings (e.g., classroom sink, cafeteria table, kitchen counter, and hallway water fountain). When designing multiple exemplar instruction, examples and non-examples are used to emphasize the boundaries of a concept and to teach discrimination between correct and incorrect responses.

5.2.2.9 Visual Support

Visual supports are visible cues that provide students with information about a routine, activity, expectations, or skill demonstration (Hume, 2013). Visual supports typically involve but are not limited to using pictures, drawings, written words, objects, graphic organizers, maps, labels, and scripts (Hume, 2013). The NPDC categorized types of visual supports into: (a) visual boundaries (e.g., arranging the environment in a systematic way, removing irrelevant materials for the activity); (b) visual schedule (e.g., first-then board, activity schedule); and (c) visual cues (e.g., visual instruction, graphic organizers, choice board, and item labels).

During academic interventions, various forms of visual supports can be used to increase independent performance and visually present key information to help students focus on important concepts. The use of *graphic organizers* is an instructional strategy that has been demonstrated to be effective for students with IDD across academic subject areas (Browder et al., 2018; Browder, Root, Wood, & Allison, 2017; Ciullo, Falcomata, & Vaughn, 2015; Roberts, Kim, Tandy, & Meyer, 2019; Stringfield, Luscre, & Gast, 2011; Zakas, Browder, Ahlgrim-Delzell, & Heafner, 2013). Browder et al. (2017) taught three elementary-aged students with ASD to identify story elements of narrative texts (i.e., character, setting, problem, solution, outcome) and organize the information on an electronic touch-based story map researcher developed using the SMART notebook© application. The electronic story map was presented on an iPad and allowed students to record their answers in various modes (e.g., speech-to-text, drawing tool, on-screen keyboard). In Roberts et al. (2019), effects of content area literacy strategies during shared reading on comprehension of high school students with moderate ID were investigated. Visual cues (i.e., STOP sign) were inserted at the end of each paragraph of the adapted science texts, and the students were prompted to find key information from the paragraph and organize the information on a graphic organizer sheet. Browder et al. (2018) evaluated effects of modified schema-based instruction that included effective practices (e.g., pictorial task analysis, graphic organizers, manipulatives, systematic prompting with feedback) on word problem solving of students with moderate ID. The students were prompted to select a graphic organizer sheet for each corresponding problem type and use manipulatives on the graphic organizer.

Manipulatives are another type of visual supports that have been used for students with IDD, typically in the area of mathematics (Spooner, Root, Saunders, & Browder, 2018). Manipulatives include any kind of concrete or virtual objects that assist students' learning process, such as blocks, buttons, stickers, and counting bears. Manipulating objects can assist students in understanding abstract concepts by visually representing the concept in a variety of ways (Barnett & Cleary, 2015). For example, clocks are commonly used to teach digit numbers and telling time for students aged 6 to 13 with mild and moderate ID (Birkan, 2005). Concrete manipulatives (e.g., toy cars, counters, number lines) can be used to teach early numeracy skills to elementary school students with severe ID (Jimenez & Staples, 2015), and 3-D virtual manipulatives can be used to teach subtraction to elementary-aged students with ASD (Bouck, Satsangi, Doughty, & Courtney, 2014).

5.2.2.10 Video Modeling

Video modeling is a method for teaching new skills with a considerable amount of support in the research base (Mason, Ganz, et al., 2012). Video modeling involves three components. First, an individual is recorded engaging in the target behavior (e.g., purchasing items at a store). Next, the video model is shown to the learner (i.e., the student learns the steps to purchase goods at a store). Finally, the learner imitates the target behavior in the natural setting. Video modeling is an effective instructional strategy that has been used to teach functional academic skills (e.g., reading instructions on a furniture assembly manual, identifying start and stop buttons, measuring food ingredients for cooking) to learners with developmental disabilities across the lifespan (Hong et al., 2016; Mason, Ganz, et al., 2012; Mason, Rispoli, et al., 2012).

Educators should consider several factors when implementing video modeling. First, educators must select an appropriate model. Models can include the target student, a peer, or an adult model (e.g., teacher, paraprofessional). Research has shown that video modeling can be effective using any of the models listed above, but greater results may be obtained with an adult model competent in the target skill (Mason, Ganz, et al., 2012). Second, current research suggests that video modeling may be more effective when used as part of a treatment package that involves multiple instructional strategies (Mason, Ganz, et al., 2012). For example, video modeling has been shown to be more effective when combined with reinforcement (Mason et al., 2012). Other instructional components may include other prompting, visual supports, or live coaching.

5.2.2.11 Technology-Aided Instruction

Technology-aided instruction (TAI) can be broadly defined as the use of electronic devices and software applications intended to teach (Odom et al., 2015). TAI has been successfully used for students with IDD across nearly all academic subject areas, including early literacy and mathematics skills (Knight, McKissick, & Saunders, 2013; Odom et al., 2015; Root, Stevenson, et al., 2017; Spooner et al., 2018; Wong et al., 2015). Various technological devices can be used in TAI, including computers, iPads, iPods, Netbooks, mobile phones, and calculators.

One common type of TAI is computer-assisted instruction (CAI). Research has reported that CAI can be effectively used to support student learning, present teaching material, and monitor student achievement (Root Browder, et al., 2017). Students with IDD may benefit from using commercially developed CAI programs, but educators can consider developing individualized materials to address the academic needs of their students as well. Several software programs (e.g., Microsoft PowerPoint®, GoTalk Now©) have been used to develop individualized programs that include visual and auditory cues to support students' learning and utilized on a computer or tablet. For example, research studies applied individualized CAI programs to teach sight words (Coleman, Cherry, Moore, Park, & Cihak, 2015; Lee &

Vail, 2004). These CAI programs were intended to deliver systematic instruction, such as constant time delay, prompting, reinforcement, and error correction. TAI is also effective for teaching academic vocabularies (Smith, Spooner, & Wood, 2013), phonics (Ahlgrim-Delzell et al., 2016), purchasing skills (Hsu, Tang, & Hwang, 2014), and geometry (Creech-Galloway, Collins, Knight, & Bausch, 2013) to students with IDD.

5.2.2.12 Peer-Mediated Instruction

Including students with developmental disabilities in the same educational setting as typically developing peers is often insufficient to guarantee meaningful engagement in learning and social opportunities that arise in the inclusive classroom (Wehmeyer, Lattin, Lapp-Rincker, & Agran, 2003). One way to promote meaningful interaction and academic engagement in the general education setting is to involve peers as mediators of instruction and learning (Carter, Sisco, Brown, Brickham, & Al-Khabbaz, 2008; Jimenez, Browder, Spooner, & Dibiase, 2012). Benefits of having peers assist in delivering instruction include increasing opportunities to engage in age-appropriate and contextually relevant social interactions (Chan et al., 2009), and potentially decreasing the overreliance on support from paraprofessionals (Giangreco, Halvorsen, Doyle, & Broer, 2004). Peer-mediated instruction has been used to teach a wide range of academic skills to students with IDD, including science content vocabulary, letter-writing, spelling, sight word recognition, and reading comprehension (Hudson, Browder, & Wood, 2013). For example, a class-wide peer tutoring intervention implemented with dyads of elementary-aged students with ASD and peer tutors in 30-minute sessions produced improvements in reading fluency and comprehension (Kamps, Barbetta, Leonard, & Delquadri, 1994). The class-wide peer tutoring intervention included three 45-min training sessions for both students with ASD and their peers as they played both the roles of the learner and the tutor in the program. Each learner read short passages and received corrective and positive feedback from the peer tutor and then their roles were reversed. Appropriate engagement with the reading activity earned them points, which resulted in public recognition of the total number of points in the class.

5.2.2.13 Behavior Skills Training

Behavioral skills training (BST) is a systematic method for teaching new skills. BST has been used to teach learners with IDD a variety of skills, including safety, employment, social, and academic (Beaulieu, Hanley, & Santiago, 2014; Brazeau et al., 2017; Sanchez & Miltenberger, 2015; Xin, Grasso, Dipipi-Hoy, & Jitendra, 2005). BST consists of four components. Step one of BST involves providing the learner with written or verbal instructions outlining how to perform the target skill. For example, in the context of teaching functional math skills, this may involve giving the learner a picture-based task-analysis that lists all steps involved in measuring ingredients for a recipe. Step two of BST involves modeling or demonstrating for the learner *how* they should complete the task. Modeling can be done live (in-vivo) or using video recordings. Step three of BST involves the learner practicing how to complete the target skill. During role-play, the educator observes the student completing the task and records their performance. After the learner demonstrates the skill independently, the educator provides feedback (Step 4) on their performance. Feedback can be categorized as supportive or corrective. Both forms of feedback are critical for skill development. Supportive feedback involves acknowledging the steps the learner performed correctly. One example of supportive feedback is an educator saying, "You did a great job measuring ½ cup!" Corrective feedback involves addressing steps that the learner performed incorrectly. For example, an educator might say, "I like the way you tried to measure ¼ cup, but you poured too much flour." The cycle of instructions, modeling, role-play, and feedback continues until the learner reaches predetermined mastery criteria. Mastery criteria will vary based on the target skill and the individual learner characteristics. In most cases, acceptable mastery criteria involve the student performing between 80 and 100% of steps correctly and independently.

5.2.2.14 Explicit Instruction

Explicit instruction involves a sequence of supports and scaffolds for guiding the learning process of students in small steps with explicit explanations and demonstrations of the targeted skills as well as for providing practice opportunities with feedback until mastery is attained (Archer & Hughes, 2011). Explicit instruction has several attributes that make it particularly suitable for students with IDD. Specifically, explicit instruction is a task-oriented and teacher-directed approach in which target concepts are presented in a direct, clear way and students receive immediate feedback during instruction (Stroizer, Hinton, Flores, & Terry, 2015). Explicit instruction has been successfully used across different content areas (e.g., science, reading, and mathematics) for students with moderate to severe IDD (e.g., Spooner et al., 2018). For instance, explicit instruction was used to teach mathematical word problem-solving to elementary students with ASD and moderate ID (Root, Browder, Saunders, & Lo, 2017) and independent purchasing skills for high school students with ASD and moderate ID (Cihak & Grim, 2008). In addition, explicit instruction was effective for teaching science descriptors (e.g., wet) within a science inquiry lesson for elementary-aged students with ASD (Knight, Smith, Spooner, & Browder, 2012).

5.3 Strategies to Improve Academic Outcomes of Students with ID and DD

Let us revisit scenarios of three students: Santiago, Alex, and Kayla (see Table 5.1). As each of the three students has different educational needs, the focus of educational goals and objectives in academic subject areas can be different for each student. For example, in early childhood settings, educators may place more emphasis on teaching emergent literacy (e.g., print awareness, narrative skills) and early numeracy skills (e.g., number identification, one to one correspondence). For school-age children, educators may want to balance between teaching standard-based academic skills (e.g., reading grade-level textbooks) and teaching functional academic skills (e.g., reading recipes).

In the previous section, we described research-based practices to teach academic skills to students with IDD. The purpose of this section is to provide case examples of academic interventions for students with IDD across academic and functional curricula in literacy, mathematics, and science.

5.3.1 Literacy Instruction

5.3.1.1 Emergent Literacy

Emergent literacy refers to the skills, knowledge, and attitudes that are developmental precursors to reading and writing (Whitehurst & Lonigan, 1998). From birth to about 6 years of age, children generally begin to understand that written language is related to oral language and it can deliver message (i.e., print awareness), identify and manipulate small units of oral language (i.e., phonological awareness), distinguish letter shape and name letters (i.e., alphabet knowledge), and describe events and tell stories (e.g., narrative skills). Although typically developing children gain emergent literacy skills by observing others and participating in informal literacy activities (Justice & Kaderavek, 2002), children with IDD may require instructional accommodations and modifications. This is needed to develop emergent literacy skills and often remain in this stage for a longer period of time than typically developing children due to their cognitive, communication, behavioral, and physical challenges.

Shared reading (sometimes called *repeated reading*, *shared stories*, or *story-based lessons*) is a research-based intervention package that uses task-analytic instruction to support students to engage in grade-appropriate reading activities (Browder, Trela, & Jimenez, 2007; Spooner, Rivera, Browder, Baker, & Salas, 2010). In shared reading activities, an adult reading partner (e.g., teacher, parent) reads a story to a student or a group of students and leads a discussion of themes, vocabulary, and events of the story (Browder, Spooner, & Ahlgrim-Delzell, 2011). Through the process, the reading partner explicitly models the reading strategies and skills of proficient readers. Common features of the shared reading intervention include: (a) attention getters, (b) repeated story lines, (c) picture symbol paired with words, (d) summarized text with controlled vocabulary, and (e) repeated reading (Hudson & Test, 2011). Typically, a shared reading lesson is divided into three segments: (a) before reading, (b) during reading, and (c) after reading, with specific instructional strategies associated with each segment (Reutzel & Cooter, 1996).

Before reading strategy supports the students to activate their prior knowledge and anticipate the topic before reading the book. The educator presents pictures or objects related to the section (e.g., presenting shiny fish scales before reading about Rainbow Fish) and show a cover page of the book. Then, the students look at the cover page, scan some pictures within the book, and answer some prediction questions (e.g., asking "what do you think this book will be about?").

During reading strategy involves reading the story aloud and sharing the information. The educator reads the story aloud and asks students to point or say new vocabulary words. The students can be asked to anticipate repeated story line (e.g., "Can you help me read our story line?"). If they are verbal, the educator may have the students read the story line and points to each word in chosen sentences while reading aloud. The educator can also pose various types of comprehension questions including literal (e.g., "What is his name?") and non-literal (e.g., "How did he feel after sharing his scales?") questions.

After reading strategy reviews the predictions and summarizes the story. The students are reminded what they had predicted the book would be about and prompted to go back and check if the prediction was correct (e.g., "Was the book about a fish? Were you right?"). Then, the educator models retelling the story and asks students to summarize the story using their own words. If necessary, picture cards inserted in the book can be used as visual cues to retell the story.

It is important to note that shared reading interventions have been successfully used not only for teaching emergent readers in early childhood settings but also for teaching elementary and secondary school students with IDD across academic subject areas (Kim, Rispoli, Lory, & Gregori, 2018; Roberts et al., 2019; Spooner, Ahlgrim-Delzell, Kemp-Inman, & Wood, 2014). Different before, during, and after reading strategies can be adopted within a shared reading intervention. In Table 5.3, a template for planning a shared reading intervention is presented.

5.3.1.2 Academic Literacy

Academic literacy is generally defined as the ability to engage in academic materials taught in school (Alberto, Fredrick, Hughes, McIntosh, & Cihak, 2007). The ability to read and comprehend written texts is one of the fundamental skills to access all academic subject areas and critical for success in school (Fluery, Miramontez, Hudson, & Schwartz, 2014). Reading involves not only decoding the written symbol but also extracting meaning (comprehending). The National Reading Panel (2000) recommended educators to teach all five reading essential components, including: (a) phonemic awareness, the ability to identify and manipulate

Table 5.3 A template for planning a shared reading intervention

Plans for shared reading	
STEP 1. Identify context	
Students	(e.g., number of students, grade, types of disabilities)
Setting	(e.g., one-on-one, small group, whole group, resource room, circle time)
Other resources	(e.g., paraprofessional, iPad, computer)
STEP 2. Select reading materials	
Title	
Type	(e.g., expository, narrative)
Adaptation (if necessary)	(e.g., pictures, shortening, highlighted keywords, repeated story line, text-to-speech)
STEP 3. Before reading strategy Activating prior knowledge and making them predict	
(e.g., pre-teach a key vocabulary word, recap the previous chapter, talk about the title/cover page, watch a video clip related to the topic)	
STEP 4. During reading strategy Reading aloud and sharing the information	
Reading aloud (e.g., use visual cues for reading one paragraph at a time, text-to-speech, point to the word to read, error correction) *Questioning* (e.g., ask literal/inferential questions, identify the main idea/story elements)	
STEP 5. After reading strategy Summarizing obtained information	
(e.g., ordering picture cards, graphic organizers, retelling, writing a summary sentence/ paragraph)	

phonemes in spoken words; b) phonics, the knowledge of the relationship between sounds and letters to read and write; (c) fluency, the ability to read a text quickly, accurately, and with proper expression; (d) vocabulary, the ability to understand words by linking the written words to spoken; and (e) comprehension, the ability to use information and understand what is read to engage in academic materials, students are required to learn and integrate all five skills.

Although research on reading instruction for students with IDD has heavily focused on sight words (Ahlgrim-Delzell et al., 2016), a growing body of research has suggested the effects of *systematic instruction* that combines stimulus prompting, time delay, and error correction to teach the five NRP reading components (Browder et al., 2011). For example, Santiago's teacher is concerned that he is unaware of letters and letter-sound relationships and may want to provide him with systematic phonics-based reading instruction. Table 5.4 describes a case example of how time delay and error correction procedures can be applied to teach phoneme identification skills to Santiago. The same procedures can be applied to teach other skills, such as blending sounds (e.g., present a written word bag with distractors, and say "/b/ /aaag/" "What word I am saying?") and decoding for matching words with pictures (e.g., present a written word *apple* and say, "Read the word and find the picture").

Table 5.4 Using time delay and error correction to teach phoneme identification to Santiago

Steps	Detailed procedures
1. Present letter cards on the table	s t b p m
2. Ask "what letter says /s/?"	
3. Use time delay	Provide gestural prompt (0-sec, 1-sec, 3-sec) after the verbal demand *Start with 0-sec delay, then gradually increase the time.
4. Use error correction procedures if necessary	*If Santiago responded correctly* Provide verbal praise (e.g., "great job finding the letter says /s/") *If Santiago did not respond or responded incorrectly* Correct errors (e.g., "no, that's the letter says /p/") Model correct response (e.g., point to the letter s and say, "this letter says /s/") Represent the verbal demands If he responded correctly, provide verbal praise If he did not respond correctly, repeat the error correction procedure

Comprehension is a meta-cognitive procedure to read and understand the information obtained from the written text. Given that standard-based curriculum typically involves learning from written information in textbooks, comprehension skills are necessary to make progress across all academic subject areas. The other four reading components identified by National Reading Panel (i.e., phonemic awareness, phonics, fluency, vocabulary) can contribute to comprehension skills. However, they are insufficient to develop comprehension and students with IDD who have advanced decoding skills may require individualized interventions to learn comprehension skills.

The first step of developing reading comprehension interventions is selecting appropriate reading materials. To increase the accessibility to grade-level reading materials, educators may consider using adapted reading materials. The Lexile Framework for Reading (http://lexile.com) provides a numerical index for the vocabulary and complexity of the text. Lexile measures for more than 100 million books can be found on their website, and the Lexile measures for the adapted texts can be obtained through the Lexile Analyzer. Depending on student ability, some books may require changes to the text itself to increase or decrease the Lexile level, for example, by varying sentence structure, sentence length, and difficulty of vocabulary. Other books may be accessible with augmentations, such as adding pictures paired with words, inserting summaries with controlled vocabulary, adding definitions and explanations for important unfamiliar words, highlighting keywords, or inserting text-to-speech (Hudson, Browder, & Wakeman, 2013; Saunders, Spooner, Browder, Wakeman, & Lee, 2013).

Questioning is one approach to improve reading comprehension skills of students with IDD (Browder et al., 2007; Browder, Lee, & Mims, 2011; Kim et al., 2018). The purpose of reading differs according to types of text (e.g., expository text, narrative text), and different types of comprehension questions (e.g., literal, inferential) can be posed to enhance students' comprehension. For example, comprehending narrative text typically starts with understanding who the main character is and what the person did (Gately, 2008). Asking "Wh"-questions, such as "Who knocked on the door?" or "What did Nate do?", can guide students to identify who-did-what. Furthermore, understanding characters' feelings, emotions, and motivations are necessary to understand why the character made certain decisions. Both literal (i.e., asking what the author stated) and inferential comprehension questions (i.e., asking what the author meant that was not directly stated) can be posed during reading to guide students to understand the structure of narrative stories. Conversely, reading expository text primarily requires factual understanding. Comprehension of students can be monitored by asking literal questions (e.g., "What are proteins made of?", "What happened after the war?") and educators can model the procedure of finding necessary information from the text. Students with IDD may comprehend one type of text but not another. Educators can pose various types of comprehension questions to guide them to use appropriate comprehension strategies to understand different types of texts.

Students with IDD often have difficulties connecting their previous knowledge with new information and focusing on main ideas or important details. *Graphic organizers*, also known as story map or concept map in the context of reading instruction, can be used to support students to visually display obtained information and show the relationships between ideas. Graphic organizers can be used to illustrate the cause and effect, classify items, compare and contrast, and describe. Educators can use an existing template or create a new template, but it is important that the template is directly aligned with the lesson objectives. For example, Alex's teacher can select a cycle web to teach the concept of evaporation and use a story map to teach him to focus on major story elements (e.g., characters, settings, problems, resolution).

5.3.1.3 Functional Literacy

It is important to remember that not all academic goals and objectives taught to students with IDD must be dictated by state academic standards (Snell & Brown, 2011). Teaching functional literacy skills that are necessary for improving a student's performance in school, home, and community is often prioritized for students with IDD if a student's Individualized Educational Plan (IEP) team considers it appropriate. For example, for some students with IDD who have extensive support needs, such as Kayla, teaching sight words that she frequently uses in her daily life (e.g., food labels, warning signs) can be part of her primary goals and objectives in reading.

Systematic instruction combined with prompting, time delay, error correction, stimulus fading, and multiple exemplars has been successfully used to teach functional literacy skills to students with IDD. If Kayla's teacher plans to increase the number of sight words she can read in a grocery store, the teacher can consider using stimulus prompting and fading procedures. For example, to teach reading the written word Cheez-it ©, a picture of a Cheez-it © box can be presented. After Kayla starts to identify a given stimuli, the visual prompts can be gradually faded out until she can read the written word (e.g., use picture – use logo – remove signature color – present plain word written in black).

Technology devices, such as computers, iPads, and SMART Boards, have been used to teach sight words to students with IDD (Lee & Vail, 2004; Mechling, Gast, & Krupa, 2007). Teaching sight words that are frequently used in the community can be primarily targeted for students with IDD who are preparing post-secondary life like Kayla. For example, an ability to read grocery aisle signs allows her to find necessary items and increase independent community functioning. Kayla's teacher can use Microsoft PowerPoint® to develop an individualized, technology-assisted intervention that includes time delay, reinforcement, and error correction features (See Fig. 5.3 for an example).

5.3.2 *Mathematics Instruction*

5.3.2.1 Early Numeracy

Generally, children start to develop mathematical concepts and skills from early ages and gain some early numeracy skills prior to formal schooling (Kilpatrick, Swafford, & Findell, 2001). Early numeracy encompasses a wide range of skill sets, including: (a) number identification, (b) rote counting, (c) one-to-one correspondence, (d) number conservation, (e) composing and decomposing numbers, (f) magnitude of numbers, (g) identifying bigger/smaller and qualities, (h) understanding the effects of operation (e.g., adding, subtracting), and (i) patterning (Browder et al., 2012). Teaching early numeracy skills are important because these skills are fundamental to learning basic math skills and developing advanced mathematical knowledge (Van Luit & Schopman, 2000), but children with IDD often show delayed early numeracy skills and require systematic direct instructions to develop age-appropriate early numeracy skills (Browder et al., 2012; Hart & Risley, 1995; Sarama & Clements, 2009).

To teach early numeracy skills to students with IDD like Santiago, manipulatives (e.g., sorting bears, Unifix © cubes, Links, counter chips, pom-poms, pattern blocks, tangrams) can be used to provide visual representation of abstract math concepts (Fraser, 2013). For example, sorting objects according to its colors, shapes, and sizes is one of the early numeracy skills that can be taught by using manipulatives.

Counting is one of the early numeracy skills that require knowing the number names and the count sequence while identifying one-to-one correspondence and

Screen	Narration/Action
1. Cereal 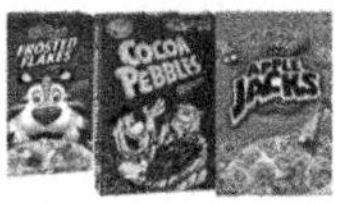	***Program says***: This is the word 'cereal.' What word is this? The student can click the speaker icon to hear the word again. The page changes when the student clicks the right arrow on the bottom.
2. Cereal Water Dairy	***Program says***: Find the word 'cereal.' The student can click the speaker icon to hear the word again.

Fig. 5.3 Example of individualized CAI for teaching sight words

cardinality (Greer & Erickson, 2019). One research-based practice to teach counting concepts to students with IDD is incorporating manipulatives into explicit instruction. Educators may consider creating a series of routines to provide students with IDD with predictable and repeated instruction (Greer & Erickson, 2019). For example, Santiago's teacher can deliver brief instruction to teach the counting of numbers 1 through 10 over ten days. A different number is introduced each day, and the teacher can use explicit counting instruction to guide Santiago to name the number, count the items, match the number with items, and compare quantities. This routine can provide Santiago with learning experiences with all of the ten numbers by the end of the cycle.

5.3.2.2 Academic Mathematics

The National Council of Teachers of Mathematics (2000) recommended that educators teach all five domains of mathematics, including (a) number and operations, (b) algebra, (c) geometry, (d) measurement, and (e) data analysis and probability (Browder, Spooner, Ahlgrim-Delzell, Wakeman, & Harris, 2008). In the research base, mathematics instruction for children with moderate to severe disabilities has focused heavily on repetitive practices of computation and has been limited to content areas such as number and money skills (Browder et al., 2012). It is crucial that students with IDD should have the opportunity to learn and meet the mathematics standards. For students who can achieve grade-level standards with minimal supports, educators may only need to provide accommodations, such as providing calculators, manipulatives, or sheets of math facts, and visual supports. Visual supports (e.g., graphic organizers) have been used to support students to understand complex math content and procedural skills by connecting math vocabulary words to visuals and enhancing their ability to recall information (Rivera & Baker, 2013).

The goal for some students with IDD who need more extensive supports in academics can be "alternate skills" which is still aligned with grade-level standards, but different in scope or complexity (Browder, Jimenez, & Trela, 2012). For example, when peers are expected to fluently multiply multi-digit whole numbers using the standard algorithm, Alex can be taught to solve one digit by one-digit multiplication that are related to his daily life. To support Alex to meet this alternative objective, teachers may consider using systematic instruction, such as task analysis, prompting, and time delay. Table 5.5 provides an example of how grade-level standards can be task-analyzed for Alex.

5.3.2.3 Functional Mathematics

In addition to academic math skills, students with cognitive, physical, or communicative disorders should receive instruction related to functional math skills. Skills in this domain are often related to activities of daily living, such as shopping, banking, and cooking (Browder, Spooner, Ahlgrim-Delzell, Wakeman & Harris, 2008). The majority of research focused on mathematics instruction for students with IDD has involved interventions to teach functional math skills (Browder, Jimenez, & Trela, 2012), which led to several empirically supported practices that can be used to teach critical functional skills. The remainder of this section will describe how to apply three specific evidence-based practices for students with IDD.

As noted earlier, reinforcement is a component of many empirically supported academic interventions because it strengthens target behaviors (Cooper et al., 2007). To be effective, reinforcement should be provided immediately following the occurrence of the desired behavior. Santiago's kindergarten teacher can use reinforcement to teach him to identify new shapes. During one-on-one instruction, Santiago's teacher may use components of systematic instruction to introduce new shapes. After his teacher has introduced these shapes, she should offer Santiago an

Table 5.5 Example of alternative objectives and task analysis for Alex

Grade-level standard	Alternative objective	Task analysis
Grade 5: Fluently multiply multi-digit whole numbers using the standard algorithm	Solve one digit by one-digit multiplication that are related to Alex's daily life (e.g., Alex bought some bags of chips for a party. If he had 8 friends coming over and he bought 2 bags of chips for each one of them, how many bags of chips did he buy?)	1. Read the problem 2. Underline the question Alex bought some bags of chips for a party. If he had 8 friends coming over and he bought 2 bags of chips for each one of them, how many bags of chips did he buy? 3. Identify the facts in story Alex bought some bags of chips for a party. If he had 8 friends coming over and he bought 2 bags of chips for each one of them, how many bags of chips did he buy? 4. Write an equation $8 \times 2 =$ 5. Solve the problem using a multiplication table $8 \times 2 = 16$ 6. Write an answer statement Alex bought 16 bags of chips.

opportunity to respond. For example, she may present a picture of a triangle and ask, "What shape?" If Santiago responds correctly, the teacher should provide brief praise (e.g., "Yes, triangle is correct!") and brief access to one of Santiago's preferred items or activities. In the future when Santiago's teacher shows him a picture of a triangle and asks, "What shape?," Santiago will be more likely to provide the correct answer.

Behavioral skills training can be used to teach functional math skills to high school students like Kayla, who are preparing for transition out of high school. Instructions, modeling, rehearsal, and performance feedback are used to teach purchasing skills to students with IDD. For Kayla, teachers can use these components on a class outing to the local grocery store. First, teachers can provide Kayla with a task analysis that lists the steps required to purchase her grocery items. These steps might include the following: (a) place item on the conveyer belt; (b) hand cashier the money; (c) collect change; (d) say "thank you"; and (e) place item back in cart.

Given that Kayla can only read 15 to 20 sight words, her teachers can use pictures to represent each skill within the task analysis. Next, Kayla's teacher would demonstrate how to purchase groceries, by first purchasing her own items. The teacher would then ask Kayla to purchase her items. As Kayla purchases the items, the teacher would provide feedback on her performance. Correct actions would be reinforced with praise ("Nice job handing the cashier the money"), and incorrect steps would be addressed using an error correction procedure. Error correction may involve stopping Kayla, providing brief corrective feedback (e.g., "That's not quite right"), and modeling how to complete the skill correctly. The teacher would then allow Kayla another opportunity to demonstrate the skill independently.

Consider how purchasing instruction may differ for Kayla if video modeling were used as the primary intervention instead of BST. As you recall from section two, video modeling is another empirically supported practice for teaching both academic and functional skills in community-based settings. Before implementing video modeling, Kayla's teacher must ensure that a series of videos have been created that align with all the steps included in the purchasing task analysis. Additionally, the videos should be filmed in the location where the student is expected to demonstrate the target skill.

As described by Ganz, Earles-Vollrath, and Cook (2011), effective implementation of video modeling requires several steps. First, Kayla's teachers should allow her to view the videos just before she purchases her grocery items. If Kayla's peers are also learning how to purchase grocery items, the students can watch the videos in a small group. After Kayla finishes viewing the videos, her teacher will ask her to demonstrate the skill. Her teacher will collect data on her performance and the data will be used to inform instruction and modify the instructional procedure as necessary.

5.3.3 Science Instruction

5.3.3.1 Academic Science

Learning science concepts involves (a) mastering a substantial amount of content area vocabulary critical to the comprehension of science text (Scruggs, Mastropieri, & Okolo, 2008) and (b) acquiring the process of inquiry as it provides a foundation for reasoning, procedural, and investigative skills, which are fundamental scientific skills (Knight, Browder, Agnello, & Lee, 2010). Fortunately, there is a range of practices to support students with IDD in accessing science curriculum. Systematic instruction, for example, can be used to teach a variety of science content within the context of inquiry-based lessons (Spooner et al., 2011). For example, an inquiry-based science lesson can involve using constant time delay to teach vocabulary; prompting and feedback to review prior knowledge and teach new knowledge, multiple exemplars to illustrate concepts; and task analysis to conduct and report an investigation (Smith, Spooner, Jimenez, & Browder, 2013).

When delivering science instruction to individuals with IDD in the general education setting, we can utilize typically developing peers to mediate instruction. For example, Alex, the fifth grader, does not need intensive supports all day and spends only a portion of his day in the special education setting. Engaging in peer-mediated cooperative learning groups will provide Alex with opportunities for context-relevant social interaction with typically developing peers and improve his comprehension of science content. Training of peers can be implemented in the form of a PowerPoint © presentation that incorporates written instructions, video modeling, and examples and nonexamples. Most importantly, peers should go through guided practice and learn how to self-monitor their implementation of instruction or supports (Jimenez et al., 2012). Note that hands-on activities are encouraged as they promote opportunities for inquiry and generalization of vocabulary and skills across stimuli (Spooner et al., 2011).

5.3.3.2 Functional Science

The National Science Education Standards (National Research Council, 1996) include functional skills (e.g., first aid skills, safety skills) under the personal and social perspectives category. Science curriculum can be aligned with socially significant goals that promote the functional outcome of individuals with IDD. See Table 5.6 for examples of how to design a functional science curriculum in alignment with national standards.

For individuals with severe IDD, such as Kayla the tenth grader, teaching her how to identify the weather and select appropriate outerwear (e.g., shorts versus long pants, sandals versus boots) can be a priority skill as it promotes her independent living skills. See Table 5.6 for an example of how you can break down this task into smaller, more manageable subtasks by creating a task analysis and using visual supports to help Kayla make decisions about what to wear and whether she needs an umbrella. The color-coded yes/kind of/no buttons provide a means for Kayla to self-monitor her behavior, which will promote maintenance of the skill when the educator or caregiver is no longer providing any prompts or cues. Depending on Kayla's familiarity with the mobile app icons, she may need to be explicitly taught to discriminate between the icons. This can be done using time delay procedures and introducing one icon at a time until each is mastered before introducing more icons.

5.4 Summary

In this chapter, we described *what to teach* and *how to teach* students with IDD in academic subject areas. Due to the increased emphasis on using EBPs to support all students to work toward grade-level academic standards, educators of students with IDD are now required to demonstrate how the students will participate and make meaningful progress in the areas of literacy, mathematics, and science. IEP team

Table 5.6 Weather identification task analysis with visual supports

Identify weather			Did I do it right?		
1	Tap		YES	KIND OF	NO
2	See picture	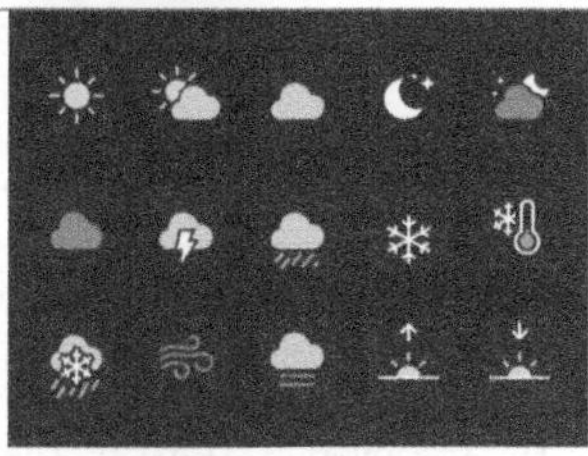	YES	KIND OF	NO
3	Rain?	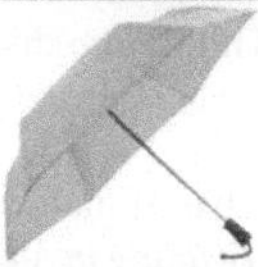	YES	KIND OF	NO
4	Cold?	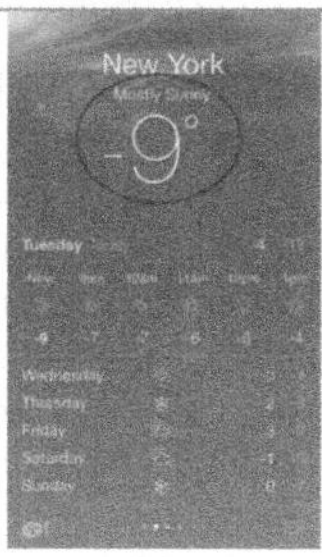	YES	KIND OF	NO

members should consider all essential factors in deciding appropriate academic goals and objectives, which can be selected from standard-based curriculum, functional curriculum, or both. Using empirically supported practices increases the likelihood that the intervention leads to positive outcomes of students. The evidence base on systematic instruction that involves prompting, time delay, task analysis, reinforcement, and/or error correction procedures suggest positive academic outcomes of students with IDD across the lifespan. Visual supports (e.g., graphic organizers, manipulatives), peer-mediated instruction, TAI, explicit instruction, self-directed instruction, and BST are also considered as research-based practices. Regardless of the approach utilized, it is important to collect data and make changes to the intervention based on student response and progress. There is a rapidly growing body of research focused on academic instruction for students with IDD. Increased academic expectations for students with IDD require educators to keep up with recent literature.

References

Ahlgrim-Delzell, L., Browder, D. M., Wood, L., Stanger, C., Preston, A. I., & Kemp-Inman, A. (2016). Systematic instruction of phonics skills using an iPad for students with developmental disabilities who are AAC users. *The Journal of Special Education, 50*, 86–97.

Alberto, P. A., Fredrick, L., Hughes, M., McIntosh, L., & Cihak, D. (2007). Components of visual literacy: Teaching logos. *Focus on Autism and Other Developmental Disabilities, 22*, 234–243.

Archer, A., & Hughes, C. A. (2011). *Explicit instruction: Efficient and effective teaching*. New York, NY: Guilford Publications.

Ayres, K. M. (2012). Reconciling ecological educational planning with access to common core: Putting the cart before the horse? A response to Hunt and McDonell. *Research and Practice for Persons with Severe Disabilities, 37*, 153–167.

Ayres, K. M., Lowrey, K. A., Douglas, K. H., & Sievers, C. (2011). I can identify Saturn but I can't brush my teeth: What happens when the curriculum focus for students with severe disabilities shifts. *Education and Training in Autism and Developmental Disabilities, 46*, 11–21.

Ayres, K. M., Lowrey, K. A., Douglas, K. H., & Sievers, C. (2012). The question still remains: What happens when the curricular focus for students with severe disabilities shifts? A reply to Courtade, Spooner, Browder, and Jimenez (2012). *Education and Training in Autism and Developmental Disabilities, 47*, 14–22.

Barnett, J. E. H., & Cleary, S. (2015). Review of evidence-based mathematics interventions for students with autism spectrum disorders. *Education and Training in Autism and Developmental Disabilities, 50*, 172.

Beaulieu, L., Hanley, G. P., & Santiago, J. L. (2014). Improving the conversational skills of a college student with peer-mediated behavioral skills training. *The Analysis of Verbal Behavior, 30*, 48–53.

Birkan, B. (2005). Using simultaneous prompting for teaching various discrete tasks to students with mental retardation. *Education and Training in Developmental Disabilities, 40*, 68–79.

Bouck, E. C., Satsangi, R., Doughty, T. T., & Courtney, W. T. (2014). Virtual and concrete manipulatives: A comparison of approaches for solving mathematics problems for students with autism spectrum disorder. *Journal of Autism and Developmental Disorders, 44*, 180–193.

Brazeau, K., Rehfeldt, R. A., Mazo, A., Smalley, S., Krus, S., & Henson, L. (2017). On the efficacy of mindfulness, defusion, and behavioral skills training on job interviewing skills in dually-diagnosed adults with developmental disorders. *Journal of Contextual Behavioral Science, 6*, 145–151.

Browder, D., Spooner, F., & Ahlgrim-Delzell, L. (2011). Literacy. In D. M. Browder & F. Spooner (Eds.), *Teaching students with moderate and severe disabilities* (pp. 125–140). New York, NY: The Guilford Press.

Browder, D. M., Ahlgrim-Delzell, L., Spooner, F., Mims, P. J., & Baker, J. N. (2009). Using time delay to teach literacy to students with severe developmental disabilities. *Exceptional Children, 75*, 343–364.

Browder, D. M., Hudson, M. E., & Wood, L. (2013). Teaching students with moderate intellectual disability who are emergent readers to comprehend text. *Exceptionality, 38*, 17–29.

Browder, D. M., Jimenez, B. A., Spooner, F., Saunders, A., Hudson, M., & Bethune, K. S. (2012). Early numeracy instruction for students with moderate and severe developmental disabilities. *Research and Practice for Persons with Severe Disabilities, 37*, 308–320.

Browder, D. M., Jimenez, B. A., & Trela, K. (2012). Grade-aligned math instruction for secondary students with moderate intellectual disability. *Education and Training in Autism and Developmental Disabilities, 47*, 373–388.

Browder, D. M., Lee, A., & Mims, P. (2011). Using shared stories and individual response modes to promote comprehension and engagement in literacy for students with multiple, severe disabilities. *Education and Training in Autism and Developmental Disabilities, 46*, 339–351.

Browder, D. M., Root, J. R., Wood, L., & Allison, C. (2017). Effects of a story-mapping procedure using the iPad on the comprehension of narrative texts by students with autism spectrum disorder. *Focus on Autism and Other Developmental Disabilities, 32*, 243–255.

Browder, D. M., Spooner, F., Ahlgrim-Delzell, L., Harris, A. A., & Wakeman, S. (2008). A meta-analysis on teaching mathematics to students with significant cognitive disabilities. *Exceptional Children, 74*(4), 407–432. Retrieved from http://search.ebscohost.com/login.aspx?direct=true&db=psyh&AN=2009-03338-002&site=ehost-live

Browder, D. M., Spooner, F., Ahlgrim-Delzell, L., Wakeman, S. Y., & Harris, A. (2008). A meta-analysis on teaching mathematics to students with significant cognitive disabilities. *Exceptional Children, 74*, 407–432.

Browder, D. M., Spooner, F., Wakeman, S., Trela, K., & Baker, J. N. (2006). Aligning instruction with academic content standards: Finding the link. *Research and Practice for Persons with Severe Disabilities, 31*, 309–321.

Browder, D. M., Spooner, F., Ya-yu, L., Saunders, A. F., Root, J. R., Davis, L. L., & Brosh, C. R. (2018). Teaching students with moderate intellectual disability to solve word problems. *The Journal of Special Education, 51*, 222–235.

Browder, D. M., Trela, K., & Jimenez, B. (2007). Training teachers to follow a task analysis to engage middle school students with moderate to severe developmental disabilities in grade appropriate literature. *Focus on Autism and Other Developmental Disabilities, 22*, 206–219.

Browder, D. M., Wood, L., Thompson, J., & Ribuffo, C. (2014). *Evidence-based practices for students with severe disabilities* (Document No. IC-3). Retrieved from University of Florida, Collaboration for Effective Educator, Development, Accountability, and Reform Center website: http://ceedar.education.ufl.edu/tools/innovation-configurations/

Carroll, R. A., Joachim, B. T., St. Peter, C. C., & Robinson, N. (2015). A comparison of error-correction procedures on skill acquisition during discrete-trial instruction. *Journal of Applied Behavior Analysis, 48*, 257–273.

Carter, E. W., Sisco, L. G., Brown, L., Brickham, D., & Al-Khabbaz, Z. A. (2008). Peer interactions and academic engagement of youth with developmental disabilities in inclusive middle and high school classrooms. *American Journal on Mental Retardation, 113*, 479–494.

Chan, J. M., Lang, R., Rispoli, M., O'Reilly, M., Sigafoos, J., & Cole, H. (2009). Use of peer-mediated interventions in the treatment of autism spectrum disorders: A systematic review. *Research in Autism Spectrum Disorders, 3*, 876–889.

Charlop, M. H., Lang, R., & Rispoli, M. (2018). *Play and social skills for children with autism spectrum disorder*. New York, NY: Springer.

Cihak, D. F., & Grim, J. (2008). Teaching students with autism spectrum disorder and moderate intellectual disabilities to use counting-on strategies to enhance independent purchasing skills. *Research in Autism Spectrum Disorders, 2*, 716–727.

Ciullo, S., Falcomata, T., & Vaughn, S. (2015). Teaching social studies to upper elementary students with learning disabilities: Graphic organizers and explicit instruction. *Learning Disability Quarterly, 38*, 15–26.

Coleman, M. B., Cherry, R. A., Moore, T. C., Park, Y., & Cihak, D. F. (2015). Teaching sight words to elementary students with intellectual disability and autism: A comparison of teacher-directed versus computer-assisted simultaneous prompting. *Intellectual and Developmental Disabilities, 53*, 196–210.

Collins, B. C., Branson, T. A., Hall, M., & Rankin, S. W. (2001). Teaching secondary students with moderate disabilities in an inclusive academic classroom setting. *Journal of Development and Physical Disabilities, 13*, 41–59.

Collins, B. C., & Griffen, A. K. (1996). Teaching students with moderate disabilities to make safe responses to product warning labels. *Educational and Treatment of Children, 19*, 30–45.

Collins, B. C., Hager, K. L., & Creech Galloway, C. (2011). Addition of functional content during core content instruction with students with moderate disabilities. *Education and Training in Autism and Developmental Disabilities, 46*, 22–39.

Cooper, J. O., Heron, T. E., & Heward, W. L. (2007). *Applied behavior analysis* (2nd ed.). Upper Saddle River, NJ: Pearson.

Courtade, G., Spooner, F., Browder, D., & Jimenez, B. (2012). Seven reasons to promote standards-based instruction for students with severe disabilities: A reply to Ayres, Lowrey, Douglas, & Sievers (2011). *Education and Training in Autism and Developmental Disabilities, 47*, 3–13.

Cox, A. W. (2013). *Prompting (PP) fact sheet*. Chapel Hill, NC: The University of North Carolina. Frank Porter Graham Child Development Institute, The National Professional Development Center on Autism Spectrum Disorders.

Creech-Galloway, C., Collins, B. C., Knight, V., & Bausch, M. (2013). Using a simultaneous prompting procedure with an iPad to teach the Pythagorean Theorem to adolescents with moderate intellectual disability. *Research and Practice for Persons With Severe Disabilities, 38*, 222–232.

Davenport, L. A., & Johnston, S. S. (2015). Using most-to-least prompting and contingent consequences to teach numeracy in inclusive early childhood classrooms. *Topics in Early Childhood Special Education, 34*(4), 250–261.

Davis, T. N., Hodges, A., Weston, R., Hogan, E., & Padilla-Mainor, K. (2017). Correspondence between preference assessment outcomes and stimulus reinforcer value for social interactions (2017). *Journal of Behavioral Education, 26*, 238–249. https://doi.org/10.1007/s10864-017-9271-x

Every Student Succeeds Act, Pub. L. No. 114-95, § 1177 Stat. (2015). Available at https://www.congress.gov/114/plaws/publ95/PLAW-114publ95.pdf, downloaded August 13, 2020.

Fiorile, C. A., & Greer, D. R. (2007). The induction of naming in children with no prior tact responses as a function of multiple exemplar histories of instruction. *The Analysis of Verbal Behavior, 23*, 71–87.

Fluery, V. P., Miramontez, S. H., Hudson, R. F., & Schwartz, I. S. (2014). Promoting active participation in book reading for preschoolers with autism spectrum disorder: A preliminary study. *Child Language Teaching and Therapy, 30*, 273–288.

Fraser, D. W. (2013). 5 tips for creating independent activities aligned with the Common Core State Standards. *Teaching Exceptional Children, 45*, 6–15.

Ganz, J. B., Earles-Vollrath, T. L., & Cook, K. E. (2011). Video modeling: A visually based intervention for children with autism spectrum disorder. *Teaching Exceptional Children, 43*, 8–19.

Gately, S. E. (2008). Facilitating reading comprehension for students on the autism spectrum. *Teaching Exceptional Children, 40*, 40–45.

Giangreco, M. F., Halvorsen, A. T., Doyle, M. B., & Broer, S. M. (2004). Alternatives to overreliance on paraprofessionals in inclusive schools. *Journal of Special Education Leadership, 17*, 82–90.

Greer, C. W., & Erickson, K. A. (2019). Teaching students with significant cognitive disabilities to count: Routine for achieving early counting. *Teaching Exceptional Children, 51*, 382–389.

Hart, B., & Risley, T. R. (1995). *Meaningful differences in the everyday experience of young American children*. Baltimore, MD: Paul H. Brookes.

Hetzroni, O. E., & Shalem, U. (2005). From logos to orthographic symbols: A multilevel fading computer program for teaching nonverbal children with autism. *Focus on Autism and Other Developmental Disabilities, 20*, 201–212.

Heward, W. L., Alber-Morgan, S. R., & Konrad, M. (2017). *Exceptional children: An introduction to special education* (11th ed.). Upper Saddle River, NJ: Pearson.

Hong, E. R., Ganz, J. B., Mason, R., Morin, K., Davis, J. L., Ninci, J., … Gilliland, W. D. (2016). The effects of video modeling in teaching functional living skills to persons with ASD: A meta-analysis of single-case studies. *Research in Developmental Disabilities, 57*, 158–169.

Hsu, G. L., Tang, J. C., & Hwang, W. Y. (2014). Effects of extending the one-more-than technique with the support of a mobile purchasing assistance system. *Research in Developmental Disabilities, 35*, 1809–1827.

Hudson, M. E., Browder, D., & Wakeman, S. (2013). Helping students with moderate and severe intellectual disability access grade-level text. *Teaching Exceptional Children, 45*, 14–23.

Hudson, M. E., Browder, D. M., & Wood, L. A. (2013). Review of experimental research on academic learning by students with moderate and severe intellectual disability in general education. *Research and Practice for Persons with Severe Disabilities, 38*, 17–29.

Hudson, M. E., & Test, D. W. (2011). Evaluating the evidence base of shared story reading to promote literacy for students with extensive support needs. *Research and Practice for Persons with Severe Disabilities, 36*, 34–45.

Hume, K. (2013). *Visual supports (VS) fact sheet*. Chapel Hill, NC: The University of North Carolina, Frank Porter Graham Child Developmental Institute, The National Professional Developmental Center on Autism Spectrum Disorders.

Jimenez, B. A., Browder, D. M., Spooner, F., & Dibiase, W. (2012). Inclusive inquiry science using peer-mediated embedded instruction for students with moderate intellectual disability. *Exceptional Children, 78*(3), 301–317. https://doi.org/10.1177/001440291207800303

Justice, L. M., & Kaderavek, J. (2002). Using shared storybook reading to promote emergent literacy. *Teaching Exceptional Children, 34*, 8–13.

Kamps, D. M., Barbetta, P. M., Leonard, B. R., & Delquadri, J. (1994). Classwide peer tutoring: An integration strategy to improve reading skills and promote peer interactions among students with autism and general education peers. *Journal of Applied Behavior Analysis, 27*, 49–61.

Kilpatrick, J., Swafford, J., & Findell, B. (2001). *Adding it up: Helping children learn mathematics*. Washington, DC: National Research Council.

Kim, S. Y., Rispoli, M., Lory, C., & Gregori, E. (2018). The effects of a shared reading intervention on narrative story comprehension and task engagement of students with autism spectrum disorder. *Journal of Autism and Developmental Disorders, 48*, 3608–3622.

Knight, V., Browder, D., Agnello, B., & Lee, A. (2010). Academic instruction for students with severe disabilities. *Focus on Exceptional Children, 42*, 1–14.

Knight, V. F., McKissick, B. R., & Saunders, A. F. (2013). A review of technology-based interventions to teach academic skills to students with autism spectrum disorder. *Journal of Autism and Developmental Disorders, 43*, 2628–2648.

Knight, V. F., Smith, B. R., Spooner, F., & Browder, D. (2012). Using explicit instruction to teach science descriptors to students with autism spectrum disorder. *Journal of Autism and Developmental Disorders, 42*, 378–389.

Leaf, J. B., Alcalay, A., Leaf, J. A., Tsuji, K., Kassardjian, A., Dale, S., … Leaf, R. (2016). Comparison of most-to-least to error correction for teaching receptive labelling for two children diagnosed with autism. *Journal of Research in Special Educational Needs, 16*, 217–225.

Lee, Y., & Vail, C. O. (2004). Computer-based reading instruction for young children with disabilities. *Journal of Special Education Technology, 20*, 5–18.

Mason, R. A., Ganz, J. B., Parker, R. I., Burke, M. D., & Camargo, S. P. (2012). Moderating factors of video-modeling with other as model: A meta-analysis of single-case studies. *Research in Developmental Disabilities, 33*, 1076–1086.

Mason, R. A., Rispoli, M., Ganz, J. B., Boles, M. B., & Orr, K. (2012). Effects of video modeling on communicative social skills of college students with Asperger syndrome. *Developmental Neurorehabilitation, 15*, 425–434.

Mayer, R. G., Sulzer-Azaroff, B., & Wallace, M. (2012). *Behavior analysis for lasting change* (3rd ed.). Cornwall on Hudson, NY: Sloan Publishing.

Mechling, L. C., Gast, D. L., & Krupa, K. (2007). Impact of SMART Board technology: An investigation of sight word reading and observational learning. *Journal of Autism and Developmental Disorders, 37*, 1869.

Morse, T. E., & Schuster, J. W. (2014). Simultaneous prompting: A review of literature. *Education and Training in Developmental Disabilities, 39*, 153–168.

National Council of Teachers of Mathematics (NCTM). (2000). *Principles and standards for school mathematics*. Reston, VA: NCTM.

National Reading Panel. (2000). *Teaching children to read: An evidence-based assessment of the scientific research literature on reading and its implications for reading instruction*. Washington, DC: Government Printing Office.

National Research Council. (1996). *National science education standards*. Washington, DC: National Academy Press.

Odom, S. L., Thompson, J. L., Hedges, S., Boyd, B. A., Dykstra, J. R., Duda, M. A., … Bord, A. (2015). Technology-aided interventions and instruction for adolescents with autism spectrum disorder. *Journal of Autism and Developmental Disorders, 45*, 3805–3819.

Pennington, R. C., Stenhoff, D. M., Gibson, J., & Ballou, K. (2012). Using simultaneous prompting to teach computer-based story writing to a student with autism. *Education and Treatment of Children, 35*, 389–406.

Reutzel, D. R., & Cooter, R. B. (1996). *Teaching children to read: From basals to books* (2nd ed.). Englewood, NJ: Merrill.

Rivera, C. J., & Baker, J. N. (2013). Teaching students with intellectual disability to solve for *x*. *Teaching Exceptional Children, 46*, 14–21.

Roberts, C. A., Kim, S. Y., Tandy, J. A., & Meyer, N. (2019). Using content area literacy strategies during shared reading to increase comprehension of high school students with moderate intellectual disabilities on adapted science text. *Education and Training in Autism and Developmental Disabilities, 54*, 147–160.

Root, J. R., Browder, D. M., Saunders, A. F., & Lo, Y. Y. (2017). Schema-based instruction with concrete and virtual manipulatives to teach problem solving to students with autism. *Remedial and Special Education, 38*, 42–52.

Root, J. R., Stevenson, B. S., Davis, L. L., Geddes-Hall, J., & Test, D. W. (2017). Establishing computer-assisted instruction to teach academics to students with autism as an evidence-based practice. *Journal of Autism and Developmental Disorders, 47*, 275–284.

Sanchez, S., & Miltenberger, R. G. (2015). Evaluating the effectiveness of an abduction prevention program for young adults with intellectual disabilities. *Child and Family Behavior Therapy, 37*, 197–207.

Sarama, J., & Clements, D. H. (2009). *Early childhood mathematics education research: Learning trajectories for young children*. New York, NY: Routledge.

Scruggs, T. E., Mastropieri, M. A., & Okolo, C. M. (2008). Science and social studies for students with disabilities. *Focus on Exceptional Children, 41*, 1–24.

Smith, B. R., Schuster, J. W., Collins, B., & Kleinert, H. (2011). Using simultaneous prompting to teach restaurant words and classifications as non-target information to secondary students with moderate to severe disabilities. *Education and Training in Autism and Developmental Disabilities, 46*, 251–266.

Smith, B. R., Spooner, F., Jimenez, B. A., & Browder, D. (2013). Using an early science curriculum to teach science vocabulary and concepts to students with severe developmental disabilities. *Education & Treatment of Children, 36*(1), 1–31.

Smith, B. R., Spooner, F., & Wood, C. L. (2013). Using embedded computer-assisted explicit instruction to teach science to students with autism spectrum disorder. *Research in Autism Spectrum Disorders, 7*, 433–443.

Snell, M. E., & Brown, F. (2011). *Instruction of students with severe disabilities*. Upper Saddle River, NJ: Person.

Snyder, S. M., Knight, V. F., Ayres, K. M., & Mims, P. J. (2017). Single case design elements in text comprehension research for students with developmental disabilities. *Education and Training in Autism and Developmental Disabilities, 52*, 405–421.

Spooner, F., Ahlgrim-Delzell, L., Kemp-Inman, A., & Wood, L. A. (2014). Using an iPad2 with systematic instruction to teach shared stories for elementary-aged students with autism. *Research and Practice for Persons with Severe Disabilities, 39*, 30–46.

Spooner, F., Knight, V., Browder, D. M., Jimenez, B., & Dibiase, W. (2011). Evaluating evidence-based practice in teaching science content to students with severe developmental disabilities. *Research and Practice for Persons with Severe Disabilities, 36*, 62–75.

Spooner, F., Rivera, C. J., Browder, D. M., Baker, J. N., & Salas, S. (2010). Teaching emergent literacy skills using cultural contextual story-based lessons. *Research and Practice for Persons with Severe Disabilities, 34*, 102–112.

Spooner, F., Root, J. R., Saunders, A. F., & Browder, D. M. (2018). An updated evidence-based practice review on teaching mathematics to students with moderate and severe developmental disabilities. *Remedial and Special Education, 40*, 150–165.

Stringfield, S. G., Luscre, D., & Gast, D. L. (2011). Effects of a story map on accelerated reader postreading test scores in students with high-functioning autism. *Focus on Autism and Other Developmental Disabilities, 26*, 218–229.

Stroizer, S., Hinton, V., Flores, M., & Terry, L. (2015). An investigation of the effects of CRA instruction and students with autism spectrum disorder. *Education and Training in Autism and Developmental Disabilities, 50*, 223–236.

U.S. Department of Education, National Center for Education Statistics. (2019). The digest of education statistics, 2017 (NCES 2018-070).

van der Meer, L., Achmadi, D., Cooijmans, M., Didden, R., Lancioni, G. E., O'Reilly, M. F., … Green, V. A. (2015). An iPad-based intervention for teaching picture and word matching to a student with ASD and severe communication impairment. *Journal of Developmental and Physical Disabilities, 27*, 67–78.

Van Luit, J. E., & Schopman, E. A. (2000). Improving early numeracy of young children with special educational needs. *Remedial and Special Education, 21*, 27–40.

Waugh, R., Fredrick, L. D., & Alberto, P. A. (2009). Using simultaneous prompting to teach sounds and blending skills to students with moderate intellectual disabilities. *Research in Developmental Disabilities, 30*, 1435–1447.

Wehmeyer, M. L., Lattin, D. L., Lapp-Rincker, G., & Argan, M. (2003). Access to the general curriculum of middle school students with mental retardation: An observational study. *Remedial and Special Education, 24*, 262–272.

Whitehurst, G. J., & Lonigan, C. J. (1998). Child development and emergent literacy. *Child Development, 69*, 848–872.

Winterling, V., Gast, D. L., Worlery, M., & Farmer, J. A. (1992). Teaching safety skills to high school students with moderate disabilities. *Journal of Applied Behavior Analysis, 25*, 217–227.

Wong, C., Odom, S. L., Hume, K., Cox, A. W., Fettig, A., Kucharczyk, S., … Schultz, T. R. (2013). *Evidence-based practices for children, youth, and young adults with autism spectrum disorder*. Chapel Hill: The University of North Carolina, Frank Porter Grahan Child Development Institute, Autism Evidence-Based Practice Review Group.

Wong, C., Odom, S. L., Hume, K. A., Cox, A. W., Fettig, A., Kucharczyk, S., … Schultz, T. R. (2015). Evidence-based practices for children, youth, and young adults with autism spectrum disorder: A comprehensive review. *Journal of Autism and Developmental Disorders, 45*, 1951–1966.

Xin, Y. P., Grasso, E., Dipipi-Hoy, C. M., & Jitendra, A. (2005). The effects of purchasing skill instruction for individuals with developmental disabilities: a meta-analysis. *Exceptional Children, 71*, 379–400.

Zakas, T. L., Browder, D. M., Ahlgrim-Delzell, L., & Heafner, T. (2013). Teaching social studies content to students with autism using a graphic organizer intervention. *Research in Autism Spectrum Disorders, 7*, 1075–1086.

Chapter 6
Improving Skills to Empower Community Access and Increase Independence

Kevin M. Ayres, Kelsie M. Tyson, Emily N. White, and Jessica L. Herrod

To empower an individual in a manner that permits them to maximize their independence and inclusion in the community requires building their individualized skill sets to meet the demands of their local environment. As educators, therapists, parents, and individuals with disabilities consider the skills that one needs to interact with their community as independently as possible, they must first examine the intersection of an individual's skills with the opportunities and barriers presented in their community. This should result in a lifelong process of revisioning of educational and support plans designed to increase and adapt skill sets across environments and technologies. Planning for the optimum curriculum requires careful consideration because, as Ayres, Lowrey, Douglas, and Sieveres (2011) pointed out, the time-limited instruction that federal law mandates has a time cap. Further, federal law emphasizes that IEP's must include "a statement of measurable annual goals, including academic and functional goals designed to—(A) Meet the child's needs that result from the child's disability to enable the child to be involved in and make progress in the general education curriculum" (IDIEA Sec. 300.320). This creates a situation where educators have to make decisions and prioritize instructional targets lest their students miss the opportunity to learn the skills they need to engage their community. As Bouck (2010) reported, access to and engagement in instruction of life skills diminishes rapidly upon exit from public school. If students do not learn these skills at home, and teachers do not teach them in school, they may not learn them when they graduate and therefore will have less engagement with their community.

This chapter focuses on programming for skill acquisition required to successfully participate in one's community across the lifespan. For shorthand, we will

K. M. Ayres (✉) · K. M. Tyson · E. N. White · J. L. Herrod
The University of Georgia, Center for Autism and Behavioral Education Research, Athens, Georgia
e-mail: kayres@uga.edu

R. Lang, P. Sturmey (eds.), *Adaptive Behavior Strategies for Individuals with Intellectual and Developmental Disabilities*, Autism and Child Psychopathology Series, https://doi.org/10.1007/978-3-030-66441-1_6

refer to these as "life skills" and these encompass everything from self-care, community navigation, workplace behaviors, domestic housekeeping/home care behaviors, and perhaps, most importantly, the social skills required in all of these environments. We will not argue about where these skills should be taught (i.e., as part of the student's school curriculum or as an extra-curricular effort as some have argued) nor will the chapter serve as a prescriptive list of all skills students need. Rather, the chapter focuses on a process for skill identification across the lifespan. This is coupled with guidance on selection of evidence-based practices for teaching skills that fall into this broad domain. While standard curricula in US education tend to focus on specific objectives that all students must learn, our approach, both in terms of curriculum and instruction, emphasizes the individual and his or her community.

Some educators might wish to rely on published curricula to help guide the process of programming for a student. Many such curricula exist that can serve as a valuable framework. For example, the *Life Center Career Education Curriculum* (Lloyd & Brolin, 1997) continues to provide a strong structure for programming related to employment. The *Assessment of Functional Living Skills* (Partington & Mueller, 2012) clearly guides educators through skills and assessment related to basic life skills, domestic chores, community-related tasks, and vocational skills. The program includes recommendations for sequencing skills in addition to instructional techniques. Similarly, *The Eden Model* (Holmes, 1998) and corresponding curriculum lays out a cogent scope and sequence of skills across life skill domains and provides assessment and instructional programming support for teachers and therapists. Each of these serves only as a starting point for program development. None of them are specific to an individual learner's context. This chapter focuses on a process for designing programs to help learners of all ages increase their access to the community by maximizing their independence with critical skills at their current level of development.

Upon completion of this chapter, readers will have a process through which they can design appropriate programming relating directly to their client or student's context. Using this as a foundation for educational planning will help ensure that their learners are equipped to maximize community engagement and live as independently as possible. Whereas this chapter focuses on program and curriculum development, drawing on other chapters within this book will help readers understand some of the best ways to approach the instruction of these skills. We encourage readers to use this process as a catalyst for matching specific skills to instructional procedures discussed elsewhere in the text.

6.1 What Are Life Skills?

What constitutes a life skill depends on the community in which one finds themselves. For a child growing up in a large urban city, learning to cross the street, hail a cab, ride public transit, operate an elevator, and grocery shop in a small bodega are all important life skills. In contrast, a child living in a rural community may likely need a different skill set that could include things as varied as safely crossing rural roads (higher speed than city streets, no crosswalks), interactions with livestock (e.g., never approach a horse from the rear or a bull from the front), and shopping in large discount stores. While learning the skills for other communities can be beneficial, it may also take instructional time away from skills that are more functional.

In the 1970s, Lou Brown described functional skills (or life skills) as those skills that, if an individual cannot do them, someone else has to do for them (Brown et al., 1979). In other words, the individual cannot independently complete the skills required and has to rely on others to support them. This support usually comes at some financial cost. With strong programming, teachers and therapists can mitigate this cost and provide individuals with a higher quality of life and greater independence. For teachers or therapist pondering whether or not a skill is critical for their student's day to day life as adults, they should examine the skills they are attempting to teach their students and ask themselves the following questions: "When was the last time I had to do this?" and "How often do I need to do this?" If the answer was today, this week, or recently and/or frequently, then these are skills that a student should learn to perform. If the answer to these questions is never or seldom, then the teacher should reconsider inclusion of the skill in the student's program unless the skill is something unique to that student's context. What constitutes a life skill will vary based on the individual and their community.

6.1.1 *Life Skill Deficits*

Many factors contribute to an individual's ability to acquire the skills they need to maximize their engagement in their community. First, a deficit of cognitive and communication skills may make some tasks complex. Therapists and teachers need to exercise vigilance with these deficits and not use them as an excuse to stop teaching a skill. If a task appears too complex, educators must evaluate whether the learner has all of the prerequisite skills necessary. For example, if a learner cannot match a picture of an item on a list to the actual object in the grocery store, can they even match identical items to one another? If not, then reprogramming to build those early foundational skills making discriminations between identical stimuli might help the learner make progress. Educators should also consider technology-based supports for complex tasks (Bereznak, Ayres, Mechling, & Alexander, 2012). Incorporating technology in day to day living can be normalizing. Typically, developing individuals often optimize the technology available to them to complete tasks on a daily basis. Giving individuals with ID the skills required to access knowledge in this way can provide opportunities for community access and greater levels of independence. Second, deficits may arise because of limited opportunity to practice the skills (Ayres, Mechling, & Sansosti, 2013). If the student has all prerequisite skills and technological support does not help achieve mastery criteria, then evaluating whether the principle of partial participation (Collins, 2012) would still permit greater engagement. (See Chap. 9, *The Role of Applied Cognitive Technology and Assistive Technology in Supporting the Adaptive Behavior of People with Intellectual Disability* by Wehmeyer, Tanis, Davies, and Stock for a comprehensive discussion of use of technology to teach and support adaptive behavior in individuals with intellectual disabilities).

If an educator succumbs to the rationale that the skill is "too hard" and fails to take steps to address potential barriers, then a second reason may explain why a learner fails to develop an adequate life-skills repertoire: they have been denied the opportunity. Lack of quality instruction can result in a learner failing to acquire the most critical of life skills. Imagine for a moment if a supervisor or boss assumes an employee already has the required skills for a job or can learn them as they work and therefore did not provide adequate training prior to the assignment beginning. Without knowledge related to specific environmental expectations, the employee will likely fail at this job. Consider this perspective when programming instruction for individuals with disabilities: They must have opportunities to learn the skills for their current and future environments.

One additional reason that life skill deficits may arise relates to other aspects of instructional quality. Wolery and Hemmeter (2011) pointed out that failure to generalize skills may occur because teachers teach skills in contexts devoid of the natural establishing operations (EOs). While the literature on generalization has focused extensively on differences between instructional materials and environments in which behaviors are expected to generalize, researchers have paid less attention to the role of EOs. For the purposes of this chapter, we will consider EOs in the sense that understanding what a learner expresses that they want to learn about should be included in their programming. For example, if a teenager expresses that they want to access the community pool, then the teacher or therapist might want to consider this as a learning objective even if the caregivers had not identified it as an important environment (but give their permission). The motivation for learning skills to access the community pool (e.g., paying for entry, using the changing facilities) would likely be high and result in more rapid learning than if the teacher structured the learners programming around less desired leisure activities.

6.1.2 Chapter Organization

The next section of the chapter provides a chronological context for program development by focusing on some of the age specific skills that learners need to maximize engagement in their community. This includes a summary of some skills that typically developing children in that age range would perform in relation to their community and a small review of extant research on teaching those skills. At each level, we focus on social skill aspects and other nonsocial life skills. These sections are not exhaustive lists of skills but rather will hopefully assist readers without experience at that age band some sense of the sorts of skills that might need to be in a student's program. The reader will notice a slight variation in how these age band sections progress and this is largely a function of the types of those skills and domains that increase in relevance across the student's school career. The third section outlines a process for developing comprehensive programming and provides the reader with an example of building a portion of a program from an ecological inventory. The chapter concludes with a summary of key points and final considerations for successful programming.

6.2 Age-Band Specific Considerations

Regardless of what age group a teacher or therapist works most frequently, a general understanding of the curricular needs across other age bands can provide perspective (where the student started, to where they should progress). Attempting to summarize all of the skills needed at each would require volumes, therefore the chapter focuses instead on how to identify those individual skills and this section attempts to put highlight some of the types of skills that students need at each age level and how educators might approach programming for them.

6.2.1 Pre-kindergarten

For many children, prekindergarten serves as the first introduction to formal schooling and provides them with new opportunities to learn and grow in independence. For many children, the focus of their programming will revolve around learning new "school behaviors" in order to succeed in the classroom environment (e.g., attending to an adult, walking in a line, sitting at a table, raising their hand, and interacting with peers). For children who had not previously received early intervention services, the learning curve can represent a large obstacle as they face the twin challenges of learning to learn and integrating into a school community for the first time. Children with Autism Spectrum Disorders and other developmental disabilities may require additional instruction on communication and functional skills to further increase independence and access to the curriculum. The ability to communicate with those in your environment creates learning opportunities and reinforcement. Behaviors such as joint attention, imitation, requesting, and play are important foundational skills (Ingersoll & Schreibman, 2006). Along with emerging communication skills, children in Pre-K are expected to demonstrate greater independence with functional skills (e. g., walking in a line, storing personal belongings, and remaining in an assigned area). Other functional skills might include self-care tasks such as using the restroom independently or washing hands. In regards to class-wide expectations, instructors expect students to follow instructions, sit and engage at a table, participate in group learning contexts, and transition between activities throughout the day. Parents and teachers generally need to provide direct teaching to ensure success with these tasks.

6.2.1.1 Communication Skills

In Pre-K, children develop relationships through communication and play. Children with complex communication needs frequently need supplemental supports and interventions to engage their environment. One area of deficit that often influences this interaction involves difficulty with joint attention and imitation (Ingersoll & Schreibman, 2006). In a review of the literature on imitation, Ledford and Wolery (2011) found that prompting strategies, embedded instruction, teaching multiple models, and reinforcement are all interventions that could increase imitation. Typically developing children at this age should also be requesting preferred items or materials they might need. Examples of requests made at this age include asking for a drink of water, a turn with a preferred toy, or assistance with buttoning their jacket. In contrast to one-to-one therapy arrangements, Pre-K instructors will often have large class sizes that may prevent them from attending to the needs of one child. To function independently in this environment, students should be able to identify the appropriate communication partner and initiate their requests. If students with disabilities have deficits in this area, instructors should prioritize instruction to increase communication skills. (See Chap. 4, *Teaching Communication Skills to People with Intellectual and Developmental Disabilities*, by Jeff Sigafoos for a full description of teaching communication skills.)

Play frequently provides the context in which children begin to explore and create their own play schemas and develop peer relationships. Typical classrooms include physical center areas with materials designed to promote various types of play such as gross and fine motor, dramatic, symbolic, or functional. Children with limited play repertoires may miss the naturally occurring opportunities for reinforcement and chances to learn from their peers. For children with Autism Spectrum Disorders, deficits are often displayed through less symbolic, variety and diversity of play behavior (Lifter, Mason, & Barton, 2011).

When programming play instruction, instructors should define target play behaviors required in the child's environment. Sometimes, observing typical peer play can provide a clear set of expectations and lend social validity to the skills targeted. If typical children engage in this sort of play, programming for that may increase the likelihood that play behaviors will generalize to interactions with peers. After observing typical children and identifying the play expectations in that environment, teachers should then evaluate the play skills that the child currently has in their repertoire, and then systematically provide intervention for the next appropriate step. Using taxonomies such as Barton (2010) could be helpful in assisting instructors as they define play behaviors and evaluate next steps in play instruction.

Building these play skills creates opportunities for socialization and interaction which may then generalize to other parallel activities with peers like taking turns and sharing classroom materials, etc. Sharing, for example, is a skill that can be difficult for all children to learn, yet programming instruction around sharing is beneficial because it can lead to increased engagement with peers and decreased dependence on adults. As students learn to share preferred items or request turns from peers, teachers may observe a decrease in problem behavior. Ideally, instructors should teach skills like sharing within the natural environment with the materials that children use. Researchers have evaluated systematic ways to teach turn taking for children with disabilities and found that interventions such as the system of least prompts, and reinforcement strategies might be effective in increasing sharing behavior (Gilley & Ringdahl, 2014; Stanton-Chapman & Snell, 2011).

In relation to developing receptive communication, at this age, children need to learn how to follow teacher or therapist instructor instructions. A teacher could give a broad classroom instruction such as "clean up your toys" or a more individualized instruction such as, "Sarah, throw away your trash". The child must attend to the instruction and complete the task with minimal guidance. Children with deficits in receptive communication may not attend to instructions, or they may not discriminate how to respond to the fleeting verbal stimuli. Additionally, if they have a deficit in expressive communication they might not ask for help or clarification. Building these communication skills will permit the child to interact similarly to his or her peers and begin to establish relationships with them which will foster later social skill development.

6.2.1.2 Other Life Skills

Along with communication skills, at the Pre-K level, children begin learning to learn behaviors that permit them to navigate their community environment with adults more easily. This includes things such as transitioning between activities or locations, using the bathroom more independently, and engaging in learning activities in group activities with minimal guidance. Depending on the child and their current or near future environments, the range of life skills will vary and require consultation with the child's family.

When we talk about transitioning, we are referring to a child leaving one activity or location and moving to another activity and/or location. These skills increase in importance as young children enter Pre-K and their teachers, etc., expect them to exhibit greater independence. Unlike many other skills, transitions look different within community and school settings. Young children often transition within the community by holding adult's hands. Tasks such as crossing a street, navigating a store, or entering vehicles require close and direct supervision to ensure safety. In contrast, safety precautions taken in school settings afford young children with the freedom to transition throughout the school with less physical guidance. Transitioning throughout the building might involve an instructor with a group of students walking in a line. Students need to attend to their instructor and walk in a line as they navigate through the building. Providing additional instruction on transition behavior for children with disabilities will increase their independence within the school setting. A literature review by Knight, Sartini, and Spriggs (2015) found that visual activity schedules could effectively support independent tool in increasing transitioning behavior, among other behaviors, for children with disabilities (Dettmer, Simpson, Myles, & Ganz, 2000; Knight et al., 2015). Multiple exemplars should be included to increase generalization when teaching transition behavior.

Examples of exemplars might include transitions inside and outside of the classroom or from preferred to non-preferred activities.

In classroom settings, Pre-K instructors expect to provide minimal prompting for children to complete bathroom routines. Prompts might include prescheduled group trips, assistance buttoning clothes, or reminders of appropriate behavior. The identification of the appropriate restroom routine, pulling down/up pants, voiding, cleaning, and washing hands are all expected to be mastered skills. Often children with disabilities require additional assistance and instruction with some or all of these toileting skills. Teachers should prioritize this as a skill to intervene on, as this greatly limits independence throughout the school day. Interventions targeting bathroom independence might include systematic prompting, reinforcement, and scheduled bathroom trips (Cocchiola, Martino, Dwyer, & Demezzo, 2012). Prapti (2018) examined the effects of a video modeling intervention on the handwashing behavior of four preschool students with Autism Spectrum Disorders and found a functional relation between the intervention and washing hands, extending that video modeling might be an appropriate intervention for hand-washing behavior. Like the aforementioned skills, instructors should evaluate the expectations of typically developing peers when programming instruction targets to ensure that they are socially valid.

Similar to the increases in bathroom expectations, Pre-K students are expected to adjust to new formats of learning and interacting. The classroom environment involves a large student/instructor ratio and children begin to adjust to learning in group environments. Group environments include circle time, small groups, or story time where the format is one adult addressing groups of children. Students are now expected to sit in a chair for periods of time, raise their hand when they want a turn to speak, and house their belongings in a specific location. Children begin to experience independence as instructors do not give specific feedback simultaneously to all children. For children with and without disabilities, this transition can be hard. Consequently, instructors should be clear in explaining expectations, reinforce appropriate behaviors, and program instruction for children who are not acquiring the skill. Barton, Reichow, Wolery, and Chen (2011) discuss that environment, material, or activity are all elements of a circle time in which adaptations can be made for children with disabilities.

Children with disabilities experience new opportunities to learn and grow in their independence within the Pre-K environment. If identified as a deficit, instructors should provide instruction on communication and functional skills. As young children transition to elementary school, skills such as sharing, following instructions, transitioning, and bathroom skills will provide foundations for new opportunities to learn.

6.2.2 Elementary School

The change from Pre-K to elementary school occurs gradually as individuals with and without disabilities begin to increase their level of independence in the home and community settings. Parent and teacher expectations evolve during this time and, for individuals with disabilities, these new expectations related to skill acquisition intensify the instructional demands and increase the importance of teaching skills in the exact environment in which they need to occur. Teaching in the environments where students need the skills can contribute to enhanced generalization. For example, the focus of instruction emphasizes certain communication skills such as social pragmatics, making and maintaining friendships with similar aged peers, and expanding the child's verbal behavior. Demands related to functional skills may shift some instruction to other settings such as at home or in the community and include a wide variety of behaviors (e.g., hygiene, simple food preparation, ordering at a restaurant, household tasks, grocery and retail shopping, and identifying community signs).

Regardless of the skills teachers target, they must consider the general instructional arrangement and who will deliver instruction. For home-based and community skills, the responsibility of teaching often falls on the parents. In some cases, when schools provide community based-instruction (CBI), teachers share the responsibility of teaching these functional skills to individuals on their caseload. As discussed throughout the chapter, skills targeted for instruction should focus on the individualized needs of each student with input from parents as necessary. When teaching community skills, parents and teachers have a unique relationship of teaching similar skills in similar environments. Setting up instruction for functional or life skills may be easier because the situations are frequently simpler to contrive in contrast with communication training. Communication or social skills often require greater coordination of communication partners and appropriate antecedent events (i.e., EOs) to set the context for prompting and modeling communication. For example, a classroom environment with few students who vocalize limits opportunities to practice conversation skills. Individuals without disabilities often learn through naturalistic approaches (i.e., as situations arise in the moment), but for individuals with disabilities, teachers need to carefully plan to increase the likelihood of success and create a sufficient number of learning opportunities. In addition, teachers need to engineer the environment to include the materials and resources that set the occasion for appropriate communication learning trials (e.g., limiting the number of scissors available in an art activity to require students to request and share).

6.2.2.1 Communication

We discussed the complex communication needs of some individuals with disabilities at the Pre-K level and naturally these will persist to an extent as the child ages even with appropriate instruction. Communication deficits vary greatly with some individuals unable to use vocal language and other individuals able to carry on conversations with few communication breakdowns (Pence Turnbull & Justice, 2012). For typically developing individuals, several social skills (e.g., empathy, joking, play skills) are learned prior to elementary school (Hansen, Frantz, Machalicek, & Raulston, 2017). Pre-K teachers often create their classroom environments to facilitate play which at the preschool age also facilitates communication. As individuals move into elementary school, the opportunity to play decreases significantly, also changing the opportunities to learn communication skills, for example, from more child- to more teacher-directed). For individuals with disabilities, several disadvantages around communication now occur simultaneously. For those individuals who did not learn comprehensive social-communication skills during Pre-K, the context and demands of elementary school will require them to focus more on teacher action (rather than following their own child-directed interests) and this may influence motivation. At this age, teachers will often focus on a broad range of communication skills and build on things learned in Pre-K. The new and broadening skills might include social pragmatics (e.g., greetings, initiating a conversation, responding, maintaining a topic of interest, displaying appropriate body language, and making social connections to create friendships; Andzik, Chung, & Kranak, 2016; Cannella-Malone, Fant, & Tullis, 2010). For individuals who do not develop speech, teachers and therapist must identify a modality of augmentative and alternative communication (e.g., sign, picture, speech-generating device, etc.) and teach the individual to functionally use that modality to access their environment (O'Neill, Light, & MacNaughton, 2017). Gevarter et al. (2013) identified multiple components of different interventions used to teach individuals how to use AAC; those components included using an individual's motivation, incorporating errorless learning, and modeling.

At the Pre-K, caregivers often focus on teaching requesting skills (manding) but as individuals mature, the demands on their communication expand. Teachers may achieve greater success teaching pragmatics to higher functioning individuals on AAC, but for individuals with moderate to severe disabilities, learning to ask for a break or for teacher attention may take priority. Most communication research for individuals with disabilities focuses on requesting, and ignores other verbal operants (i.e., commenting, responding to a question, imitating language). At the elementary school age, however, instruction should extend from requests to more complex communication. Explicit communication training may need to occur in multiple settings with multiple people for the skills to generalize to new, untrained situations, and maintain over time (Ingersoll & Schreibman, 2006; Stokes & Osnes, 1989). Implementing naturalistic training approaches (e.g., milieu teaching, shaping, linguistic mapping, etc.) provide opportunities for the student to practice the skill in the environment it will naturally occur and under those exact circumstances (Ingersoll & Schreibman, 2006).

6.2.2.2 Functional Life Skills

For home-based functional skills, individuals may now perform certain aspects of their health and hygiene (e.g., independent toileting including locating the appropriate restroom, brushing their teeth, taking a bath, putting on clean clothes, etc.) or prepare a small meal or snack independently (e.g., making a sandwich, making a simple meal with the microwave, etc.) Expectations to complete household tasks increases during this time with age-appropriate tasks such as making their bed, emptying the dishwasher, putting away clothes, cleaning up their toys, or helping put groceries away. Meal-related skills could include ordering their own food at a restaurant (with pictures or adult help), taking appropriately-sized bites of food, and identifying the correct utensil needed for different food items (i.e., a spoon for applesauce instead of a fork). (See Chap. 2, *Interventions to Support Feeding in People with Intellectual and Developmental Disabilities, by* Penrod, Silbaugh, Page and Moseman for a comprehensive discussion of teaching eating skills.)

The transition to elementary school frequently provides additional services not often available in preschool settings, such as CBI. This creates an opportunity to visit different locations (e.g., grocery stores, retail stores, restaurants, etc.) within their surrounding community. These trips afford individuals with a chance to explicitly practice newly taught life skills in each setting. Targeting different community skills within the corresponding setting promotes independence on future trips. Teachers and therapists can program instruction of the new skills into CBI trips. Where and what teachers decide to teach should reflect their use of ecological inventories (discussed later in this chapter).

In a review of the literature, Walker, Uphold, Richter, and Test (2010) identified that teachers instruct community skills in a combination of three ways (i.e., in the classroom only or before going into the community, in the community only, and a video modeling or picture prompt simulation). Common strategies used to teach targeted skills include prompting, constant time delay, modeling (including video modeling and picture prompts), progressive time delay, sequencing, task analyses, contingent reinforcement, and least-to-most prompting (Walker et al., 2010). For elementary school students, Walker et al. (2010) identified social skills and safety skills important domains to focus on. Another suggestion was to teach prerequisite skills first before advancing on targeted community skills and they provided the example of teaching money value before teaching how to purchase items (Walker et al., 2010). Identification and programming for all of these skills relies on sound inventories of the student's current and future environments.

For example, children who spend considerable time in the community with their parents need to develop skills related to walking beside or remaining in close proximity to their caregiver as most individuals at this age have outgrown being able to ride in a grocery cart or stroller. Individuals must learn to discriminate settings in which they can run and play (i.e., at a playground) and when they must walk, speak at a quieter level, and remain near a familiar adult (i.e., in a grocery store). Identifying, locating, and knowing what key community signs, such as "stop", "exit", etc., mean also become important skills during this period as individuals might need to identify an exit is crucial to their safety.

Other skills that teachers and therapists target in elementary commonly focus around grocery or retail shopping which include several smaller components to be considered a success. Ecological inventories, as discussed later, will help teachers identify how to break down skills into component parts and group them for more efficient instruction. Some of these skills for younger individuals might include locating and discriminating between items on a shelf (i.e., milk). Older individuals' programs might include more advanced skills like, assisting in creating the list of items needed or assist with picking out clothing items they prefer. Morse and Schuster (2000) evaluated instructional strategies commonly used to teach grocery shopping skills during CBI for 5- to 12-year-old children. Procedures included the use of a task analysis, in vivo training, constant time delay, and pictures. Intervention also continued in the classroom on days trips to the grocery store did not occur and consisted of completing a storyboard activity related to going to the grocery store. Following intervention, participants successfully learned the steps of the task analysis to purchase the items on their grocery list, suggesting the instructional strategies used effectively taught grocery shopping to elementary aged students.

6.2.2.3 Academics

At the Pre-K level, academic instruction primarily consists of letter and number recognition, letter sound identification, and basic math concepts such as rote counting, spatial awareness, and classifying objects by attributes. In elementary school, academic instruction expands greatly, however, for this purpose, the focus will surround emergent literacy and numeracy skills. (See Chap. 5, *Teaching Academic Skills to People with Intellectual and Developmental Disability* by Kim et al., for a detailed discussion of teaching academic skills).

Phonics instruction incorporates many foundational skills and simultaneously teaching sounds, letters, writing, and spelling rules (i.e. silent /e/) allows students to enhance their literacy comprehension (Ehri & Flugman, 2018). According to Chall (1983), individuals in elementary school progress through three phases of literacy development: (1) decoding, (2) fluency, and (3) gaining new information from reading. As previously stated, individuals with disabilities often require explicit training on simplified targeted skills. Phonics instruction for individuals with disabilities may differ slightly from the general curriculum to specify on related functional skills (i.e. vocabulary words related to grocery shopping) ensuring meaningful and individualized instruction.

Some foundational numeracy skills taught in early elementary school include computational procedures (i.e., addition, subtraction, multiplication) and concepts of time and money. Teachers can program these skills into CBI trips, allowing for the instruction of math concepts to occur in functional situations. Incorporating numeracy skills provides the chance to teach and expand in similar contexts over multiple lessons. A teacher could plan a lesson on identifying the price of an item (building on number identification taught in Pre-K) and then plan a lesson on adding the prices of two items together, targeting addition. Similarly, to teaching communication and functional life skills, the instruction of academic skills requires identifying the individuals' current and future needs.

Individuals in elementary school experience a range of increasing independence. To minimize negative effects of learning new skills, parents and teachers need to prepare to explicitly teach most new skills for individuals with disabilities. Planning for generalization at the beginning will bring the most success for the skills to occur in multiple settings and increase the likelihood of them maintaining over time.

6.2.3 Middle and High School

All children experience significant life changes when entering middle school; these changes include things like new social freedoms, physical development, and new opportunities for asserting independence. These changes may have accompanying difficulties, yet permit students to access to novel reinforcers. Individuals with ID have a right to engage in those activities and contact age appropriate reinforcers just as their typically developing peers. Moreover, as a matter of dignity, parents and teachers have to be sensitive to these changes and opportunities for their children. As students mature, they enter a critical time period where intentional life skills curriculum and instruction can have a drastic impact on their futures; failure to program for these may result in restricted access to their community. For example, given that individuals with disabilities are at higher risk to be victims of crime and injury (Agran & Krupp, 2010), teachers need to focus attention on skills that will keep them safe as they engage the community more independently.

As individuals reach young adulthood, additional options emerge to engage and contribute to their communities. Explicit instruction on appropriate community behaviors may allow young adults to access reinforcement in community settings and could potentially lead to greater independence in the form of employment, for example. Instructors should combine academic with vocational instruction to promote successful postschool outcomes (Phelps & Hanley-Maxwell, 1997). Further, having the social and communication skills to navigate their environments and access age-appropriate leisure activities with peers allow for community involvement. When considering curriculum to teach young adults skills to navigate their communities, teachers must individualize instruction based on individual needs as they relate to the community.

Age appropriate leisure activities for young adults can vary greatly depending on their individual lifestyles. Factors such as socioeconomic status, community geography, and social climate can contribute to these differences. Though the recreational activities may differ, there are certain social skills that are essential to appropriate leisure access. These skills may require explicit instruction from teachers and therapists to increase the likelihood that individuals will engage in appropriate social behaviors in the community. Age-appropriate recreational activities could include social media, social gatherings, movies, sporting events, meals with peers, or a variety of other, individually-preferred activities. Though the activities may differ, individuals must acquire a comprehensive set of life skills that allow them to succeed in social circumstances. When selecting social life skills for instruction, teachers and therapists may benefit from observing same aged peers in similar environments to determine what skills will promote independence and acceptance in the community. In this section of the chapter, we will discuss functional academics, social etiquette, sexual maturation, and problem behavior because as students age, mastery of these skills becomes more important and stand apart as somewhat unique from those skills required at early ages to successfully engage the community.

6.2.3.1 Academics

Selecting life skills that have functional utility and contact meaningful reinforcement is likely to increase engagement and performance maintenance over time. Instructors should consider the naturally occurring reinforcers that maintain academic behaviors when designing curriculum. For example, consider the reinforcing consequences for identifying numbers. Examples could include making purchases, calling a friend on the phone, or finding a television channel. Instruction using simplified stimuli, such as note cards with numbers on them, is often essential to the skill acquisition process. However, including naturally occurring stimuli with the target information, such as a remote control, increases the likelihood of generalization while ensuring the instructional focus remains the applied utility of the skill. Phelps and Hanley-Maxwell described this functional academics curriculum as the combination of academics and vocational education (Phelps & Hanley-Maxwell, 1997).

The role of functional academics evolves through the lifetime. As individuals reach the age of young adulthood, the goals for each individual post-graduation or aging out of school need to sharpen in focus. Foundational literacy in mathematics and language skills will benefit individuals in a variety of community circumstances. As young adults progress, instructors must continuously monitor with their growth and continue to add life skills that will benefit the individual across community settings. Many evidence-based practices exist that can serve as the basis for instructional programming. If students do not progress sufficiently after multiple attempts at implementing evidence-based practices, instructors should further adapt the skills to the individual's needs or add supports to the current instruction.

Literacy skills drastically influence an individual's access to community engagement. As previously suggested with younger age groups, phonics instruction is an important focus for all individuals, including those who have ID. By teaching individuals phonemic skills, they potentially have the ability to access novel words throughout the community. This can benefit them in a variety of circumstances, including shopping for specific items, navigating means of public transportation, or even socializing using various forms of social media. As young adults progress through middle and high school, cater literacy instruction to an individual's specific post-education plans. Teachers and caretakers should collaborate to determine the prioritized literacy skills, such as necessary vocabulary, for students to achieve their goals and highest potential of independence. For example, if a student is working to become a part of the custodial staff, vocabulary words related to cleaning materials or locations around their place of employment should be explicitly taught. If a student is working to become a cashier, instructors may prioritize words related to menu items (Browder et al., 2009).

Numeracy skills also contribute to an individual's independence. Educators must think about the functional use of mathematics in the community. Life skills such as checking the price of an item and paying for an item (Cihak & Grim, 2008), making change (Burton, Anderson, Prater, & Dyches, 2013), and depositing a check serve functionally relevant and meaningful purposes. However, skills such as identifying numbers on a hundreds chart or naming quadrilaterals are often irrelevant to life skills, though they are part of the general curriculum for typically developing individuals. Teaching core math skills such as number identification, money value, and one to one correspondence are catalysts to individuals acquiring higher levels of independence in the community.

6.2.3.2 Etiquette and Social Skills

Engaging in social skills accepted by members of the community increases the likelihood that individuals will be accepted, included, and engaged with by others. Appropriate social skills are regularly targeted from a young age, but as individuals mature, new experiences and expectations are introduced that can require explicit instruction. Other important social skills in the community include identification of community personnel. Generally speaking, the ability to identify people such as store employees can provide individuals with greater access to the community with facilitators of support and help in various settings. Likewise, identifying figures such as police officers and paramedics as helpful community members who can offer assistance in emergencies could keep individuals safe.

As many life skills do, this will vary greatly depending upon the individual's environment. Social media represents an important way for individuals of all abilities to interact and create meaningful relationships. Cihak, Wright, McMahon, Smith, and Kraiss (2015) demonstrated that using direct instruction can teach individuals with ID digital literacy skills, such as email. However, one of the issues that warrants consideration relates to online relationships and how that evolves with technology. Instructors should think about teaching explicit discrimination skills regarding which individuals are appropriate to interact with and which are not. Other aspects of community interaction may also require instruction in discrimination (e.g., code switching). For example, individuals with ID may need direct instruction on etiquette standards such as who is appropriate to hug, joke with, call on the phone, or ask personal questions.

Individuals also need to exhibit certain soft skills such as good conversational manners, punctuality, and work ethic to maintain various forms of community involvement such as volunteering or paid work. A 2014 study by Ju, Pacha, Moore, and Zhang concluded that employability skills that were valued by both educators and employers included skills such as "ability to be on time, ability to show respect for others, demonstrating personal integrity/honesty in work, and ability to follow directions" (Ju, Pacha, Moore, & Zhang, 2014, p. 209). Instructors must take into account that naturally occurring consequences for these skills, such as maintaining a job, may not serve as reinforcers for all individuals. Creating a program of instruction which involves contrived edible or tangible reinforcers may be necessary.

6.2.3.3 Hygiene/Sexual Behavior

In addition to appropriate social etiquette, teaching individuals with ID to engage in sanitary hygiene skills can increase the likelihood of community engagement. As adolescents reach the age of puberty, explicit instruction about skills such as deodorant application and shaving can decrease stigmatization in the community while promoting dignity. Hygiene skills are an excellent catalyst to encourage self-management and routines. Supports such as visual schedules and task analyses can assist with educating young adults on hygienic life skills.

Some programming for individuals who are anatomically female will need to focus on menstruation once reaching the age of puberty. Teachers and therapists need to design instruction for this important life skill for females to maintain their health. Not only are the hygiene skills involved with period maintenance important but skills such as monitoring and predicting menstruation makes self-care in community settings possible. Caring for menstruation safely and independently increases the likelihood that females will engage in activities in the community, such as prolonged leisure activities or employment. (See Chap. 3, *Empirically Supported Strategies for Teaching Personal Hygiene Skills to People with Intellectual Disabilities* by McLay, van Deurs, Gibbs, and Whitcombe-Dobbs for further discussion of teaching these skills).

In addition, sexual changes occur once individuals become young adults and often, students with disabilities require explicit instruction about these changes though comprehensive curriculum addressing these issues is lacking. McDaniels and Fleming (2016) noted that poor education about sex and sexuality likely contributes to individuals with developmental disabilities being at increased risk for abuse and sexually transmitted infection. These individuals have every right to have sexual experiences as their typically developing peers do; however, the socially appropriate practices and legal boundaries should be emphasized to ensure community access is maintained (Travers & Tincani, 2010). Students may start to identify that they have novel feelings developing that differ from those previously experienced toward family or a platonic peer. Educators must consider that sexual attraction is something experienced by all individuals, regardless of IQ or ability, and they have the same rights to be attracted to individuals of the same or another gender. They also have the same rights to engage in sexual behavior, including masturbation or intercourse. Similar to teaching individuals to differentiate between whom they can and cannot hug, teaching the discrimination skills involved with confirming sexual consent is a necessary component of comprehensive sex education. Engaging in inappropriate sexual behavior in community settings will greatly restrict access to age-appropriate social or leisure activities and decrease chances of employment opportunities. For example, masturbation in a public bathroom could result in arrest. Therefore, students need to learn appropriate locations for sexual activity, such as private bedrooms.

6.2.3.4 Problem Behavior

We opted to only address problem behavior in this age band because, as a young adult, engaging in problem behavior may place even greater limits on their access to community settings (Myrbakk, 2008). As they get older and grow physically, instructors must note the challenges this can present in a variety of settings. Though teachers and therapists must address problem behavior as early as possible, reduction of problem behavior may continue to be a high priority as students age. If neglected, individuals engaging in behaviors such as aggression, self-injury, disruption, or elopement may restrict access to school settings, where many individuals receive life skill instruction.

Instances of problem behavior in the community could result in dangerous situations for students and members of the community. The physical growth that comes with maturing may introduce new risks for individuals engaging in aggression, for example. Though many younger, and smaller, individuals engage in problem behavior, community members rarely view them as threatening. However, young adults engaging in problem behavior in public may pose larger threats to those surrounding them. This can impede their ability to access reinforcement in community settings and in the worst-case scenarios result in interaction with law enforcement.

When working with young adults who engage in problem behaviors, teachers and therapists must follow best assessment and treatment methods that have been established as evidence-based practices. This may include reviewing or reconducting functional assessment. Older assessments may not apply in new environments that consist of different antecedents and consequences than previously noted. Further, intervention practices that helped to reduce problem behavior previously may no longer sufficiently suppress the behavior. Therefore, revisiting previous assessments and current treatment components to ensure that an appropriate function-based treatment is in place will promote independence and community access.

6.3 Recommendations for Practitioners

As this chapter has focused more on curriculum than instructional methods, this section, provides practitioners with a process by which to approach curriculum development. While curriculum should be student specific, students living in the same community should have overlap in their objectives. This process, building an ecological inventory (see Table 6.1 adapted from Spriggs, Ayres, Trump, & Taylor, 2018), can require a significant investment in time initially, but in the long term provides a structure that will guide individualized curriculum planning. To the extent that the teacher or therapist invests time in a thorough examination of the learner's community they can use this inventory to assess skills of multiple students who happen to access or need to access those same parts of the community.

Table 6.1 An ecological inventory

Environment: fast food restaurant					
Sub-environments	Skills	Social engagement	Key Vocabulary[a]	Special supports	Notes
Parking lot	Cross streets Walk down aisles Locate building	Minimal	**N/A**		
Cashier	Identify food choice Order food Pay for food Take food	Verbal interaction with staff, ordering Waiting a turn	**Cheeseburger** **Hamburger** **French fries** **Large** **Medium** **Small** **Drink**	AAC One dollar bills to use dollar plus	
Condiment/drink/napkin counter	Pour fountain drink Get napkins Get ketchup	Waiting a turn			
Dining room	Locate an empty/clean table Consume meal Clean up area Dispose of trash	Interaction with friends	**Reserved**	AAC	
Bathroom	Wash hands Use toilet	Minimal	**Women/men**		

Typical scenario. An individual without a disability would enter the restaurant and get in the queue. They would read the menu and prepare to order. When his or her turn came, the individual would vocally place their order with the cashier and respond to any questions (e.g., what size? do you want ketchup on that?). They would move to the order pick-up area and await their food. They would listen for their order number to be called (and or match the order number to their receipt). Once the employee called the order, the individual would pick up their tray and check their order. They would then take their tray to the condiment counter to get napkins, a drink and any condiments they need. This may require a brief wait for space to open up at the counter. After getting their napkin, drink, etc., they would move to the dining area to locate an empty table. This would require scanning the dining room. If their friends had already taken a seat, they would have to locate them and move to their table. Once seated, the individual would consume their meal and interact with their friends. When they complete their meal, they would pick up their trash and dispose of it in the trash receptacle. After this they would exit the building and move to their vehicle or the bus. At any point, while in the restaurant, the individual might use the restroom. This would involve locating the correct restroom (men's/women's) and the associated skills inside.

The following information represents a probable scenario that may have led to the development of these ecological inventories and illustrate how that information is incorporated into learning objectives. Typically, the student's program would include objectives related to many more environments than this which span the larger community in which they interact.

Interviews

Interviews with the parent and student indicated that eating at a fast food place with friends is a preferred leisure activity and that he enjoyed eating at a particular chain hamburger fast food restaurant. Both Jaquez and his parents indicated that when he is living in a more independent situation after high school he would like to go to do these things with his friends. Because this was of interest to Jaquez and it was something that he currently needed help with doing, the ecological inventory was conducted.

(continued)

Table 6.1 (continued)

Informal Performance Evaluation

Relative to the expected standard, Jaquez is able to do all tasks at criterion levels except:

- Navigating the parking lot
- Paying for any item
- Reading the menus
- Locating an appropriate seat
- Vocally interacting with anyone.

Present Level of Performance

1. Navigating the parking lot. Currently Jaquez knows to look both ways as he is moving through the lot, but on trials requiring a traverse of the lot of a distance over 100 yards, he stops looking in both directions and is not picking out cars that are backing up. On the last three trials, he made at least five errors each trial.
2. Jaquez can pay for items less than $1. On dollar amounts from $1–10, he pays correctly at chance levels (typically overpaying). Most frequently he looks to the cashier to cue him.
3. Of the sight words associated with the restaurant (i.e., the ones that are specific words), he can only identify MEN with 100% accuracy (in vivo and on flashcards). On probe trials of the other words, presented one at a time in simulation, he is at 0%. He is able to identify WOMEN in the community 100% of the time.
4. He can communicate with his device the items he wants but does not vary responding and would not be able to respond differently if something he requested were not available.
5. In the dining room, Jaquez sits at the nearest table regardless of whether anyone else is sitting there that he knows.

Objectives (listed in order of priority)

The objectives are listed in order of priority based on the critical nature of the skill (safety) and on the frequency with which the skill shows up in other settings.

1. Given direct instruction, in vivo practice and video modeling, Jaquez will improve his parking lot navigation from an average of five errors per trial (on a 100 yd parking lot) to 0 errors per trial across six consecutive trials (i.e., three trips and two trials per trip).
2. Given direct instruction in the form of computer-based simulation and in vivo practice on the dollar more strategy (using 10 one dollar bills), Jaquez will improve his ability to pay to 100% accuracy (never paying more than $0.99 than an item costs and without prompts from a cashier).
3. Given simulation practice with flash cards and in vivo direct instruction, Jaquez will increase accuracy of reading sight words (Men, Women, Large, Small, Medium, Cheeseburger, Fries) in vivo (across at least two environments) and on flash cards. He will improve from 0% in vivo for all words except Men and Women to 100% and from 9% (Men) to 100% with the words in simulation.
4. Given direct instruction in vivo and in simulation, Jaquez will improve (from 0% in vivo) identifying an appropriate place to sit by sitting at an empty table in 100% table across least 3 sessions when the nearest tables to the food pick up are occupied.
5. Given a cashier saying "sorry we are out of ______" Jaquez will make an appropriate communicative response with his Augmentative and Alternate Communication within 5 s of being told the item is not available. He will master this when he can perform the task on three separate trials across at least two cashiers.

[a]Bold faced words are sight vocabulary

In 1979, Brown et al. outlined one of the model ways to develop ecological inventories. In sum, the teacher or therapist examines the learner's current and future environments, breaks those environments into sub-environments, and within those sub-environments identifies the skills needed to operate independently. After identifying the skills required and evaluating the learner's level of independence across skills, the teacher can prioritize skills and group skills according to common features (e.g., locating cashiers).

6.3.1 Surveying the Environment

Prior to beginning a survey of a student's environment, the teacher or therapist must learn from the student and his or her family about the student's current and future planned community (where will they live, with whom will they live, etc.) This can take the form of an informal interview whereby the teacher inquires about things such as where the family shops for groceries, clothes, etc., where they spend their leisure time, if they attend religious organizations, if they eat out at restaurants where do they dine. All of this information about the student's current environment helps the teacher to create an outline of locations where he or she must visit in order to create more detailed summaries. In addition to where in the community the family visits, the teacher needs to learn how they travel there. Do they take the bus, the train, do they walk, take a taxi or drive their own car? This helps to inform the curriculum.

A detailed and well-structured survey of the immediate community can provide a curricular foundation for many students. The teacher or therapist must, however, be mindful of differences between families and their expectations and not unnecessarily recycle material that does not apply. In classroom contexts, where teachers might be focused on CBI, comprehensive community surveys, combined with quality family interviews, can help the teacher organize training sights to maximize utility for the whole of the class.

After identifying community locations and breaking them into sub-environments (which allows the teacher or therapist to program for generalization across similar sub-environments), the teacher must identify and task analyze the skills required to navigate that environment as independently as possible. Frequently this involves a combination of motor and academic type tasks (e.g., physically moving or navigating through an environment and reading/decoding signs or other stimuli to determine what to do). Within the academic tasks, breaking down the skills into cogent domains like reading and math can assist with organizing programming around things like sight vocabulary, counting, and social communication. Sometimes scripting out a typical sequence of activities in that environment and how someone would typically experience or navigate that environment will help to draw the teacher or therapist's attention to critical features of the setting that they should include in their programming.

6.3.2 Developing Skill Inventories

Organizing skills within environments around academic, motor/chained, and overlapping social skills (which often take into accompany chained and discrete academic tasks) helps a teacher or therapist design effective programming. Many detailed resources exist that describe the process for task analyzing a skill (Cooper, Heron, & Heward, 2019; Ledford, Lane, & Barton, 2019). When exploring the community to develop task analysis, the teacher or therapists should consider a few important things. First, observe others doing the skill. Relying only on their own performance, the teacher or therapist may overlook important steps that others take for executing a skill. Seeing others perform the skill may help the teacher or therapist recognize permissible variation. For example, with drying hands using a blow drier in the bathroom, on task analysis may specify that the learner use one of their hands to depress the button. Upon observations of others pushing the button, successful response variations may emerge (pushing the button with an elbow or shoulder) which can translate into task analyses that are more accommodating to the learner.

Frequently while building task analyses, the teacher or therapist will recognize some portion of the academic skills required to succeed in the environment. This can include everything from reading signage, counting money, identifying employees, matching (e.g., from a list to an object), discriminating feature/function/class (e.g., flour is located in the "Baking" aisle) and social skills associated with these community tasks. Cataloging the critical stimuli (e.g., printed words) and require responses for social interaction allows for design of a comprehensive curriculum that the teacher or therapist can implement in the community setting and other training environments (e.g., home, school) to provide sufficient repetition on all aspects of community engagement.

Ultimately, the teacher or therapist completes this process with a very explicit set of expectations and behavioral definitions that represent how a person without a disability engages the environment and performs the skills. This becomes the criteria against which the teacher will evaluate the learner's performance and establish instructional targets with an aim of proficiency at least equivalent to the typical learner. While developing this set of criteria, if the teacher can attend to ways that they could modify skills or provide supplemental supports, then he or she can adapt the criteria later to meet the learner's needs as they strive to parallel the performance of their peers without disabilities. For example, a student may have difficulty reading the labels on the dial of a washing machine, so the teacher could modify the skill so that the learner does not have to read a written mark on the dial but instead matches the dial to a specific color. In this way the learner can still do a portion of the skill while acquiring the rest of the response.

6.3.3 Assessment

To fully assess student performance of community skills, the teacher or therapist has to consider several factors. First, assuming that he or she has distilled the skills to include only those the family and learner deem most relevant, the teacher has to find a way to assess those skills in vivo. Whether or not a student can perform the skills in the classroom likely has only marginal relevance as to whether or not they can perform them in the natural environment. For example, Ayres, Langone, Boon, and Norman (2006) reported on a group of students who could accurately count money for a purchase in a classroom simulation but could not execute the skill in the natural environment. Had they relied solely on classroom observation they would have wrongly concluded that the students could effectively navigate a purchase in the community.

Ideally a teacher or therapist will go into the community with the learner and evaluate each of the skills required for that environment to identify the individual's present level of performance. Essentially, the assessment process aims to identify a discrepancy between the environmental expectations and the learner's present level of performance. Once this is identified, the teacher or therapist can establish mastery criterion and consider how long they will need to teach the skill (i.e., how many learning trials, trip to the community, etc.) From there, they can design the instructional programming (response prompting; see Ledford, Lane, & Barton, 2019) and begin implementation. Assessment must continue across implementation to ensure that instructional procedures meet the learner's needs and, if they do not make progress, the teacher or therapist can adjust. (See Jimenez, Mims, & Browder, 2012 who provide a good overview of data-based decision making for contexts like this). As students master objectives, the teacher has to continually return to his or her ecological inventory to find new skills to incorporate into programming. By checking in with the learner and his or her family, the teacher can make certain they are prioritizing the skills that will maximize the learner engagement in their community.

6.4 Summary and Future Directions

Maximizing a learner's skill set so they can participate fully in their community should be the primary objective of all educational enterprises. Teachers and therapists take a leading role in developing curriculum to meet the needs of their students. Strong curriculum design reflects the teachers' attention to the intersection of the learner and his or her community. This chapter has emphasized that individualization. While acknowledging the benefits of "ready-made" curricula, the chapter has outlined how teachers should approach curriculum design. The chapter organizes some of the discussion around skills students may need to either engage their community at different ages and around skills that may serve as prerequisites for future environments. The intention was not to catalog all of the skills a student would need to access their community; this would have been impossible. Rather, this portion of the chapter aimed to help readers less familiar with some age bands learn about the types of community demands that teachers can program at each of those levels.

We know that post-school outcomes for individuals with developmental disabilities, namely that upon graduation from school students with severe disabilities, have poor outcomes related to quality of life (Shogren, Garnier Villarreal, Dowsett, & Little, 2016). In 2012, Bouck and Joshi reported little relationship between the type of curriculum students with mild ID received in school and their post-school outcomes. These findings were consistent with Bouck's (2012) report on students with moderate to severe disabilities where focus of educational curriculum failed to predict post-school outcomes. In 2015, Bouck and Joshi reported additional findings focused on individuals with Autism Spectrum Disorders that aligned with previous data on intellectual disability (ID). If all these data reflect little correlation between what teachers teach in schools and what happens after school in the community, what should educators and therapists do? The first thing to consider is that these studies are all correlational. They cannot determine causality. A well designed randomized controlled trial would require first that researchers randomly assign students to receive, from Pre-K, either a life skill-based curriculum or a strict general academic curriculum and that the assigned curriculum remain static throughout their education. Then, the researchers would have to follow these students post-graduation to evaluate for immediate and delayed effects. Even in the best research funding climate, this audacious experiment would require resources well beyond what government agencies could allot. The logistics would present researchers with a tremendous barrier. In addition, this sort of dichotomy (general curriculum vs. life skills; that which scholars have set up) does not represent reality. Rarely, if ever, would a teacher design an individualized curriculum for a student that exclusively focuses on general curriculum or life skills. Moreover, as students' needs change and as they learn, they may require the balance of their educational programming to shift between the two to different degrees. In the end, an answer to the question "What curriculum best prepares students to engage their community post-school?" will remain elusive. Perhaps the best move forward arises from findings put forth by Bouck (2010) where she reported that when students do not receive instruction in a particular domain (e.g., life skills) in school, they are unlikely to receive instructional support in that domain later. Ultimately, if teachers and therapists fail to teach students skills when they are school aged, the student likely will enter adulthood with little chance to acquire those skills. If educators know that a particular environment requires specific skills to optimize access and engagement, they have a moral obligation to prepare students for those environments regardless of how they categorize those skills.

References

Agran, M., & Krupp, M. (2010). A preliminary investigation of parents' opinions about safety skills instruction: An apparent discrepancy between importance and expectation. *Education and Training in Autism and Developmental Disabilities, 45*, 303–311.

Andzik, N. R., Chung, Y., & Kranak, M. P. (2016). Communication opportunities for elementary school students who use augmentative and alternative communication. *Augmentative and Alternative Communication, 32*(4), 272–281. https://doi.org/10.1080/07434618.2016.1241299

Ayres, K. M., Langone, J., Boon, R. T., & Norman, A. (2006). Computer-based instruction for purchasing skills. *Education and Training in Developmental Disabilities, 41*(3) 253–263.

Ayres, K. M., Lowrey, K. A., Douglas, K. H., & Sievers, C. (2011). I can identify Saturn but I can't brush my teeth: What happens when the curricular focus for students with severe disabilities shifts. *Education and Training in Autism and Developmental Disabilities, 46*(1) 11–21.

Ayres, K. M., Mechling, L. M., & Sansosti, F. (2013). The use of mobile technologies to assist with life skills/independence of students with moderate/severe intellectual disability/autism spectrum disorder. *Psychology in the Schools, 50*, 259–271. https://doi.org/10.1002/pits.21673

Barton, E. E. (2010). Development of a taxonomy of pretend play for children with disabilities. *Infants & Young Children, 23*(4), 247–261.

Barton, E. E., Reichow, B., Wolery, M., & Chen, C. (2011). We can all participate! Adapting circle time for children with autism. *Young Exceptional Children, 14*(2), 2–21. https://doi.org/10.1177/1096250610393681

Bennett, K., Reichow, B., & Wolery, M. (2011). Effects of structured teaching on the behavior of young children with disabilities. *Focus Autism Other Developmental Disabilities, 26*(3), 143–152. https://doi.org/10.1177/1088357611405040

Bereznak, S., Ayres, K. M., Mechling, L., & Alexander, J. (2012). Video self-prompting and mobile technology to increase daily living and vocational independence for students with autism spectrum disorders. *Journal of Developmental and Physical Disabilities, 24*, 269–285.

Bouck, E. C. (2010). Reports of life skills training for students with intellectual disabilities in and out of school. *Journal of Intellectual Disability Research, 54*(12), 1093–1103.

Bouck, E. C. (2012). Secondary students with moderate/severe intellectual disability: Considerations of curriculum and post-school outcomes from the National Longitudinal Transition Study-2. *Journal of Intellectual Disability Research, 56*(12), 1175–1186.

Browder, D., Gibbs, S., Ahlgrim-Delzell, L., Courtade, G. R., Mraz, M., & Flowers, C. (2009). Literacy for students with severe developmental disabilities: What should we teach and what should we hope to achieve? *Remedial and Special Education, 30*, 269–282.

Brown, L., Branston, M. B., Hamre-Nietupski, S., Pumpian, I., Certo, N., & Gruenewald, L. (1979). A strategy for developing chronological-age-appropriate and functional curricular content for severely handicapped adolescents and young adults. *The Journal of Special Education, 13*(1), 81–90.

Burton, C. E., Anderson, D. H., Prater, M. A., & Dyches, T. T. (2013). Video self-modeling on an iPad to teach functional math skills to adolescents with autism and intellectual disability. *Focus on Autism and Other Developmental Disabilities, 28*, 67–77.

Cannella-Malone, H. I., Fant, J. L., & Tullis, C. A. (2010). Using the picture exchange communication system to increase the social communication of two individuals with severe developmental disabilities. *Journal of Developmental and Physical Disabilities, 22*(2), 149–163.

Chall, J. S. (1983). *Stages of reading development*. New York, NY: McGraw-Hill.

Cihak, D. F., & Grim, J. (2008). Teaching students with autism spectrum disorder and moderate intellectual disabilities to use counting-on strategies to enhance independent purchasing skills. *Research in Autism Spectrum Disorders, 2*, 716–727.

Cihak, D. F., Wright, R., McMahon, D., Smith, C. C., & Kraiss, K. (2015). Incorporating functional digital literacy skills as part of the curriculum for high school students with intellectual disability. *Education and Training in Autism and Developmental Disabilities, 50*, 155–171.

Cocchiola, M. A., Martino, G. M., Dwyer, L. J., & Demezzo, K. (2012). Toilet training children with autism and developmental delays: An effective program for school settings. *Behavior Analysis in Practice, 5*(2), 60–64.

Collins, B. C. (2012). *Systematic instruction for students with moderate and severe disabilities*. Chelsea, MI: Brookes Publishing.

Cooper, J. O., Heron, T. E., & Heward, W. L. (2019). *Applied behavior analysis* (3rd ed.). Upper Saddle River, NJ: Pearson.

Dettmer, S., Simpson, R. L., Myles, B. S., & Ganz, J. B. (2000). The use of visual supports to facilitate transitions of students with autism. *Focus on Autism and Other Developmental Disabilities, 15*(3), 163–169.

Ehri, L. C., & Flugman, B. (2018). Mentoring teachers in systematic phonics instruction: Effectiveness of an intensive year-long program for kindergarten through 3rd grade teachers and their students. *Reading and Writing, 31*(2), 425–456.

Gevarter, C., O'Reilly, M. F., Rojeski, L., Sammarco, N., Lang, R., Lancioni, G. E., & Sigafoos, J. (2013). Comparisons of intervention components within augmentative and alternative communication systems for individuals with developmental disabilities: A review of the literature. *Research in Developmental Disabilities, 34*(12), 4404–4414. https://doi.org/10.1016/j.ridd.2013.09.018

Gilley, C., & Ringdahl, J. E. (2014). The effects of item preference and token reinforcement on sharing behavior exhibited by children with autism spectrum disorder. *Research in Autism Spectrum Disorders, 8*(11), 1425–1433.

Hansen, S., Frantz, R., Machalicek, W., & Raulston, T. (2017). Advanced social communication skills for young children with autism: A systematic review of single-case intervention studies. *Review Journal of Autism and Developmental Disorders, 4*(3), 225–242. https://doi.org/10.1007/s40489-017-0110-8

Holmes, D. L. (1998). *Autism through the lifespan: The Eden model.* Bethesda, MD: Woodbine House.

Ingersoll, B., & Schreibman, L. (2006). Teaching reciprocal imitation skills to young children with autism using a naturalistic behavioral approach: Effects on language, pretend play, and joint attention. *Journal of Autism and Developmental Disorders, 36*(4), 487–505. https://doi.org/10.1007/s10803-006-0089-y

Jimenez, B. A., Mims, P. J., & Browder, D. M. (2012). Data-based decisions guidelines for teachers of students with severe intellectual and developmental disabilities. *Education and Training in Autism and Developmental Disabilities, 47*, 407–413.

Ju, S., Pacha, J., Moore, K., & Zhang, D. (2014). Employability skills for entry-level employees with and without disabilities: A comparison between the perspectives of educators and employers. *Journal of Vocational Rehabilitation, 40*, 203–212.

Knight, V., Sartini, E., & Spriggs, A. D. (2015). Evaluating visual activity schedules as evidence-based practice for individuals with autism spectrum disorders. *Journal of Autism and Developmental Disorders, 45*(1), 157–178.

Ledford, J. R., & Wolery, M. (2011). Teaching imitation to young children with disabilities: A review of the literature. *Topics in Early Childhood Special Education, 30*(4), 245–255. https://doi.org/10.1177/0271121410363831

Ledford, J., Lane, J. D., & Barton, E. E. (2019). *Methods for teaching in early education: Contexts for inclusive classrooms*. New York: Routledge.

Lifter, K., Mason, E. J., & Barton, E. E. (2011). Children's play: Where we have been and where we could go. *Journal of Early Intervention, 33*(4), 281–297.

Lloyd, R. J., & Brolin, D. E. (1997). *Life Centered Career Education: Modified curriculum for individuals with moderate disabilities*. Revised Edition Reston, VA: Council for Exceptional Children.

McDaniels, B., & Fleming, A. (2016). Sexuality education and intellectual disability: Time to address the challenge. *Sexuality and Disability, 34*, 215–225.

Morse, T. E., & Schuster, J. W. (2000). Teaching elementary students with moderate intellectual disabilities how to shop for groceries. *Exceptional Children, 66*(2), 273–288.

Myrbakk, E. (2008). Psychiatric disorders and behavior problems in people with intellectual disability. *Research in Developmental Disabilities, 29*, 316–332.

O'Neill, T., Light, J., & McNaughton, D. (2017). Videos with integrated AAC visual scene displays to enhance participation in community and vocational activities: Pilot case study with an adolescent with autism spectrum disorder. *Perspectives of the ASHA Special Interest Groups, 2*(12), 55–69.

Partington, J. W., & Mueller, M. M. (2012). *The assessment of functional living skills guide.* Pleasant Hill, CA: Behavior Analysts, Inc..

Pence Turnbull, K. L., & Justice, L. M. (2012). *Language development from theory to practice* (2nd ed.). Cranbury, NJ: Pearson Education.

Phelps, L. A., & Hanley-Maxwell, C. (1997). School-to-work transitions for youth with disabilities: A review of outcomes and practices. *Review of Educational Research, 67*, 197–226.

Prapti, N. (2018). *Using a video modeling-based intervention package to teach hand washing to children with autism.* University of Kentucky, Unpublished Masters Thesis. https://orcid.org/0000-0002-7675-3338

Shogren, K. A., Garnier Villarreal, M., Dowsett, C., & Little, T. D. (2016). Exploring student, family, and school predictors of self-determination using NLTS2 data. *Career Development and Transition for Exceptional Individuals, 39*(1), 23–33.

Spriggs, A., Ayres, K. M., Trump, C., & Taylor, C. (2018). Building programs focused on daily living and adult independence. In H. Chiang (Ed.), *Curricula for teaching students with autism spectrum disorders* (pp. 195–224). Cham, Switzerland: Springer.

Stanton-Chapman, T. L., & Snell, M. E. (2011). Promoting turn-taking skills in preschool children with disabilities: The effects of a peer-based social communication intervention. *Early Childhood Research Quarterly, 26*(3), 303–319.

Stokes, T. F., & Osnes, P. G. (1989). An operant pursuit of generalization. *Behavior Therapy, 20*(3), 337–355.

Travers, J., & Tincani, M. (2010). Sexuality education for individuals with Autism Spectrum Disorders: Critical issues and decision making guidelines. *Education and Training in Autism and Developmental Disabilities, 45*, 284–293.

Walker, A. R., Uphold, N. M., Richter, S., & Test, D. W. (2010). Review of the literature on community-based instruction across grade levels. *Education and Training in Autism and Developmental Disabilities, 45*(2), 242–267.

Wolery, M., & Hemmeter, M. L. (2011). Classroom instruction: Background, assumptions, and challenges. *Journal of Early Intervention, 33*, 371–380.

Chapter 7
Community Safety Skills of People with Intellectual and Developmental Disabilities

Robert Didden, Femke Jonker, Monique Delforterie, and Henk Nijman

7.1 Definitions

Safety skills can be defined as preventive or reactive verbal or nonverbal behaviors which establish or maintain a person's safety. Preventive skills serve to avoid potentially dangerous situations, whereas reactive skills allow escape from or termination of occurring situations (Clees & Gast, 1994). Individuals with intellectual and developmental disabilities (IDD) have an increased risk in dangerous situations due to their deficiencies in social and communication skills, judgment, and intellectual ability (Dixon, Bergstrom, Smith, & Tarbox, 2010). For example, it appears that children with disabilities are overrepresented among children involved in road accidents (Strauss, Shavelle, Anderson, & Baumeister, 1998; Wright & Wolery, 2011). Many children with autism between the ages of 4 and 10 engage in elopement (e.g., leaving an area without permission) and a significant number of parents reported that their child could not answer questions about their name, address, and phone number (Carlile, DeBar, Reeve, Reeve, & Meyer, 2018). Deficits in safety skills place individuals with IDD at an increased risk of injury, abduction, getting lost, or

R. Didden (✉)
Behavioural Science Institute of the Radboud University at Nijmegen,
Nijmegen, The Netherlands
e-mail: r.didden@pwo.ru.nl

F. Jonker
Pro Persona, and The Netherlands Institute for Forensic Psychology and Psychiatry,
Nijmegen, The Netherlands

M. Delforterie
Trajectum, Zwolle, The Netherlands

H. Nijman
Behavioural Science Institute of the Radboud University at Nijmegen,
Nijmegen, The Netherlands

R. Lang, P. Sturmey (eds.), *Adaptive Behavior Strategies for Individuals with Intellectual and Developmental Disabilities*, Autism and Child Psychopathology Series, https://doi.org/10.1007/978-3-030-66441-1_7

even death in community settings. Also, individuals themselves highly value safety skills instructions (Agran, Krupp, Spooner, & Zakas, 2012). For these and other reasons, teaching safety skills is important to increase their participation in the community while maintaining their safety (Carlile et al., 2018; Dixon et al., 2010). This chapter provides a review of studies on teaching community safety skills to individuals with intellectual disabilities and/or autism.

7.2 Review

7.2.1 Method

Electronic search engines, such as PsychInfo, Web of Science, and Eric, were used to find studies that were published between 2000 and 2019. Studies were included if they fulfilled the following criteria: The primary aim of the intervention was to teach a safety skill, at least one of the recipients of the intervention had IDD and lived in a community-based setting, the study was published in an English language peer-reviewed journal, and the study provided quantitative data on outcomes of interventions. Excluded were qualitative studies, focus group studies, study protocols, and studies targeted at improving knowledge regarding safety skills. Studies were also excluded if the intervention was primarily directed at parents or teachers, if a curriculum was evaluated, and if the target skill was related to the prevention of sexual or physical abuse. A total of 15 studies were retained.

7.2.2 Results

The retained studies were grouped into the following categories: Respond to lures of strangers (5), lost in the community (4), road crossing skills (2), first aid skills (2), respond to bullying (1), and extinguishing a fire (1).

7.2.2.1 Respond to Lures from Strangers

Most studies were conducted on interventions for teaching individuals with IDD to respond to lures from strangers. Three 7- to 11-year-old children with autism and mild to moderate ID were taught to protect themselves to the lures of strangers (Akmanoglu & Tekin-Iftar, 2011). A two-step task analysis was developed for teaching the target skill: Verbal response (e.g., saying "No") and a motor response (e.g., going 4–5 steps away from the stranger) within 4 s after s/he was delivered a lure. The skills were taught in daily sessions in which video modeling and graduated guidance were used. Graduated guidance consisted of full physical prompts, partial physical prompts, and shadowing. During video modeling, the participant watched a video in which a stranger (an adult volunteer) and a model (a peer without IDD) appeared and in which the stranger delivers a lure to the model who provided either a correct or an incorrect response to the lure. During intervention, the teacher and participant watched the videotape and the teacher used instruction and graduated guidance. Then, the teacher left the room and a stranger came in and approached the participant and delivered a lure (e.g., "Would you like to come with me to McDonald's"?). The teacher returned immediately and delivered the instruction with graduated guidance. Correct responses were followed by verbal and edible reinforcements that were gradually faded out as soon as criterion was met (i.e., 100% correct during three consecutive sessions). Generalization sessions were conducted in a range of other settings on the university campus where the study was conducted (e.g., a park, different streets, market). Participants learned to show correct responses across a large number of different strangers and scenarios. The intervention was effective in increasing the percentage of correct responses, an effect which was maintained at follow-up. Training time to reach criterion varied between 30 and 60 min. All participants successfully generalized the target skill to other settings.

Child abduction is a serious problem and may be highly traumatic for the child and others. Perpetrators typically use lures to abduct children and many children would leave with a stranger. Behavioral skills training have been shown effective in teaching children and adults with IDD abduction prevention skills. In a study by Fisher, Burke, and Griffin (2013), these skills were taught to five adults with mild ID in the classroom followed by in situ training. Results showed that responding was inconsistent and only two showed mastery level at follow-up. Behavioral skills training was also used by Sanchez and Miltenberger (2015) to teach four young adults (18–21 years old) with moderate to mild ID to respond appropriately to an abduction lure. The participants lived at home with their parent(s) and were very social but did not seem to be able to identify potential dangers of strangers. One-to-one training was provided in the participants' school and several locations were used as training sites. The three-step task analysis consisted of: (1) Say "No," (2) get away from stranger by walking or running to the teacher within 10 s of the lure, and (3) tell an adult about the situation within 10 s of reaching the adult. During training different types of lures were presented to the participants (e.g., an authority figure, someone asking for assistance). Behavioral skills training consisted of education, modeling, rehearsal, verbal reinforcement, and corrective feedback. The trainer practiced the target skill in role plays, and the training continued until participant displayed the target skill without any prompts and showed correct responses in five different role plays. In situ assessment and training started immediately following mastery of the target skills in the training setting. During in situ training, the same instructional procedures were used. Behavioral skills training did not result in the acquisition and across setting generalization of the target skill in three out of the four participants. In situ training was effective in increasing correct responding although mastery level was not attained in two out of four participants. The results are consistent with those of the study by Fisher et al. (2013). There were large differences between participants in the target skills learning rate. The step that had the most errors was the final step of the task analysis – telling an adult about the lure. The authors speculated that this might have been caused by the teachers who these participants reported to did not provide enough and consistent verbal reinforcement, and/or a history of punishment for interruption the teacher while s/he was busy in the classroom (also see *Response to bullying* below).

Some individuals with IDD may be especially vulnerable to the lures of strangers. For example, individuals with William Syndrome are known for their social approach behaviors towards strangers. William Syndrome is a rare genetic disorder resulting in borderline to moderate ID. The behavioral phenotype consists of overly friendly behavior whereby individuals are too trusting of other people. Fisher (2014) evaluated a group behavioral skills training program to teach 21 adults aged16–48 years old with William Syndrome to respond to a stranger's lure. Training was given in groups of 4 to 6 participants. Throughout the intervention, confederate strangers who were unknown to the participants conducted in situ assessments in various community settings (e.g., cafeteria, hair salon) to explore whether the participants would generalize the target skills being taught in the intervention. Intervention consisted of three consecutive days of 30-min behavioral skills training and the sessions had a fixed sequence of instruction, modeling, role play, and feedback. Multiple exemplars of lures were used and participants were trained the target skill in response to a lure. The three-step task analysis was: (1) say "no," (2) immediately walk at least five steps away, and (3) tell a trusted adult about the stranger. During sessions, the trainer and counselors modeled correct and incorrect responses to lures. Then, correct responses were practiced during role plays and trainers provided physical and verbal prompts if participants showed incorrect responses. Verbal reinforcement was provided in case of correct responses. All participants rapidly acquired the target skills during role play, but in situ assessment revealed that not all participants showed the skill in generalization settings. That is, after training, 14% of participants agreed to leave with the stranger following a lure. This result was not related to the participants' IQ, gender, or age, or gender of stranger, type of lure, or time of day.

Women with IDD may also have an increased risk for becoming a victim of strangers. Spivey and Mechling (2016) taught three young women with IDD a range of social safety skills, such as responding to strangers who requested personal information or money and who entered the woman's personal space. A training package consisting of video modeling and a constant time delay procedure was effective in increasing and producing generalization of the women's responses to strangers' request for money and personal information to novel settings. However, the women did not generalize their responses to strangers entering their personal space.

7.2.2.2 Being Lost in the Community

Four studies have been conducted on strategies that teach individuals with IDD what to do when lost in the community. Studies have explored the feasibility and effectiveness of strategies that make use of technology such as cell phones. For example, Taber, Alberto, Hughes, and Seltzer (2002) showed that a treatment package, consisting of prompting and total task presentation, was effective in teaching middle school students with moderate ID to identify when they were lost and use their cell phone to call for assistance. Similarly, Purrazzella and Mechling (2013) used an iPhone4 with which three adults with moderate ID learned to take and send video captions of their location when lost in the community. Intervention consisted of video modeling, picture prompts, and verbal prompts. The newly learned skills generalized to unfamiliar settings.

In a recent study by Bassette et al. (2018), three youths (13–15 years old) with moderate to mild ID were taught how to use a cell phone when lost. Participants received training in the same junior high school and across five settings: Classroom, hallway, library, and a familiar and an unfamiliar community location. A task analysis was developed that consisted of 15 steps from flipping the phone open, to clicking on a button to send a picture, and wait in place until the teacher arrives. The target skills were to take a picture of the situation where the participant was and to send it to her teacher. To teach participants the target skill, a system of least-to-most prompts was used to deliver in the following order: Verbal, verbal and gesture, verbal and model, verbal and partial physical, and verbal and full physical prompt. Next, a video model was used providing a model demonstrating the following steps. The model: (1) acknowledged that she was lost, (2) noted that she could take a picture to send to help her instructor where she was, and (3) pointed directly to a key identification point (e.g., a sign) to help her teacher identify her location.

Also, the participant then immediately watched a second video that showed, from the cell phone's perspective, the sequences of buttons that needed to be touched on the phone to successfully take and send a picture based on the steps of the task analysis. The second video showed the phone and finger demonstrating the buttons to be pressed. Auditory prompts detailing the steps of the task analysis were also given. The trainer used the system of least prompts if a participant could not complete a step correctly and independently. The results showed that all three participants increased their ability to perform the task independently and all generalized the target skill across settings, including to an unfamiliar community setting. All participants learned the skill relatively quickly within two to four sessions. The gesture plus verbal prompt was the most intrusive prompt required for all participants. The authors noted several advantages of acquiring the target skill. Using a cell phone does not require locating an adult for assistance, or describing their location over the phone. It also does not require Internet access.

In another study addressing being lost in the community, Carlile et al. (2018) used video modeling to teach low- and high-tech help-seeking responses to six males with autism who were between 3 and 14 years old. Training was given in a setting located in a public school, and pre- and postintervention sessions were conducted in a variety of community settings (stores) such as ToysRUs, Michaels, and Home Depot. The task analysis for the low-tech response consisted of six steps, while the high-tech response consisted of nine steps. The difference between the two types of responses was that in the high-tech response the use of a camera was added to the task analysis. The task analysis of the low-tech response consisted of the following six steps: (1) identify lost; (2) scan area for a store employee; (3) walk up to store employee; (4) say “Excuse me, I am lost”; (5) hand over identification card; and (6) remain within 1.5 m of store employee. Intervention consisted of video modeling in which a point-of-view video model of the target response was shown to the participant. Then the participant was escorted to an area of the classroom that was arranged in a manner similar to the store (the generalization setting) and then the trainer moved out of view. Common stimuli were used by incorporating a variety of items (e.g., uniform shirts, name tags, baskets) from the stores into the classroom. The participant could then complete the steps of the task analysis. Following an incorrect response, the behavior was interrupted by the trainer and a video model of the step was re-presented after which the participant was given an opportunity to engage in the modeled response with no additional prompts. If the response was correct, the participant continued in the task analysis. If the response was incorrect, the trainer provided manual guidance and/or vocal prompts. This procedure was repeated until the participant completed the task analysis without errors. The treatment package resulted in a successful generalization across settings and people. That is, the participants showed correct responses in different stores and with novel people.

7.2.2.3 Road Crossing Skills

Two studies had addressed road-crossing skills. In the first, Brown and Gillard (2009) compared in vivo training with a classroom based program to teach road-crossing skills to a 15-year-old boy with Down syndrome and severe ID. The participant was taught the target skill in an 8-step task analysis: (1) walk to the side of the road; (2) stop; (3) look left; (4) look right; (5) say “no car” if the road is clear; (6) if a car is coming, wait until it has passed, return to step 3; (7) if the road is clear, then cross the road; and (8) look left and right while crossing the road. During in vivo training, the boy was taught the skill outside on a road and each of the above steps was modeled by a trainer and he was verbally prompted to imitate the trainer’s behavior. Correct responses were verbally reinforced. During the classroom-based instruction, the participant was taught to sequence pictures of the above road safety behaviors. The correct order of steps was taught using backward chaining. Results showed that the number of correct responses (i.e., road safety behaviors on the street) was much higher during the classroom-based program than during in vivo training. The participant generalized the skill to another trainer and maintained the skill at a high level at 6 weeks’ follow-up. Progress during in vivo training was slow as there were many distractions in the outdoor environment. Also, it was difficult to organize the teaching as two instructors were needed to support the participant. Overall, the results were disappointing as the participant never became fully independent as a pedestrian.

In the second study to address road crossing skills, Bicakci and Gul (2019) taught road crossing skills to three 7- to 9-year-old students with IDD who visited a primary school in the Turkish region of Anatolia of whom two had autism and one had mild ID. The students were trained by peers without IDD in a one-to-one training format. The peers used social stories (road crossing), modeling, and feedback to teach the students how to safely cross a street. Following the intervention, results showed that all three participants acquired the target skill and were able to generalize the skill to an untrained street. The skills were maintained at a 2-week follow-up.

7.2.2.4 First Aid Skills

Knowing how to respond during an emergency is considered an essential safety skill. Kearney, Brady, Hall, and Honsberger (2018) taught basic first aid skills to three 15- to 17-year-old participants who had autism and below average intelligence. The intervention used a story book and other interventions and was implemented in the school cafeteria in which a sink and a first aid kit were present. Prior to starting the intervention, a task analysis was developed for the first aid skills of cleaning and dressing a wound on another person. The task analysis consisted of 14 steps: (1) wash hands with soap and water, (2) get first aid kit, (3) put on gloves, (4) open gauze pad, (5) use gauze to clean around wound, (6) open new gauze pad, (7) apply gauze pad to clean, dry skin, fully covering the wound, (8) wrap gauze roll three to five wraps over wound and body and cut the roll, (9) tape gauze roll to itself, (10) take one glove off from bottom, (11) throw away used pad, trash, and gloves, (12) take other glove off from bottom and throw it away, (13) wash hands with soap and water, and (14) show or tell an adult. After developing the task analysis, a storybook was written which contained 14 pages, with each page for each step of the task analysis. On each page, a simple sentence written in the first person was shown, together with a picture of the step.

During intervention, a peer sat next to the participant and read aloud the sentence on the page, pointed to the picture, and gestured to the items (e.g., gloves, gauze pad). After the peer finished all steps, the trainer pointed to a simulated cut on the peer and asked the participant: "He's hurt. Can you do first aid?" A prompt was delivered in case of an incorrect response to a step, or not making an attempt at the step within 30s. A peer delivered the non-specific prompt, "Remember what the story said," while turning to the page of the story, and reading the page again. As progress was slow during the first half of the intervention condition, a correction procedure was added in which the peer and/or trainer modeled the correct response of the step or gave a specific verbal prompt (e.g., "Wash hands"). The intervention was effective in teaching the basic first aid skills to all participants, particularly following the introduction of the correction procedure.

Sudden cardiac arrest has gained much worldwide public attention in the last years. Individuals with cardiac arrest are more likely to survive if cardiopulmonary resuscitation (CPR) is given. In a study by Kearny et al. (2019), three adolescents (19–23 years old) with mild ID were taught to perform CPR/AED (see below) using a treatment package that consisted of modeling, 24-step task analysis, and simultaneous prompting. Training sessions were held in a conference room of a university building in which also an automated external defibrillator (AED) was present.

The first phase in the training was mastering the 14-step CPR task (chain) during which the trainer modeled the task first and the trainer and participant practiced the chain together using simultaneous prompting on two separate manikins. The task analysis of the CPR skill consisted of the following 14 steps: (1) Assess the scene, (2) Attempt to wake the victim and check for signs of life, (3) Tell someone to call 911 and identify location, (4) Retrieve gloves and face shield, (5) Put on gloves, (6) Put face shield on manikin, (7) Open airway and give two rescue breaths, (8) Provide 30 chest compressions, (9) Open airway and give two rescue breaths, (10) Repeat 30 chest compressions (trainer says "He's breathing now"), (11) Take face shield off, (12) Place person in recovery position, (13) Remove gloves and throw in trash, and (14) Wash hands with soap and water.

Following mastering of the CPR task (i.e., 93% correct unprompted responses during three consecutive sessions) the 10-step AED task was trained using the same instructional procedures. Results show that the three participants' correct responses increased to mastery level quickly after the start of the training and their CPR/AED skills generalized to an untrained second setting. Also, skill level was maintained between 7 and 17 days follow-up during which no instructional procedures were in effect.

7.2.2.5 Responding to Bullying

Many people with IDD may become victim of bullying. Bullying consists of physical and/or verbal aggressive behavior or other actions intended to harm a victim. For the victim, bullying has a range of adverse consequences, such as mental health problems or injury. It is, therefore, important to teach individuals with IDD skills to respond to bullying. While there are many studies including individuals without IDD, we could find only one study in which responses to bullying were taught to individuals with IDD (Stannis, Crosland, Miltenberger, & Valbuena, 2019). In that study, response to bullying was taught to four adult (34–64 years old) males with severe to mild ID who were residents of a community-based group home. The target skill consisted of a 4-step task analysis: (1) refrain from retaliating against the bully by avoiding physical contact or vocal statements other than those learned during the training; (2) state only a short comment of disapproval, such as "I do not like that"; (3) walk away from the bully; and (4) tell a staff member about the interaction. Three confederates (men with mild ID) implemented the bully statements to the participants in the in situ assessments. The training was conducted in the participants' group home and at a therapy center. Two sessions were held with participants. Behavioral skills training consisted of instructions, modeling, rehearsal, and feedback. During instruction, the trainer told the participant to respond to bullying. They were told to refrain from retaliation (e.g., "Do not hit"), say a short statement of disapproval, walk away, and tell a staff member. During modeling, the trainer and assistants modeled the correct target skill in a role play when a bully statement was presented. In rehearsal three to five, role play situations were conducted, whereby the trainer acted as bully and participants could demonstrate mastery level of the

4-step target skill. Finally, during feedback, correct responses were followed by verbal reinforcement, incorrect responses were followed by corrective feedback, including prompts for correct responses.

In situ assessments in the natural setting were done following participants reaching mastery level. That is, participants showed 100% correct responding on all steps of the target skill in role plays during the two training sessions. Booster sessions which included the same procedures as during behavioral skills training were held if the participant did not demonstrate all steps of the skill during in situ assessments. Data were collected in a multiple probe design. Results showed that the skills training were effective in two participants. In one case, behavioral skills training was ineffective and for this participant in situ training was effective. For the fourth participant, (the person with severe ID), adding a reinforcer (highly preferred item) resulted in an increase in correct responding, though mastery level was not attained. For the other three participants, results were maintained at a 3-week follow-up. Interestingly, one participant (a 48-year-old man with mild ID) never displayed the final step of the task analysis (telling a staff member). Criteria for mastery level were modified for this participant after he stated that he did not want to tell staff because staff were present, had observed the bullying statement, but did not respond to the incident. This outcome is similar to one of the outcomes of the study by Sanchez and Miltenberger (2015; also see *Respond to lures of strangers* above), in which teachers ignored the final step of the trained target skill (i.e., telling an adult about a lure by strangers).

7.2.2.6 Extinguishing a Fire

Mechling, Gast, and Gustafson (2009) taught three young adults with moderate ID how to extinguish a cooking-related fire. The study took place in the kitchen and barbeque areas of an apartment rented by the school for training. The students learned to extinguish fires with a lid, with flower, and with a fire extinguisher. Intervention consisted of video modeling and prompting. During baseline, students performed no steps independently and post-training performed 100% of steps correctly for each of the three skills. The effects of the intervention also generalized to novel examples of cooking-related fires and were maintained for 22–52 days.

7.2.3 Conclusions Regarding the Evidence Base

In the past 20 years, several reviews have been published on safety skills in individuals with IDD. Dixon et al. (2010) provided a review on the efficacy of interventions for safety skills in individuals with ID. They included 27 studies published in the last 30 years. The authors concluded that behavioral procedures, such as reinforcement, prompting, and role-play, were effective across a variety in participants, target skills, and settings. Results of the review in the present chapter extended and corroborated these findings. A meta-analysis of 11 single case studies on teaching safety skills to individuals with autism (5–24 years old) revealed that studies reported medium to large effect sizes. Interventions included were video modeling, response and stimulus fading procedures, role play, and verbal explanation of rules. There were no significant differences in effectiveness of interventions between categories of interventions or settings. Large effect sizes were found for generalization studies, while follow-up effect sizes were in the low range. Many studies lacked data on treatment fidelity and thus it remains unclear if interventions were implemented as intended.

Recently, a comprehensive review of 82 studies was conducted by Giannakakos, Vladescu, Kisamore, Reeve, and Fienup (2020) on the effectiveness of safety response training. Individuals with autism (16%) and developmental disability (25%) were included in the studies. A range of target skills were trained, such as fire safety, abduction prevention, firearm safety, seeking help when lost, and pedestrian safety. Interventions that were found effective were behavioral skills training (instruction, modeling, role play, feedback), in situ training (in vivo role play and feedback), prompting procedures (errorless learning), video modeling, discrete trail training, virtual reality, and differential reinforcement. The authors concluded that behavioral skills training plus in situ training is the most effective strategy for teaching safety skills.

The review in the present chapter shows that a range of behavioral interventions have shown positive results in the sense that safety skills can be taught to children, adolescents, and adults with IDD relatively quickly. A consistent finding across studies is that untrained generalization may occur but that it often needs to be promoted in situ.

7.3 Practitioner Recommendations

Studies in which the opinions of parents and teachers of children with IDD of safety skills instruction was explored revealed that while both groups found such skills important, they rarely discussed this topic with each other and expressed a lack of knowledge and expertise on how to teach safety skills to children with IDD (see e.g., Sirin & Tekin-Iftar, 2016). The topic of teaching safety skills is often overlooked by practitioners and parents (see Dixon et al., 2010). They may assume that individuals with IDD are incapable of learning a variety of safety skills. The results of the present review as well as previous reviews show that individuals with IDD can learn safety skills as a result of behavioral approaches.

As a first step, practitioners should explore which types of safety skills a given individual may be lacking and which safety skill(s) should be targeted. Following the choice of a safety skill, an assessment of prerequisite skills for teaching that safety skill may be necessary. For example, Alevriadou (2010) explored relationships between attention, cognitive style, and identification of safe and dangerous road-crossing sites in 40 boys with mild ID. Attention and field (in)dependence were assessed using visual attention and embedded figures tests. Results showed that boys with better test scores performed better in identifying safe road crossing sites than boys with lower test scores. The author concluded that attention and cognitive style should be assessed prior to teaching of road safety skills to individuals with ID.

At the start of an intervention, a further assessment may be needed as to the entry level of an intervention. For example, prior to teaching a help-seeking response when lost, Carlile et al. (2018) assessed if participants discriminated between video examples of "lost" and "not lost." If they could not discriminate between these two situations, their task analysis changed in that they were taught to wait for a store employee who approached them and asked them if they were lost. After this question (prompt) they were taught to hand over a communication card that notified that s/he was lost. As in other studies, Carlile et al. did a brief multiple stimulus without replacement preference assessment with which reinforcers were identified for each participant prior to the start of the intervention. Pre-training assessment should be considered in case participants are going to use for example virtual environments. In the study by Saiano et al. (2015) one participant did not complete the familiarization phase prior to training because of problems with depth perception.

When teaching safety skills, it is important to consider adding visual supports to the training procedures. Manualized information and prompts may be delivered through the support by drawings, video-based materials (video modeling), and/or photographs (see Akmanoglu & Tekin-Iftar, 2011). It is also important to reinforce each step of the skill and to respond to the final step of the learned target skill. If practitioners do not respond adequately, consistently, and frequently to the final step of the target skill, – especially in the beginning of the training – the skill will not be learned or extinguished (Sanchez & Miltenberger, 2015; Stannis et al., 2019).

A commonly noted dilemma in the studies on safety skills is the question whether skills should be taught in vivo/in situ or in an analogous setting (also see Dixon et al., 2010). An advantage of training in an actual environment is the strong stimulus control from the start of the intervention. A disadvantage is that precautions should be taken. Training in an analogue setting has the advantage that it may be relatively easy to organize and that errors and incorrect responses have no adverse consequences. Results of the studies included in the present review show that generalization may be stimulated by using common stimuli, multiple exemplars, task analyses, technology, etc.

The present reviews revealed that few family members such as parents and siblings were involved in the training of safety skills. Generalization of safety skills across settings and individuals should be promoted through training of multiple trainers, including parents or teachers and other caregivers. Several studies have shown that parents may be taught to implement a safety skill training to their child. For example, in the study by Harriage, Blair, and Miltenberger (2016) trained parents of three adolescents with ASD to implement behavioral skills training (i.e., in situ training) and a most-to-least prompting (full physical to verbal prompt) procedure to teach their child to use pedestrian safety skills in community settings. The intervention resulted in high levels of correct implementation of training procedures across different street locations. All three participants learned to cross different streets safely. However, it should be noted that for both the parents and their child the results of the intervention did not generalize spontaneously to other streets. Thus, while the intervention was effective in increasing the participants' safety skills and implementation of intervention procedures by parents, the skills did not generalize to untrained streets. The lack of spontaneous generalization was probably due to the differences in street types in that generalization streets were viewed as dangerous as a result of high-volume traffic. Parents may have felt less confident in their child's ability to cross the street, resulting in higher prompt levels than needed. In general, it is recommended to start teaching road crossing skills on low traffic streets until the participant shows independent responding and mastery before promoting generalization of the skills to high traffic streets (Matson, 1980; Wright & Wolery, 2011).

Practitioners should consider if booster training sessions are needed after the completion of an intervention. Some types of skills, such as road crossing or food safety skills, may come under strong natural stimulus control because individuals frequently practice the skills. Other skills, such as first aid skills or responding to lures of strangers, that have been taught may need booster training as situations in which the learned may be put into practice do not or only seldom occur. Maintenance of learned skills over many months has not been assessed in intervention studies and we do not know how well safety skills are maintained long-term and if yes, in whom. Thus, practitioners need to assess safety skills' mastery levels on a regular basis, especially in skills that are seldom or never put into practice.

7.4 Case Example

To illustrate the application of teaching community safety skills we report an illustrative case study.

Jan was a 32-year-old male with moderate to mild ID who lived in a group home in a small village. On a daily basis, he visited a daytime activity center located across the street near his group home. He needed to cross the street several times a day and Jan and other participants were brought to the center by a staff member. Before moving to the group home, he lived in a residential facility and he could walk to the activity center without having to cross the street. Now he had to learn how to cross the street which was a short and low-traffic street.

Prior to training, assessment indicated that he could discriminate between a street which was clear (with no car) and a street that was not clear (car in sight). He was taught that he was allowed to cross the street only if no traffic was in sight and the street was clear. He had no visual or physical impairment and had sufficient expressive and receptive communication skills. Additionally, the village's council agreed to make a sign on the street where Jan and other residents of the group home could cross the street (stimulus control). Jan and his parents agreed that independently crossing that street would be an important safety skill to learn.

The task analysis consisted of 8 steps similar to the task analysis used by Brown and Gillard (2009; see *Road crossing skills* above.) As Jan already had some experience in crossing the street albeit with support from a staff member of the group home, a least-to-most prompting procedure (see Duker, Didden, & Sigafoos, 2004) was thought appropriate to teach him to safely and independently cross the street and walk to the activity center or group home. Prompts and verbal reinforcement and presence of the staff member were faded out as the number of correct responses increased. Prompt levels were verbal instruction and modeling. Verbal reinforcement were given by staff at the activity center or group home immediately after he arrived at the location (see Sect. 7.3) which was given only intermittently after several weeks of training. Next to this, as the street was short and had low traffic, in situ training was chosen instead of training in a simulated setting. Training was conducted five consecutive times each time Jan had to cross the street. During the training, there were four daily sessions, including return to group home at lunchtime, which consisted of a total of 20 opportunities for street crossing. Jan learned the skill very quickly and reached mastery level within 2 days of training. The presence of the staff member at the road site was quickly faded out. To regularly check mastery level, a staff member would walk with Jan until the end of the street and observed while he crossed the street. Jan maintained the target skill and booster training was not needed. The training yielded effect very quickly and in no opportunity had his safety been at stake.

7.5 Summary and Future Directions

Recent decades have shown an increased rate of individuals with IDD living in community settings. As a result, issues of safety are much debated by caregivers, parents, and individuals themselves. Agran et al. (2012) have shown that safety skills instruction is highly valued by people with ID. Although strategies for safety skills often are embedded into curricula for students with IDD, there is a need for exploring the effectiveness and prerequisites of interventions for teaching safety skills to individuals with IDD (Bassette et al., 2018; Brown & Gillard, 2009). The present review included a relatively narrow range of types of safety skills. In future research, other types of safety skills should be investigated, such as helmet use, bike safety, firearm safety, food safety, public transportation, social media, and water safety (Caton & Chapman, 2016; Giannakakos et al., 2020; Lee et al., 2019; Lindsay & Lamptey, 2019). A pilot study on incorporating the topic of food safety in a classroom curriculum of a school for special education shows that children with a range of disabilities may improve their knowledge on food safety (e.g., hygiene, food storage, food preparation, and handling) (Madaus et al., 2010).

Results of studies published in the past 20 years show that interventions are effective in teaching a variety of safety skills to these individuals (see e.g., Wiseman et al., 2017). The learned safety skill does not always spontaneously generalize to other settings and persons, and therefore treatment approaches need to incorporate strategies for promoting generalization. Fisher (2014) pointed to the need of research in which the effects of incorporating in situ training in a treatment package is explored. In many studies, target skills are taught in a training setting and generalization of the skill is assessed in situ. A safe alternative option is the use of technology, such as virtual reality or virtual environments, in teaching safety skills. Josman, Ben-Chaim, Friedrich, and Weiss (2008) showed that six 12- to 13-year-old children with autism learned to cross a virtual street via a desktop street-crossing virtual environment. Three of the children showed some generalization of their pedestrian skills in an outside protected street sidewalk. In the study by Saiano et al. (2015) seven adult males (19–44 years old) with autism spectrum disorder and of whom three also had mild ID were taught to follow road signs and to cross streets with and without traffic lights in a virtual environment. The virtual environment represented a city (streets, buildings, etc.) which was continuously displayed on a wide screen and a motion capture device recorded participants' movements. Participants stood in front of the screen and a trainer provided reinforcement and corrective feedback, while participants completed different paths by following arrows and signs. Data were collected through questionnaires and the motion capture device. Results show that six participants improved their navigation performance although the number of errors in street crossing did not decrease. One participant was excluded because during familiarization with the apparatus it appeared that he had problems with depth perception. Data on questionnaires completed by parents and other caregivers indicated an improvement in the participants' street crossing skills suggesting generalization of skills to natural settings. More research should be conducted on the feasibility and effectiveness of interventions with virtual reality environments for teaching of safety skills in potentially dangerous situations.

A last area that deserves attention in future research is training of parents, teachers, and other caregivers in implementing teaching safety skills to persons with IDD (Harriage et al., 2016). An interesting topic is whether parents who have intellectual disability are able to teach their child home safety skills. Llewellyn, McConnell, Honey, Mayes, and Russo (2003) conducted a randomized controlled trial to evaluate the effectiveness of home-based training provided to 40 families, in which one or both parents had intellectual disability. They were parents of children younger than 5 years old. The intervention consisted of ten weekly 60–90 min sessions that were held in the family's home. During home visits, the trainer worked through a set of illustrated booklets with color, graphics, and simplified language added. Each session addressed one topic such as fire, electrical, and cooking dangers and relevant safety precautions. The aim of the intervention was to increase parents' knowledge on how to improve and maintain home safety and their child's health. Results show that this intervention improved the parents' ability to recognize home dangers, their understanding of health and symptoms of illness, and knowledge of how to manage emergencies, etc. Secondary analyses revealed that parents' IQ, health, and literacy skills did not influence the outcomes of the intervention.

References

Agran, M., Krupp, M., Spooner, F., & Zakas, T. (2012). Asking students about the importance of safety skills instruction: A preliminary analysis of what they think is important. *Research and Practice for Persons with Severe Disabilities, 37*, 45–52.

Akmanoglu, N., & Tekin-Iftar, E. (2011). Teaching children with autism how to respond to the lures of strangers. *Autism, 15*, 205–222.

Alevriadou, A. (2010). Promoting road safety for boys with mild intellectual disabilities: The effect of cognitive style and the role of attention in the identification of safe and dangerous road-crossing sites. *International Journal of Special Education, 25*, 127–135.

Bassette, L., Taber-Doughty, T., Gama, R., Alberto, P., Yakubova, G., & Cihak, D. (2018). The use of cell phones to address safety skills for students with a moderate ID in community-based settings. *Focus on Autism and Other Developmental Disabilities, 33*, 100–110.

Bicakci, M., & Gul, S. (2019). Effect of peer delivered social stories on the crossing skills of primary school students with developmental disabilities. *Education and Science, 44*, 257–278.

Brown, F., & Gillard, D. (2009). Learning road safety skills in the classroom. *British Journal of Learning Disabilities, 37*, 228–231.

Carlile, K., DeBar, R., Reeve, S., Reeve, K., & Meyer, L. (2018). Teaching help-seeking when lost to individuals with autism spectrum disorder. *Journal of Applied Behavior Analysis, 51*, 191–206.

Caton, S., & Chapman, M. (2016). The use of social media and people with intellectual disability: A systematic review and thematic analysis. *Journal of Intellectual and Developmental Disability, 41*, 125–139.

Clees, T., & Gast, D. (1994). Social safety skills instruction for individuals with disabilities: A sequential model. *Education and Treatment of Children, 17*, 163–185.

Dixon, D., Bergstrom, R., Smith, M., & Tarbox, J. (2010). A review of research on procedures for teaching safety skills to persons with developmental disabilities. *Research in Developmental Disabilities, 31*, 985–994.

Duker, P., Didden, R., & Sigafoos, J. (2004). *One-to-one training: Instructional procedures for learners with developmental disabilities*. Austin, TX: Pro-Ed.

Fisher, M. (2014). Evaluation of a stranger safety training programme for adults with Williams syndrome. *Journal of Intellectual Disability Research, 58*, 903–914.

Fisher, M., Burke, M., & Griffin, M. (2013). Teaching young adults with disabilities to respond appropriately to lures from strangers. *Journal of Applied Behavior Analysis, 46*, 528–533.

Giannakakos, A., Vladescu, J., Kisamore, A., Reeve, K., & Fienup, D. (2020). A review of the literature on safety response training. *Journal of Behavioral Education, 29*, 64–121.

Harriage, B., Cho Blair, K., & Miltenberger, R. (2016). An evaluation of a parent implemented in situ pedestrian safety skills intervention for individuals with autism. *Journal of Autism and Developmental Disorders, 46*, 2017–2027.

Josman, N., Ben-Chaim, H., Friedrich, S., & Weiss, P. (2008). Effectiveness of virtual reality for teaching street-crossing skills to children and adolescents with autism. *International Journal on Disability and Human Development, 7*, 49–56.

Kearney, K., Brady, M., Hall, K., & Honsberger, T. (2018). Using peer-mediated literacy-based behavioral interventions to increase first aid safety skills in students with developmental disabilities. *Behavior Modification, 42*, 639–660.

Kearny, K., Dukes, C., Brady, M., Pistorio, K., Duffy, M., & Bucholz, J. (2019). Using an instructional package to teach cardiopulmonary resuscitation with automated external defibrillator to college students with intellectual disability. *Journal of Special Education, 53*, 142–152.

Lee, N., Vladescu, J., Reeve, K., Peterson, K., & Giannakakos, A. (2019). Effects of behavioral skills training on the stimulus control of gun safety responding. *Journal of Behavioral Education, 28*, 187–203.

Lindsay, S., & Lamptey, D. (2019). Pedestrian navigation and public transit training interventions for youth with disabilities: A systematic review. *Disability and Rehabilitation, 41*, 2607–2621.

Llewellyn, G., McConnell, D., Honey, A., Mayes, R., & Russo, D. (2003). Promoting health and home safety for children of parents with intellectual disability: A randomized controlled trial. *Research in Developmental Disabilities, 24*, 405–431.

Madaus, J., Pivarnik, L., Patnoad, M., Scarpati, S., Richard, N., Wright Hirsch, D., ... Gable, R. (2010). Teaching food safety skills to students with disabilities. *Teaching Exceptional Children, 42*, 44–51.

Matson, J. (1980). A controlled group study of pedestrian-skill training for the mentally retarded. *Behaviour, Research and Therapy, 18*, 99–106.

Mechling, L., Gast, D., & Gustafson, M. (2009). Use of video modeling to teach extinguishing of cooking related fires to individuals with moderate intellectual disabilities. *Education and Training in Developmental Disabilities, 44*, 67–79.

Purrazzella, K., & Mechling, L. (2013). Use of an iPhone 4 with video features to assist location of students with moderate intellectual disability when lost in community settings. *Education and Training in Autism and Developmental Disabilities, 48*, 179–189.

Saiano, M., Pellegrino, L., Casadio, M., Summa, S., Garbarino, E., Rossi, V., ... Sanguineti, V. (2015). Natural interfaces and virtual environments for the acquisition of street crossing and path following skills in adults with autism spectrum disorders: A feasibility study. *Journal of Neuroengineering and Rehabilitation, 12*, 17.

Sanchez, S., & Miltenberger, R. (2015). Evaluating the effectiveness of an abduction prevention program for young adults with intellectual disabilities. *Child and Family Behavior Therapy, 37*, 197–207.

Sirin, N., & Tekin-Iftar, E. (2016). Opinions of Turkish parents and teachers about safety skills instruction to children with autism spectrum disorders: A preliminary investigation. *Journal of Autism and Developmental Disorders, 46*, 2653–2665.

Spivey, C., & Mechling, L. (2016). Video modeling to teach social safety skills to young adults with intellectual disability. *Education and Training in Autism and Developmental Disabilities, 51*, 79–92.

Stannis, R., Crosland, K., Miltenberger, R., & Valbuena, D. (2019). Response to bullying (RTB): Behavioral skills and in situ training for individuals diagnosed with intellectual disabilities. *Journal of Applied Behavior Analysis, 52*, 73–83.

Strauss, D., Shavelle, R., Anderson, T., & Baumeister, A. (1998). External causes of death among persons with developmental disability. *American Journal of Epidemiology, 147*, 855–862.

Taber, T., Alberto, P., Hughes, M., & Seltzer, A. (2002). A strategy for students with moderate disabilities when lost in the community. *Research and Practice for Persons with Severe Disabilities, 27*, 141–152.

Wiseman, K., McArdell, L., Bottini, S., & Gillis, J. (2017). A meta-analysis of safety skill interventions for children, adolescents, and young adults with autism spectrum disorder. *Review Journal of Developmental Disorders, 4*, 39–49.

Wright, T., & Wolery, M. (2011). The effects of instructional interventions related to street crossing and individuals with disabilities. *Research in Developmental Disabilities, 32*, 1455–1463.

Chapter 8
Training Parents and Staff to Implement Interventions to Improve the Adaptive Behavior of Their Children with Intellectual and Developmental Disability

Sarah G. Hansen, Jessica DeMarco, and Hannah Etchison

Training of natural change agents such as parents, teachers, and staff to improve socially important behavior is an evidence-based practice for individuals with intellectual and developmental disabilities (IDD; Wong et al., 2015; Gerow, Rispoli, Ninci, Gregori, & Hagan-Burke, 2018). For children, adolescents, and adults with IDD, parents, teachers, staff, and peers are key natural change agents who, if trained with fidelity, can significantly improve outcomes. A growing library of literature indicates the benefit of capitalizing on naturally available interventionists to improve the social validity, generalizability, and maintenance of behavior change for communication, social skills, reduction of challenging behavior, and others (Gunning et al., 2019; Machalicek, Lang, & Raulston, 2015; Tarbox, Garcia, & Clair, 2016). All skills seem to benefit from intervention implemented by individuals readily available in the natural environment. Due to their applied nature, however, adaptive skills in particular may benefit from training of natural change agents in order to increase opportunities and decrease barriers to generalization.

Adaptive skills are practical, everyday skills that for most individuals are learned in the context of the everyday environment by interacting with caregivers and experiencing typical antecedents and consequences. For example, learning to get dressed independently gives a young child more immediate access to playing with friends, learning to operate the stove gives an individual more immediate access to a meal. Although typical childhood development may involve some difficulty with particular adaptive skills (e.g., potty training; Schum et al., 2002) requiring specific intervention, most individuals develop a socially appropriate repertoire of self-help and vocational skills by early adulthood. For individuals with IDD, however, these skills may require specific, targeted, and intensive intervention (Matson, Rivet, Fodstad,

S. G. Hansen (✉) · J. DeMarco · H. Etchison
Georgia State University, Atlanta, GA, USA
e-mail: shansen@gsu.edu

R. Lang, P. Sturmey (eds.), *Adaptive Behavior Strategies for Individuals with Intellectual and Developmental Disabilities*, Autism and Child Psychopathology Series, https://doi.org/10.1007/978-3-030-66441-1_8

Dempsey, & Boisjoli, 2009; Thompson et al., 2009). Adaptive skills are some of the most predictive skills for success in adulthood (Anderson, Liang, & Lord, 2014), and yet intervention methods are relatively under-researched in comparison to communication or academic domains (Flynn & Healy, 2012; Palmen, Didden, & Lang, 2012). Fortunately, many evidence-based practices for skill acquisition in individuals with IDD are also effective to teach adaptive and vocational skills (Hume, Loftin, & Lantz, 2009; Matson, Hattier, & Belva, 2012).

In addition to the potential barriers to independence and inclusion, deficits in adaptive skills can also impact other people in their immediate environment. Surveys of parent stress, for example, often point to problems in early adaptive skills as key stressors for parents of children with disabilities (Krakovich, McGrew, Yu, & Ruble, 2016; Norton, Dyches, Harper, Roper, & Caldarella, 2016). In an intervention aimed at reducing parenting stress for parents of adolescents and adults with developmental disabilities, parents reported a primary source of stress to be their continued involvement in daily living concerns of their adolescent and adult children, such as toileting, basic hygiene, and other life skills (Lunsky, Robinson, Reid, & Palucka, 2015). Surveys of staff directly mirror these findings, with staff reporting predictors of burnout and workplace stress to include high amounts of physical care demands (Outar & Rose, 2017).

Despite established evidence-based practices for teaching adaptive skills, much of the available literature on adaptive skills feature a trained interventionist in a clinical or simulated setting (Fahmie & Luczynski, 2018; Hong et al., 2016). Although these environments might initially be helpful for training skills needing direct and intensive instruction, pre-existing barriers to generalization and maintenance of skills may mean that skills taught in isolation do not sufficiently generalize to improve overall quality of life. Individuals with IDD may require explicit technology of generalization to be able to apply them to the environments in which they are typically used. Recent reviews of teaching adaptive skills have illustrated failure of the literature to successfully account for generalization and maintenance, including the training of stakeholders in the environment (Neely et al., 2016). In a meta-analysis on generalization and maintenance of functional living skills for individuals with autism, Neely and colleagues found large differential effects for studies that planned for generalization by training in the natural environment or training with multiple exemplars (Neely et al., 2016). It is clear that by teaching in the natural environment under typically occurring contingencies, outcomes of interventions can be improved. Training parents and staff to implement intervention is one way to ensure more successful teaching in the natural environment.

For young children with IDD, parents and other caregivers are the most natural choices to teach children adaptive behaviors. Parent-mediated studies have been shown as effective for teaching skills and reducing challenging behavior (Fettig, Schultz, & Sreckovic, 2016; Kasari, Gulsrud, Paparella, Hellemann, & Berry, 2015). Parent-mediated intervention is considered an evidence-based practice for intervention in autism spectrum disorders (ASD) and developmental disabilities (Wong et al., 2015). Especially for early developing adaptive skills (e.g., toileting, sleep, basic hygiene), parents are typically available to teach the skill in the natural environment in a way that service providers are not. Systematic reviews of the literature have indicated that parents, when trained appropriately, can provide effective intervention to maintain and generalize findings across skills. Despite the evident utility of training parents, previous systematic reviews on adaptive skills have found low rates of parent-mediated intervention, and typically parents are included as an additional trainer and not the sole trainer (Kroeger & Sorensen-Burnworth, 2009). There is a need to evaluate best practices for training parents to support children with IDD to develop adaptive skills.

As children grow and develop, their dependence on parents decreases over time. Although this separation from family support may be delayed in children with IDD, individuals with IDD can access greater independence, but may require supports which typically come from staff working in specialized settings or programs such as paraprofessionals in the classroom, job support professionals, residential support staff, and other daily living support (e.g., respite care). Although there is a critical need for these professionals, these individuals are often working in high demand settings without sufficient training or supports. Untrained staff can be barriers to skill acquisition. Across all skill domains, there is little information available about how best to train staff to meet the needs of individuals with IDD and this is reported by staff as a key barrier to high quality care for their clients (Genik, McMurtry, & Breau, 2017).

It is evident that across the lifespan of individuals with IDD, there is a benefit to training natural change agents to implement evidence-based practices, and that there may be particular benefit to empowering parents and staff to teach adaptive skills in order to program for generalization and maintenance of these skills. In addition to the evident importance of training parents and staff to support adaptive skills in individuals with IDD, recent research in special education and behavior analysis has pointed to new, more efficient and effective ways of training natural change agents. These novel training methodologies are designed to improve access to, fidelity, and maintenance of skills needed by parents and staff to improve independence in individuals with IDD. Therefore, this chapter will provide: (a) a review of the current available literature on training parents and staff to teach adaptive skills, including which skills were targeted, who implemented trainings, and how training was delivered; (b) discussion of commonly implemented training methods, including example cases, useable data sheets, and procedural fidelity checklists; and (c) discussion of limitations of the available literature and ideas for future research and practice.

8.1 Literature Review

Previous literature reviews in the area of adaptive skills and individuals with IDD have focused on individual skills, such as toileting (Francis, Mannion, & Leader, 2017), feeding (Hamre, Dorrance, & Ausderau, 2017), cooking and food skills (McGowan et al., 2017), and vocational skills (Seaman & Cannella-Malone, 2016).

Other reviews have focused on intervention method, such as video modeling (Hong et al., 2016) and technological prompting (e.g., alerts on a phone or tablet; Cullen & Alber-Morgan, 2015). We also identified several general reviews of the literature on adaptive skills (Burns, Lemon, Granpeesheh, & Dixon, 2019; Neely et al., 2016). To our knowledge, however, there was no review found with a specific focus on the training of parents and staff to implement adaptive skill interventions with developmental disabilities across the lifespan. In order to inform the practices presented here, we have conducted a brief review of the literature on parent and staff training to support adaptive skills across the lifespan in order to determine: (a) the frequency of parent involvement; (b) the frequency of staff involvement; (c) the quality of the effects of parent and staff training in the available literature; (d) the scope of skills taught via parent and staff mediated interventions; and (e) the types of training used to train parents and staff.

8.1.1 Method

Searches were conducted in two academic databases. Academic search premier and Educational Recourses Information Center (ERIC) were searched using the following search terms: "(Adaptive skills or life skills or vocational or daily living or hygiene or self-help) AND (intellectual disability or autism or developmental disability or mental retardation) AND (parent training or staff training or performance feedback or supervision or coaching)". Following these initial searches, historical searches were conducted by: (a) reviewing the reference pages of the included studies and (b) searching through literature reviews on commonly occurring topics for parent-implemented studies.

8.1.1.1 Inclusion and Exclusion Criteria

From the results of this search, studies were retained that: (a) included an individual with an intellectual or developmental disability; (b) training on an adaptive skill; (c) reported the results of an intervention that also included parent or staff training; and (d) published in a peer reviewed journal between the years of 2009 and 2019. Both group and single case research designs were retained. Studies in grey literature (e.g., dissertations, magazine articles) were not retained. Qualitative studies and surveys of parent and staff perceptions were retained to inform other portions of this chapter, but were not included in the results reported here. Table 8.1 presents the results of the search, including author, year, intervention, skill, agent, and effectiveness.

8.2 Results

Fifteen studies were returned following these searches of databases, including ten single case studies, four quasi-experimental designs, and one non-experimental study. Three of the included studies were found using historical search procedures. Of these studies, 11 (73%) focused on the results of parent training. Within the parent training studies, six studies focused on training of parents to implement procedures related to feeding (i.e., food refusal, variability of food choices, mealtime skills; Johnson et al., 2015; Muldoon & Cosbey, 2018; Murphy & Zlomke, 2016; Najdowski et al., 2010; Seiverling et al., 2012; Tarbox et al., 2010), one study taught parents to intervene on self-care and hygiene skills (Cavkaytar & Pollard, 2009), one taught adherence to routines (i.e., Gerencser et al., 2018), and three taught toileting (Drysdale et al., 2015; Ozcan & Cavkaytar, 2009; Rinald & Mirenda, 2012). The remaining four studies (26%) trained staff or classroom paraprofessionals to implement procedures. Of the staff implemented studies, one trained staff to implement toilet training procedures (Cocchiola et al., 2012), one taught exercise skills (Henwood et al., 2013), one taught routines (Palmen, Didden, & Lang, 2012; Palmen, Didden, & Verhoeven, 2012), and one taught healthcare procedures (Garst et al., 2019). Twelve of the 15 studies (80%) showed at least a moderate effect, with two studies only demonstrating a weak effect, and two studies demonstrating strong effects.

8.2.1 *Participants*

There was a total of 130 participants with IDD across the 15 included studies. The age range of participants in the included studies was 2–90 years. Despite the importance of adaptive skills across the lifespan of individuals with IDD, most research was done in the early childhood age range (80% [12] of studies featured children under the age of 8 years), with relatively few studies found in adolescence or adulthood (three studies, 20%). Additionally, 80% of studies (12 studies) featured an individual with intellectual disability, two studies featured participants with developmental disabilities but no intellectual disability noted, and one study did not report the disability of the individual. Only six (43%) interventionists across studies had any demographic factors reported. Of trainer participants, 64% were parents, and 21% were staff; 16% of participants were neither parent nor staff. Parent participants were made up of 77% mothers and 23% fathers. Staff participants were 14% respite workers or residential care workers, and 7% paraprofessionals or personal aides. No job coaches or independent living support workers were interventionists in the included studies.

Table 8.1 A summary of parent training studies reviewed in this chapter

	Methodology	Participants		Skill	Training	Agent	
	Design	*N*	Ages				Treatment effectiveness
Cavkaytar and Pollard (2009)	Multiple probe	3	3–7	Self-care/ hygiene	Parent-therapist collaboration	Parent	Moderate
Cocchiola, Martino, Dwyer, and Demezzo (2012)	Concurrent multiple-baseline	5	3–5	Toilet training	Not reported	paraprofessional	Moderate
Drysdale et al. (2015)	Concurrent multiple-baseline	2	4–5	Toilet training	Not reported	Parent	Weak
Garst, Gagnon, and Brawley (2019)	Quasi-experimental	55	18–24	Healthcare	Online Training	Staff	Weak
Gerencser, Higbee, Akers, and Contreras (2018)	Non-concurrent multiple baseline	3	3–4	Routines	interactive computerized training (ICT)	Parent	Moderate
Henwood, Wooding, and De Souza (2013)	Quasi-experimental	23	63–90	Exercise	Exercise program	Staff	Moderate
Johnson, Foldes, DeMand, and Brooks (2015)	Quasi-experimental	14	2–7	Feeding	Workshop	Parent	Strong

Muldoon and Cosbey (2018)	Quasi-experimental	4	3–5	Feeding	Parent training	Parent	Strong
Murphy and Zlomke (2016)	Non-experimental	1	6	Feeding	Parent training	Parent	Weak
Najdowski et al. (2010)	Concurrent multiple-baseline	3	2–4	Feeding	Not reported	Parent	Moderate
Ozcan and Cavkaytar (2009)	Multiple probe	3	3–6	Toilet training	Parent training	Parent	Strong
Palmen, Didden, and Verhoeven (2012)	Multiple baseline	4	14–23	Routines	Performance feedback	Staff	Strong
Rinald and Mirenda (2012)	Multiple baseline	6	3–5	Toilet training	Parent training	Parents	Strong
Seiverling et al. (2012)	Multiple-baseline	3	4–8	Feeding	Parent training	Parent	Moderate
Tarbox, Schiff, and Najdowski (2010)	Multiple baseline	1	3	Feeding	Parent training	Parent	Moderate

8.2.2 Skills

The largest percentage of both parent and staff training studies focused on feeding (6 studies,40% of studies; Johnson et al., 2015; Muldoon & Cosbey, 2018; Murphy & Zlomke, 2016; Najdowski et al., 2010; Seiverling et al., 2012; Tarbox et al., 2010). Four studies taught toileting skills (27%; Cocchiola et al., 2012; Drysdale et al., 2015; Rinald & Mirenda, 2012), two taught adherence to routines (13%; Gerencser et al., 2018; Palmen, Didden, & Lang, 2012; Palmen, Didden, & Verhoeven, 2012), one taught hygiene (7%; Cavkaytar & Pollard, 2009), one study taught exercise skills (7%; Henwood et al., 2013), and one study taught health skills (7%; Garst et al., 2019). Notably absent in skills covered in this review were household chores, direct vocational skills, safety skills, and skills related to adolescence and sexuality.

8.2.3 Setting

The largest percentage of the included studies took place in the home (nine studies, 60%; Murphy & Zlomke, 2016; Najdowski et al., 2010; Ozcan & Cavkaytar, 2009; Seiverling et al., 2012; Tarbox et al., 2010). Outside the home, the most frequent setting was a clinic (i.e., a clinic, day treatment center, or rehab center; Henwood et al., 2013; Johnson et al., 2015; Muldoon & Cosbey, 2018; Palmen, Didden, & Lang, 2012; Palmen, Didden, & Verhoeven, 2012), which made up 27% of the included studies (four studies). There was also a study in a school bathroom (Cocchiola et al., 2012, 7% of studies), and a daycare (Henwood et al., 2013, 7% of studies).

8.2.4 Training Method

A range of different training methodologies was used. The most frequent training methodology used was behavioral parent training or modified behavioral parent training (sometimes labeled behavior skills training [BST] for parents), which was used in 40% of included studies (Najdowski et al., 2010; Ozcan & Cavkaytar, 2009; Seiverling et al., 2012; Murphy & Zlomke, 2016; Johnson et al., 2015; Tarbox et al., 2010). Online training was used in two studies (Garst et al., 2019; Gerencser et al., 2018; 13% of studies). A group workshop was used in one of the studies (Rinald & Mirenda, 2012, 7% of studies), a train the trainer approach was used in one study (Muldoon & Cosbey, 2018, 7% of studies), and one study (Cocchiola et al., 2012, 7% of studies) did not report their training methodology.

8.3 Practitioners' Recommendations

The rest of this chapter will discuss effective training practices appropriate for parent and staff training. For each training method, we will provide a brief vignette, overview the training process, and rationale for its effectiveness. Additionally, we will provide a data sheet or hypothetical data and conclude the scenario.

8.3.1 Behavior Skills Training

James is a paraprofessional working with students in a self-contained classroom for individuals with multiple and severe disabilities. The teacher in the classroom where James is working, Henry, wants James to learn a forward chaining procedure so he is able to improve hygiene skills in the students in his care. Henry has given James written materials on teaching hygiene skills, but James has not been successful in improving hygiene skills. Henry uses the steps of BST to teach James how to implement the procedure with fidelity.

BST is a method of skills training with a robust body of literature supporting its effectiveness (Sarokoff & Sturmey, 2004; Rosales, Stone, & Rehfeldt, 2009; Nigro-Bruzzi & Sturmey, 2010). Typically, BST includes skill rehearsal with feedback and prompting (Parsons, Rollyson, & Reid, 2012) and is aimed at training personnel to implement behavior change procedures (Parsons et al., 2012). BST is made up of eight key steps: (a) Provide and explain rationale for the target skill being trained; (b) describe steps of the target skill; (c) provide a written artifact of the skill steps; (d) model the skill; (e) rehearse the target skill with the trainee; (f) take data on correct steps of the trainee; (g) provide corrective feedback; and (h) repeat steps (f)–(h) until the trainee demonstrates mastery to a given criteria (Nigro-Bruzzi & Sturmey, 2010; Parsons, Rollyson, & Reid, 2012).

BST has been successfully used to teach child safety skills (Holcombe, Wolery, & Katzenmeyer, 1995; Pan-Skadden et al., 2009), professional-implemented teaching strategies (Nigro-Bruzzi & Sturmey, 2010; Rosales et al., 2009), parent-implemented feeding techniques (Mueller et al., 2003; Seiverling, et al., 2012), and child compliance strategies (Miles & Wilder, 2009). It is a technique that has been demonstrated to be effective across trainees and target skill. BST may be particularly useful for transfer of skill to novice stakeholders working directly with individuals with IDD, because it allows for sufficient practice and opportunity for feedback (Parsons et al., 2012). Figure 8.1 shows the steps that Henry will take to train James on the chaining procedure.

James is able to implement the forwards chaining procedure with fidelity, improving the hygiene skills of the students he works with. James maintains treatment fidelity over time, and is able to apply the principles he learned to other skills. James' ability to consistently implement procedures over time leads to increased student maintenance of hygiene skills.

Component	*Definition*	*Example*
Rationale for skill taught	Trainer defines skill being taught, why it is important, and why the learner needs to know how to use it.	Henry explains to James why improving hygiene skills is important for his students, and why forward chaining is an effective way to teach it.
Steps described	Trainer outlines steps of the skill.	Henry explains the steps of teaching via forward chaining.
Written artifact included	Trainer provides task analysis with steps of implementation.	Henry gives James a laminated checklist for the teaching procedure.
Skill modeled	Trainer models correct use of the skill.	Henry models the teaching procedure for James.
Skill rehearsed	Trainer and trainee practice the skill together with feedback from the trainer.	James practices the skill with Henry and role-plays. Henry gives James feedback on his implementation of the teaching procedure.
Data collected	Trainer observes trainee implement skill and takes data.	Henry watches James use the forwards chaining procedure with his student. Henry takes data on the steps James completes correctly.
Feedback provided	Trainer provides corrective feedback and praise as needed.	Henry provides James with feedback on any missed steps in the procedure. He also praises James for the steps he completed correctly.
Skill practiced with feedback	Trainer continues to provide feedback and rehearse with trainee as necessary until appropriate level of fidelity is reached.	Henry continues to observe James using the forward chaining procedure in class until his data shows that James can consistently use the procedure with fidelity.

Fig. 8.1 Steps of behavior skills training as applied in an adaptive skill teaching setting

8.3.2 Behavioral Parent Training

Sandy is working with Angie and her son Bobby. Angie has stated that Bobby, who has ASD and moderate intellectual disability, is not toilet trained at age four and she is concerned because she wants him to attend preschool in the fall. Sandy has worked with the family to improve Bobby's toileting skills, but when Sandy does not regularly visit their home Bobby begins having frequent accidents or refusing to use the toilet. Angie gets discouraged and goes back to use of diapers with Bobby. Sandy is looking for a way to teach Angie how to maintain the progress they have made working with Bobby on her own. Sandy decides to use behavioral parent training to teach Angie skills that will help her maintain Bobby's progress with toileting.

Behavioral parent training or parent mediated intervention is a systematic and evidence-based method of training parents to implement interventions aimed at improving skills and reducing challenging behavior in their children (Feldmen & Werner, 2002; Wainer & Ingersoll, 2015). Evidence shows that parents are able to both learn and implement evidence-based interventions with their children (Dunlap, Ester, Langhans, & Fox, 2006; Kashinath et al., 2006) and can improve generalization and maintenance of intervention effects. Benefits to this practice include use of the child's natural setting (Dunlap et al., 2006; Dunst, Hamby, Trivette, Raab, & Bruder, 2000; McCollum & Hemmeter, 1997; Sandall, Hemmeter, Smith, & McLean, 2005) and increased frequency of training sessions (McWilliam, 2000).

Components of behavioral parent training typically mirror BST, including didactic instruction on key principles of interventions, some level of direct coaching and/or performance feedback, and supports for maintenance of skills in absence of trainer. Behavioral parent training methods differ in terms of intensity and delivery method depending on the needs of the parents and the time availability of the trainer. The following components are important for evidence-based behavioral parent training: (a) Content training; (b) role play and modeling; (c) practice with child with input from trainer; (d) coaching that includes error correction procedures and praise; and (e) insurance of a minimum level of fidelity prior to ending coaching sessions. Figure 8.2 shows a task fidelity checklist that Sandra and Angie can use.

Sandra creates parent friendly materials for Angie to review about the toilet training methodology they selected together. Then, Sandra practiced the steps of the intervention together and rehearsed key strategies such as prompting hierarchies and use of a token economy. Sandra coaches Angie using behavioral parent training coaching practices that include error correction, least to most prompting of Angie's skills and praise. Angie reports better understanding of the content and more confidence implementing the procedures. The next time Sandra checks in with Angie, she finds that Bobby has reduced levels of toileting accidents and is consistently using the toilet independently with support from Angie.

8.3.3 Performance Feedback

Julie runs a job coaching program for adults with IDD. She has a new job coach, Emma, who has been trained but is just starting to work independently in the field. Julie uses a combination of text-message based and in-vivo *performance feedback to ensure that Emma is continuing to have good treatment fidelity as she works on job skills with her clients.*

In the special educator training context, performance feedback refers to the ongoing communication between an educator (such as a paraprofessional or teacher) and a supervisor or other person who has delivered training in educational or

Fidelity Checklist
Toileting Intervention

I discussed importance of toilet training with parent	**Y**	**N**
I taught parent about prompting	**Y**	**N**
I taught parent about token economies	**Y**	**N**
I checked to be sure parent understands procedures	**Y**	**N**
I modeled the steps of the toileting intervention for the parent	**Y**	**N**
I watched the parent rehearse with their child and provided feedback	**Y**	**N**
I used least to most prompting with the parent when needed	**Y**	**N**
I completed error correction procedure with parent if they errored	**Y**	**N**
I gave positive praise throughout	**Y**	**N**

Fig. 8.2 Task fidelity checklist for parent training on toileting

behavioral strategies to the educator. Studies have shown that performance feedback leads to greater gains in the educator's ability to teach the strategies to students and their long-term maintenance of the teaching skills. For example, Leblanc, Ricciardi, and Luiselli (2005) showed that training in Discrete Trial Intervention delivered to paraprofessionals serving children with ASD had greater efficacy when paired with abbreviated performance feedback (8–10 minute feedback sessions with the supervisor-trainer). Performance feedback is related to longer maintenance of skill use (Brock et al., 2016).

Implementation of performance feedback can also be implemented using technology. Studies where supervisors use text messages or emails to provide immediate and distilled feedback to teachers and paraprofessionals working in the field (Barton, Rigor, Pokorski, Velez, & Domingo, 2018; Oborn & Johnson, 2015). Further research is needed on the student outcomes of staff-delivered teaching strategies which employ performance feedback to improve staff effectiveness. However, the results of existing research suggest this approach improves fidelity in the delivery of evidence-based strategies. Figure 8.3 shows hypothetical data on Emma's task fidelity, while teaching job skills to individuals with disabilities.

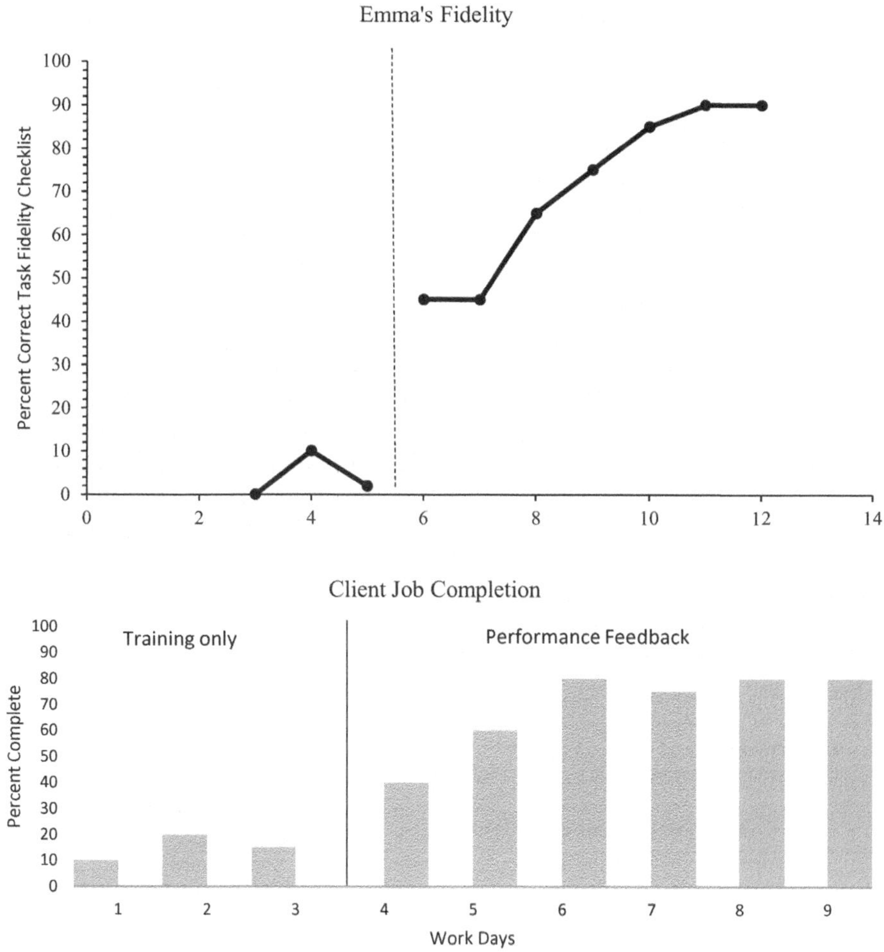

Fig. 8.3 Top tier shows Emma's increase in fidelity following performance feedback from manager. Bottom tier shows example related increase in client job completion

Emma's fidelity increases through receiving immediate performance feedback via *text message from her supervisor Julie. Emma sometimes sends Julie videos of her training procedures for feedback. Emma's clients show better rates of independent task completion over time.*

8.3.4 Digital or Telehealth Training of Parents or Staff

Max is an early intervention provider in a rural area. Max has a few clients working on feeding and food refusal. Max needs to train parents to complete a gradual extinction intervention in their young children with developmental disabilities. Max does not have

the capacity to see the families in his care frequently enough to teach them the procedure only during visits. Max needs a way to have more frequent contact with these families in order to support them in acquiring the skills they need to help their children.

Telehealth refers to the provision of healthcare or therapy by means of telecommunication. This includes text, visuals, video, audio, and multimedia information broadcast from a distance. In most contexts, the practice utilizes internet capabilities, although telephone and other communication means are acceptable options. For the parents of young children with disabilities, telehealth may offer treatment options that were previously difficult or impossible to access (Higgens et al., 2017; Wacker et al., 2013). Several studies have shown the efficacy of these telehealth programs on various issues impacting young children with disabilities, including behavioral and educational concerns (Neely et al. 2017; Tomlinson, Gore, & McGill, 2018).

Telehealth is not limited to clinics with video conferencing capabilities, however. Some telehealth interventions have utilized web-based, self-guided tutorials on delivering therapy to children with disabilities, or to train staff on teaching procedures (Garst et al., 2019). Digitally delivered training practices have promise to address barriers to service delivery and improve access to evidence-based practices for those in rural or otherwise removed settings (Traube, Hsiao, Rau, & Hunt-O'Brien, 2019). Web-based modules have also gathered momentum as potential parent training methodology, and have been moderately effective at increasing parent knowledge (McGoron et al., 2018). Figure 8.4 shows a task fidelity checklist Max can use to coach parents over telehealth.

Instructions:
For observed behavior(s) code a "+". If a behavior is not observe code a "-".

Fidelity for Coaching Sessions			
	Observed	Not observed	N/A
**DON'T FORGET TO RECORD YOUR SESSION **			
1. I began the videoconference meeting with a "warm" greeting and introduction.			
2. I reviewed teaching procedures of the session.			
3. I asked the parent if they have any questions before they get started.			
4. I offered to role play with the parent.			
5. I provided descriptive feedback after parent error. If the parent identified the error correctly, the I provided descriptive praise for the error identification.			
6. If the parent did not identify the error, I provided explanation of the error and/or modeling of the skill if necessary.			
7. I provided immediate descriptive praise for the targeted behavior.			
8. I talked to the parent after the session to answer any additional questions or provide additional feedback if needed.			
9. I thanked the parent and reviewed next steps if needed.			
Total fidelity = Observed/Observed + Not observed x 100			

Fig. 8.4 Self-monitoring checklist for telehealth session with parent

Max sets families up with secure software and is able to teleconference more frequently. More frequent connection with the parents on his caseload makes it easier for Max to use a parent training package to improve parent fidelity on the feeding intervention he has selected to address food refusal. Parents report better luck with feeding protocols now that they have a mechanism for consistent support and feedback from professionals.

8.4 Summary and Future Directions

This chapter has introduced key issues in the training of parents and staff to implement interventions to address adaptive skills for individuals with IDD. We have also illustrated different methods and aspects of training parents and staff with examples and hypothetical outcomes. Altogether, this chapter shows the value of teaching natural change agents to intervene on adaptive skills. A systematic review of the literature indicated only modest amounts of parent or staff training studies despite the growing body of literature on adaptive skills (Palmen, Didden, & Lang, 2012). Despite systematic reviews in other areas of intervention showing a hearteningly robust body of research involving parents and staff in intervention (Wong et al., 2015), adaptive skills are less prevalent in the literature, and even more so with parent and staff interventionists.

Within the available literature, there is a need to further examine the best practices for training parents and staff to intervene on these skills. In the small body of literature on parenting training for adaptive skills, parent training skills were largely concerned with feeding, and tapered off early in the child's lifespan. The typical parent training study in this review featured a feeding intervention for a young child by a parent taught using BST or modified BST. Staff training had very little representation outside of residential settings or rehabilitation clinics, including little available literature on paraprofessional training for these skills. Para-professionals often are charged with supporting their students across all areas of their school day, and would benefit from explicit instruction on teaching adaptive skills. A recent review of teacher use of paraprofessional training materials indicated teachers were often unsure what materials to select and how to train paraprofessionals in general (Douglas, Uitto, & Reinfelds, 2019). Training for teachers on how to train paraprofessionals using a pyramidal model (i.e., train the trainer) would be of benefit.

Although a variety of training methodologies were used in the studies included in this review, most studies employed a parent-centered BST package. For the few staff studies, most studies used BST or a coaching intervention either standalone or in combination with other forms of training. The largest group of studies was on feeding skills followed by toileting, hygiene, and routines. Noticeably missing from studies training parents and staff were safety skills, vocational skills, and sexual education. Studies focused on these topics were constrained to researcher mediated and clinical formats.

Parents were seldom agents in studies with children over the age of eight, and conversely staff training studies were almost completely restricted to adolescents or adults. Additionally, studies with children over eight for the most part did not take place in community settings, but rather in home or clinical settings. Because older individuals with IDD are more likely than young children to be placed outside the home (Friedman, 2014), there is a need to train staff in elementary educational settings, or community based vocational or educational programs. Further, while some individuals with IDD may be living independently with supports, many live at home with their parents through late adolescence and adulthood, meaning that parents and families are in need of supports for continuing to teach life skills as children age.

One example of this is education related to sexuality and adolescence. While this is an emerging area of research (Bornman & Rathbone, 2016; Harflett & Turner, 2016), there is little guidance given to parents as to how to best prepare their children with IDD for typical adolescent concerns. In a qualitative study of parents of children with ASD between the ages of 6–13, researchers found that parents were deeply concerned about potential risk related to sexuality for their children with ASD, including engaging in inappropriate sexual behavior and being in risky sexual relationships (Ballan, 2012). Parents are often uniquely able to teach adolescents with IDD about sensitive subjects, where school staff may not provide sufficient information or be able to identify individual risk factors. Future research should continue to expand parent training in these areas.

In addition to the need to consider parent and staff training throughout the lifespan of individuals with IDD, further research is needed on specific parent and staff training practices for adaptive behavior. We suggest that BST, behavioral parent training, performance feedback, and telehealth training may all be viable ways to improve the capacity of parents and staff to teach adaptive skills. Although these are all training methods with fairly robust evidence bases in other areas, it should be noted that the results of our review did not indicate most of these strategies had been studied in detail for this set of skills and this population. Future research should work to increase capacity of trainers of parents and staff through use of effective training methods.

The results of the included studies are largely promising, but there was little follow-up data collected, leaving little insight as to whether these effects sustained over time and across settings. Technology that will continue to maintain the fidelity of the intervention (e.g., self-monitoring, performance feedback) and is flexible enough for extremely applied settings (e.g., technology-based prompting, telehealth) will help to improve available interventions for parents and staff to support the adaptive skills of individuals with IDD. Promising technology can also reduce cost of interventions by reducing travel, increasing maintenance of skills, and supporting generalization of parent and staff skills to new child skills. Future research and practice should continue to search out innovative technology to reduce cost and improve sustainability of interventions.

8.5 Conclusion

This chapter discussed issues related to parent and staff training to improve adaptive skills. We presented the results of a brief review of the literature, including participant demographics, settings, trainings used, intervention targets, and effectiveness of the intervention. Next, this chapter provided several vignettes of likely problems encountered by individuals attempting to improve parent and staff capacity to improve adaptive skills in individuals with IDD. We suggested a training methodology to address the problem identified, and present artifacts that can be modified to be used by practitioners with similar dilemmas. Finally, this chapter identified areas for future grown in research and practice. Reference.

References

Anderson, D. K., Liang, J. W., & Lord, C. (2014). Predicting young adult outcome among more and less cognitively able individuals with autism spectrum disorders. *Journal of Child Psychology and Psychiatry, 55*(5), 485–494.

Ballan, M. S. (2012). Parental perspectives of communication about sexuality in families of children with autism spectrum disorders. *Journal of autism and developmental disorders, 42*(5), 676–684.

Bornman, J., & Rathbone, L. (2016). A sexuality and relationship training program for women with intellectual disabilities: A social story approach. *Sexuality and Disability, 34*(3), 269–288.

Bozkurt, F., & Gursel, O. (2005). Effectiveness of constant time delay on teaching snack and drink preparation skills to children with mental retardation. *Education and Training in Developmental Disabilities, 40*(4), 390–400.

Brock, M. E., Cannella-Malone, H. I., Schaefer, J. M., Justin Page, E., Andzik, N. R., & Seaman, R. L. (2016). Efficacy of training job coaches to implement evidence-based instructional strategies. *Journal of Vocational Rehabilitation, 45*(3), 351–364.

Burns, C. O., Lemon, J., Granpeesheh, D., & Dixon, D. R. (2019). Interventions for daily living skills in individuals with intellectual disability: A 50-year systematic review. *Advances in Neurodevelopmental Disorders*, 201*(3)* 1–11.

Cavkaytar, A., & Pollard, E. (2009). Effectiveness of parent and therapist collaboration program (PTCP) for teaching self-care and domestic skills to individuals with autism. *Education and Training in Developmental Disabilities, 44*(3), 381–395.

Cocchiola, M. A., Martino, G. M., Dwyer, L. J., & Demezzo, K. (2012). Toilet training children with autism and developmental delays: An effective program for school settings. *Behavior Analysis in Practice, 5*(2), 60–64.

Cullen, J. M., & Alber-Morgan, S. R. (2015). Technology mediated self-prompting of daily living skills for adolescents and adults with disabilities: A review of the literature. *Education and Training in Autism and Developmental Disabilities, 50*(1), 43–55.

Douglas, S. N., Uitto, D. J., Reinfelds, C. L., & D'Agostino, S. (2019). A systematic review of paraprofessional training materials. *The Journal of Special Education, 52*(4), 195–207.

Drysdale, B., Lee, C. Y. Q., Anderson, A., & Moore, D. W. (2015). Using video modeling incorporating animation to teach toileting to two children with autism spectrum disorder. *Journal of Developmental and Physical Disabilities, 27*(2), 149–165.

Dunlap, G., Ester, T., Langhans, S., & Fox, L. (2006). Functional communication training with toddlers in home environments. *Journal of Early Intervention, 28*(2), 81–96.

Dunst, C. J., Hamby, D., Trivette, C. M., Raab, M., & Bruder, M. B. (2000). Everyday family and community life and children's naturally occurring learning opportunities. *Journal of Early Intervention, 23*(3), 151–164.

Fahmie, T. A., & Luczynski, K. C. (2018). Preschool life skills: Recent advancements and future directions. *Journal of Applied Behavior Analysis, 51*(1), 183–188.

Fettig, A., Barton, E. E., Carter, A., & Eisenhower, A. (2016). Using e-coaching to support an early intervention provider's implementation of a functional assessment-based intervention. *Infants and Young Children, 29*(2), 130–147.

Feldman, M. A., & Werner, S. E. (2002). Collateral effects of behavioral parent training on families of children with developmental disabilities and behavior disorders. *Behavioral Interventions: Theory & Practice in Residential & Community-Based Clinical Programs, 17*(2), 75–83.

Friedman, C. (2019). The relationship between disability prejudice and institutionalization of people with intellectual and developmental disabilities. *Intellectual and Developmental Disabilities, 57*(4), 263–273.

Flynn, L., & Healy, O. (2012). A review of treatments for deficits in social skills and self-help skills in autism spectrum disorder. *Research in Autism Spectrum Disorders, 6*(1), 431–441.

Francis, K., Mannion, A., & Leader, G. (2017). The assessment and treatment of toileting difficulties in individuals with autism spectrum disorder and other developmental disabilities. *Review Journal of Autism and Developmental Disorders, 4*(3), 190–204.

Garst, B. A., Gagnon, R. J., & Brawley, A. M. (2019). Efficacy of online training for improving camp staff competency. *Journal of Adventure Education and Outdoor Learning, 19*(1), 12–27.

Genik, L. M., McMurtry, C. M., & Breau, L. M. (2017). Caring for children with intellectual disabilities part 1: Experience with the population, pain-related beliefs, and care decisions. *Research in Developmental Disabilities, 62*(1), 197–208.

Gerencser, K. R., Higbee, T. S., Akers, J. S., & Contreras, B. P. (2018). Evaluation of interactive computerized training to teach parents to implement photographic activity schedules with children with autism spectrum disorder. *Journal of Applied Behavior Analysis, 50*(3), 567–581.

Gerow, S., Rispoli, M., Ninci, J., Gregori, E. V., & Hagan-Burke, S. (2018). Teaching parents to implement functional communication training for young children with developmental delays. *Topics in Early Childhood Special Education, 38*(2), 68–81.

Gunning, C., Holloway, J., Fee, B., Breathnach, Ó., Bergin, C. M., Greene, I., & Bheoláin, R. N. (2019). A systematic review of generalization and maintenance outcomes of social skills intervention for preschool children with autism spectrum disorder. *Review Journal of Autism and Developmental Disorders, 6*(2), 1–28.

Haberlin, A. T., Beauchamp, K., Agnew, J., & O'Brien, F. (2012). A comparison of pyramidal staff training and direct staff training in community-based day programs. *Journal of Organizational Behavior Management, 32*(1), 65–74.

Hamre, M., Dorrance, K., & Ausderau, K. (2017). Feeding interventions for children with developmental disabilities: A systematic review. *American Journal of Occupational Therapy, 71*(4), 71–18.

Harflett, N., & Turner, S. (2016). Supporting people with learning disabilities to develop sexual and romantic relationships bath, UK: National Development Team for Inclusion (NDTi).

Henwood, T., Wooding, A., & De Souza, D. (2013). Center-based exercise delivery: Feasibility of a staff-delivered program and the benefits for low-functioning older adults accessing respite day care. *Activities, Adaptation, & Aging, 37*(3), 224–238.

Higgins, W. J., Luczynski, K. C., Carroll, R. A., Fisher, W. W., & Mudford, O. C. (2017). Evaluation of a telehealth training package to remotely train staff to conduct a preference assessment. *Journal of Applied Behavior Analysis, 50*(2), 238–251.

Holcombe, A., Wolery, M., & Katzenmeyer, J. (1995). Teaching preschoolers to avoid abduction by strangers: Evaluation of maintenance strategies. *Journal of Child and Family Studies, 4*(2), 177–192.

Hong, E. R., Ganz, J. B., Mason, R., Morin, K., Davis, J. L., Ninci, J., ... & Gilliland, W. D. (2016). The effects of video modeling in teaching functional living skills to persons with ASD: A meta-analysis of single-case studies. *Research in Developmental Disabilities, 57*, 158–169.

Hume, K., Loftin, R., & Lantz, J. (2009). Increasing independence in autism spectrum disorders: A review of three focused interventions. *Journal of Autism and Developmental Disorders, 39*(9), 1329–1338.

Johnson, C. R., Foldes, E., DeMand, A., & Brooks, M. M. (2015). Behavioral parent training to address feeding problems in children with autism spectrum disorder: A pilot trial. *Journal of Developmental and Physical Disabilities, 27*(5), 591–607.

Kasari, C., Gulsrud, A., Paparella, T., Hellemann, G., & Berry, K. (2015). Randomized comparative efficacy study of parent-mediated interventions for toddlers with autism. *Journal of Consulting and Clinical Psychology, 83*(3), 554.

Krakovich, T. M., McGrew, J. H., Yu, Y., & Ruble, L. A. (2016). Stress in parents of children with autism spectrum disorder: An exploration of demands and resources. *Journal of Autism and Developmental Disorders, 46*(6), 2042–2053.

Kroeger, K. A., & Sorensen-Burnworth, R. (2009). Toilet training individuals with autism and other developmental disabilities: A critical review. *Research in Autism Spectrum Disorders, 3*(3), 607–618.

Leblanc, M. P., Ricciardi, J. N., & Luiselli, J. K. (2005). Improving discrete trial instruction by paraprofessional staff through an abbreviated performance feedback intervention. *Education and Treatment of Children, 28*(1), 76–82.

Lunsky, Y., Robinson, S., Reid, M., & Palucka, A. (2015). Development of a mindfulness-based coping with stress group for parents of adolescents and adults with developmental disabilities. *Mindfulness, 6*(6), 1335–1344.

Machalicek, W., Lang, R., & Raulston, T. J. (2015). Training parents of children with intellectual disabilities: Trends, issues, and future directions. *Current Developmental Disorders Reports, 2*(2), 110–118.

Matson, J. L., Hattier, M. A., & Belva, B. (2012). Treating adaptive living skills of persons with autism using applied behavior analysis: A review. *Research in Autism Spectrum Disorders, 6*(1), 271–276.

Matson, J. L., Rivet, T. T., Fodstad, J. C., Dempsey, T., & Boisjoli, J. A. (2009). Examination of adaptive behavior differences in adults with autism spectrum disorders and intellectual disability. *Research in Developmental Disabilities, 30*(6), 1317–1325.

McCollum, J. A., & Hemmeter, M. L. (1997). Parent-child interaction intervention when children have disabilities. In M. J. Guralnik (Ed.), *The effectiveness of early intervention* (pp. 549–576). Baltimore, MD: Brooks.

McGowan, L., Caraher, M., Raats, M., Lavelle, F., Hollywood, L., McDowell, D., ... Dean, M. (2017). Domestic cooking and food skills: A review. *Critical Reviews in Food Science and Nutrition, 57*(11), 2412–2431.

McGoron, L., Hvizdos, E., Bocknek, E. L., Montgomery, E., & Ondersma, S. J. (2018). Feasibility of internet-based parent training for low-income parents of young children. Children and youth services review, 84, 198-205.

Miles, N. I., & Wilder, D. A. (2009). The effects of behavioral skills training on caregiver implementation of guided compliance. *Journal of Applied Behavior Analysis, 42*(2), 405–410.

Mueller, M. M., Piazza, C. C., Moore, J. W., Kelley, M. E., Bethke, S. A., Pruett, A. E., ... Layer, S. A. (2003). Training parents to implement pediatric feeding protocols. *Journal of Applied Behavior Analysis, 36*(4), 545–562.

Muldoon, D., & Cosbey, J. (2018). A family-centered feeding intervention to promote food acceptance and decrease challenging behaviors in children with ASD: Report of follow-up data on a train-the-trainer model using EAT-UP. *American Journal of Speech-Language Pathology, 27*(1), 278–287.

Murphy, J., & Zlomke, K. R. (2016). A behavioral parent-training intervention for a child with avoidant/restrictive food intake disorder. *Clinical Practice in Pediatric Psychology, 4*(1), 23.

Najdowski, A. C., Wallace, M. D., Reagon, K., Penrod, B., Higbee, T. S., & Tarbox, J. (2010). Utilizing a home-based parent training approach in the treatment of food selectivity. *Behavioral Interventions: Theory & Practice in Residential & Community-Based Clinical Programs, 25*(2), 89–107.

Neely, L. C., Ganz, J. B., Davis, J. L., Boles, M. B., Hong, E. R., Ninci, J., & Gilliland, W. D. (2016). Generalization and maintenance of functional living skills for individuals with autism spectrum disorder: A review and meta-analysis. *Review Journal of Autism and Developmental Disorders, 3*(1), 37–47.

Neely, L., Rispoli, M., Gerow, S., Hong, E. R., & Hagan-Burke, S. (2017). Fidelity outcomes for autism-focused interventionists coached via telepractice: A systematic literature review. *Journal of Developmental and Physical Disabilities, 29*(6), 849-874.

Nigro-Bruzzi, D., & Sturmey, P. (2010). The effects of behavioral skills training on mand training by staff and unprompted vocal mands by children. *Journal of Applied Behavior Analysis, 43*(4), 757–761.

Norton, M., Dyches, T. T., Harper, J. M., Roper, S. O., & Caldarella, P. (2016). Respite care, stress, uplifts, and marital quality in parents of children with Down syndrome. *Journal of Autism and Developmental Disorders, 46*(12), 3700–3711.

Outar, C., & Rose, J. (2017). Is there a relationship between role identity, work demands, and burnout in direct care staff working with individuals with intellectual disability?. *Journal of Intellectual & Developmental Disability, 42*(2), 123–130.

Ozcan, N., & Cavkaytar, A. (2009). Parents as teachers: Teaching parents how to teach toilet skills to their children with autism and mental retardation. *Education and Training in Developmental Disabilities, 44*(2), 237–243.

Palmen, A., Didden, R., & Lang, R. (2012). A systematic review of behavioral intervention research on adaptive skill building in high-functioning young adults with autism spectrum disorder. *Research in Autism Spectrum Disorders, 6*(2), 602–617.

Palmen, A., Didden, R., & Verhoeven, L. (2012). A personal digital assistant for improving independent transitioning in adolescents with high-functioning autism spectrum disorder. *Developmental Neurorehabilitation, 15*(6), 401–413.

Pan-Skadden, J., Wilder, D. A., Sparling, J., Severtson, E., Donaldson, J., Postma, N., … Neidert, P. (2009). The use of behavioral skills training and in-situ training to teach children to solicit help when lost: A preliminary investigation. *Education and Treatment of Children, 32*(3), 359–370.

Parsons, M. B., Rollyson, J. H., & Reid, D. H. (2012). Evidence-based staff training: A guide for practitioners. *Behavior Analysis in Practice, 5*(2), 2–11.

Rinald, K., & Mirenda, P. (2012). Effectiveness of a modified rapid toilet training workshop for parents of children with developmental disabilities. *Research in Developmental Disabilities, 33*(3), 933–943.

Rosales, R., Stone, K., & Rehfeldt, R. A. (2009). The effects of behavioral skills training on implementation of the picture exchange communication system. *Journal of Applied Behavior Analysis, 42*(3), 541–549.

Sandall, S., Hemmeter, M. L., Smith, B. J., & McLean, M. E. (2005). *The division for early childhood [DEC]-recommended practices: A comprehensive guide for practical application in early intervention/early childhood special education*. Longmont, CO: Sopris West.

Sarokoff, R. A., & Sturmey, P. (2004). The effects of behavioral skills training on staff implementation of discrete-trial teaching. *Journal of Applied Behavior Analysis, 37*(4), 535–538.

Schum, T. R., Kolb, T. M., McAuliffe, T. L., Simms, M. D., Underhill, R. L., & Lewis, M. (2002). Sequential acquisition of toilet-training skills: A descriptive study of gender and age differences in normal children. *Pediatrics, 109*(3), e48–e48.

Seaman, R. L., & Cannella-Malone, H. I. (2016). Vocational skills interventions for adults with autism spectrum disorder: A review of the literature. *Journal of Developmental and Physical Disabilities, 28*(3), 479–494.

Seiverling, L., Williams, K., Sturmey, P., & Hart, S. (2012). Effects of behavioral skills training on parental treatment of children's food selectivity. *Journal of Applied Behavior Analysis, 45*(1), 197–203.

Tarbox, J., Garcia, M. L., & Clair, M. S. (2016). Parent training and support. In J. K. Luiselli (Ed.), *Behavioral health promotion and intervention in intellectual and developmental disabilities* (pp. 231–255). New York: Springer.

Tarbox, J., Schiff, A., & Najdowski, A. C. (2010). Parent-implemented procedural modification of escape extinction in the treatment of food selectivity in a young child with autism. *Education and Treatment of Children, 33*(2), 223–234.

Thompson, J. R., Bradley, V. J., Buntinx, W. H., Schalock, R. L., Shogren, K. A., Snell, M. E., ... & Yeager, M. H. (2009). Conceptualizing supports and the support needs of people with intellectual disability. *Intellectual and Developmental Disabilities, 47*(2), 135–146.

Tomlinson, S. R., Gore, N., & McGill, P. (2018). Training individuals to implement applied behavior analytic procedures via telehealth: A systematic review of the literature. *Journal of Behavioral Education, 27*(2), 172–222.

Traube, D. E., Hsiao, H. Y., Rau, A., Hunt-O'Brien, D., Lu, L., & Islam, N. (2020). Advancing home based parenting programs through the use of telehealth technology. *Journal of Child and Family Studies, 29*(1), 44–53.

Wacker, D. P., Lee, J. F., Dalmau, Y. C. P., Kopelman, T. G., Lindgren, S. D., Kuhle, J., ... Waldron, D. B. (2013). Conducting functional communication training via telehealth to reduce the problem behavior of young children with autism. *Journal of Developmental and Physical Disabilities, 25*(1), 35–48.

Wainer, A. L., & Ingersoll, B. R. (2011). The use of innovative computer technology for teaching social communication to individuals with autism spectrum disorders. *Research in Autism Spectrum Disorders, 5*(1), 96–107.

Wong, C., Odom, S. L., Hume, K. A., Cox, A. W., Fettig, A., Kucharczyk, S., ... & Schultz, T. R. (2015). Evidence-based practices for children, youth, and young adults with autism spectrum disorder: A comprehensive review. *Journal of Autism and Developmental Disorders, 45*(7), 1951–1966.

Chapter 9
The Role of Applied Cognitive Technology and Assistive Technology in Supporting the Adaptive Behavior of People with Intellectual Disability

Michael L. Wehmeyer, Shea Tanis, Daniel K. Davies, and Steven E. Stock

Today technology impacts every aspect of a person's life. This is true for people with intellectual disability, but a myriad of barriers to technology access and use for this population remain. In recognition of barriers to universal access to technology, the University of Colorado Coleman Institute for Cognitive Disabilities convened a national group of stakeholders to craft a declaration titled *The Rights of People with Cognitive Disabilities to Technology and Information Access* (henceforth *Declaration*; Braddock, Hoehl, Tanis, Ablowitz, & Haffer, 2013). The full declaration is in Fig. 9.1.

The *Declaration* has been endorsed by 645 organizations and over 3000 individuals, including more than 50 international organizations and individuals. (Readers can learn more about the *Declaration* at http://www.colemaninstitute.org/). The *Declaration* communicates that to function successfully in advanced technology-driven societies, people must not only have access to technology and information, but to *accessible* technology and information, and that people with cognitive disabilities too often do not have such access. There is also recognition that without intentional inclusion of people with cognitive disabilities in the design and deployment of mainstream technologies, barriers will remain. This chapter examines the role of technology to support people with intellectual disability to function across life domains. We examine technology under two broad categories: *Applied Cognitive Technology* and *Assistive Technology*. We then look at features

M. L. Wehmeyer (✉)
University of Kansas, Lawrence, KS, USA
e-mail: wehmeyer@ku.edu

S. Tanis
University of Colorado, Boulder, CO, USA

D. K. Davies · S. E. Stock
AbleLink Smart Living Technologies, LLC, Colorado Springs, CO, USA

R. Lang, P. Sturmey (eds.), *Adaptive Behavior Strategies for Individuals with Intellectual and Developmental Disabilities*, Autism and Child Psychopathology Series, https://doi.org/10.1007/978-3-030-66441-1_9

WHEREAS:

Twenty-eight million United States citizens have cognitive disabilities such as intellectual disability; severe, persistent mental illness; brain injury; stroke; and neurodegenerative disorders such as Alzheimer'sdisease;

People with cognitive disabilities are entitled to inclusion in our democratic society under federal laws such as the Americans with Disabilities Act (ADA), the Developmental Disabilities Assistance and Billof Rights Act (DD Act), the Individuals with Disabilities Education Act (IDEA), Section 504 of the Rehabilitation Act, and under state and local laws;

The disruptive convergence of computing and communication technologies has substantially altered how people acquire, utilize, and disseminate knowledge and information;

Access to comprehensible information and usable communication technologies is necessary for all people in our society, particularly for people with cognitive disabilities, to promote self-determination and to engage meaningfully in major aspects of life such as education, health promotion,employment, recreation, and civic participation;

The vast majority of people with cognitive disabilities have limited or no access to comprehensible information and usable communicationtechnologies; People with cognitive disabilities must have access to commercially available devices and software that incorporate principles of universal design such as flexibility and ease of use for all;

Technology and information access by people withcognitive disabilities must be guided by standards and best-practices, such as personalization and compatibility across devices and platforms, and through the application of innovations including automated and predictive technologies; Security and privacy must be assured and managed to protect civil rights and personal dignity ofpeople with cognitive disabilities;

Enhanced public and private funding is urgently required to allow people with cognitive disabilities to utilize technology and access information as a natural consequence of their rights to inclusion in oursociety;

Ensuring access to technology and information for the 28 million people with cognitive disabilities in the United States will create new markets and employment opportunities; decrease dependency on public services; reduce healthcare costs; and improve the independence, productivity, and quality oflife of people with cognitive disabilities.

Fig. 9.1 The rights of people with cognitive disabilities to technology and information access declaration

that enable cognitive access and we provide a broad look at the application of technology to support people with intellectual disability across multiple life domains.

9.1 Applied Cognitive Technologies and Assistive Technology

We begin this chapter with a discussion of how to think about technology and information access for people with intellectual disability.

9.1.1 Assistive Technology

Historically, technology to benefit people with disabilities has been, as a class, referred to as assistive technology (AT). In the U.S., the federal special education law (*Individuals with Disabilities Education Act*, or IDEA) defines *assistive technology devices* as "any item, piece of equipment, or product system, whether acquired commercially off the shelf, modified, or customized, that is used to increase, maintain, or improve the functional capabilities of a child with a disability (§300.5, 20 U.S.C. 1401(1)). This definition came from the 1988 *Technology-Related Assistance Act for Individuals with Disabilities*, which is the basis for virtually all U.S. federal definitions of AT.

We highlight the AT definition in U.S. federal statutes to point out that AT has been understood in a disability-only context and, specifically, as technology that in some way mitigates the impairments associated with a particular type of disability (Wehmeyer & Shogren, 2013). The AT definition does refer to "any item, piece of equipment, or product system, whether acquired commercially off the shelf, modified, or customized," thus one might argue that AT should be more broadly cast than just something to mitigate the impact of a disability, but consider the last part of the definition… "that is used to increase, maintain, or improve the functional capabilities of a child with a disability." AT is definitionally tied to improving the functioning of a child with a disability and is almost always referring to technology that addresses a specific deficit. If children cannot walk or have mobility difficulties, they use a wheelchair. If a student cannot speak verbally, they use an alternative or augmentative communication (AAC) device, and so on.

Edyburn (2004) noted that the definition's requirement that AT "increase, maintain, or improve" (p. 17) functional capabilities is directly linked to deficits or impairments in performance. Further, Edyburn noted, in most schools, the AT system is distinct from the school's instructional or educational technology infrastructure. The Coleman Institute *Declaration* recognizes that in the twenty-first century, technology use is ubiquitous and is tied directly with information access and use. Access to the World Wide Web through internet browsers would not typically be considered in the context of AT, but if one wants to apply for many jobs in today's employment context, that process begins with filling out a form that is online. If the web browser or computer lacks accessibility, then one cannot complete the form. This has nothing to do with increasing, maintaining, or improving functional capacity. AT will remain important to people with disabilities, but increasingly other types of technology are becoming as or more important and, indeed, a great many functions previously performed by AT are migrating to information and electronic technology platforms commonly used by all people. For example, standalone AAC devices are being replaced with AAC apps and software operating off mobile and virtual platforms.

Thus, in this chapter, we distinguish between AT and applied cognitive technology (see next section) to broaden the focus of technology for people with intellectual disability. Traditional AT domains have included mobility, hearing and vision, communication, adaptive behavior support, home adaptation and accessibility, and environmental control and independent living/working. But, in terms of their utilization, AT and the ubiquitous types of technology referenced by the *Declaration* are merging, smart phone are now important beyond disability access, as are environmental controls, augmented and virtual reality, applications of artificial intelligence and digital content.

9.1.2 Applied Cognitive Technology

If AT is too restrictive with regard to conceptualizing technology that benefits people with intellectual disability, how might we describe such technology? The discipline of cognitive technologies has existed for years. Focused on how technology impacts cognition (Walker & Hermann, 2005), this field explores issues pertaining to artificial intelligence (AI), symbolic learning theories, knowledge representation, and the semantic web. But, the field of cognitive technologies is not an applied discipline and while issues such as robotics and AI will impact the lives of people with intellectual disability, referring to the emerging understanding of technology that improves the lives of people with intellectual disability under the cognitive technologies umbrella has limitations, not the least of which is that research in cognitive technologies has paid little attention to people with cognitive impairments.

Wehmeyer and Shogren (2013) recommended that the disability sector begin to utilize the term *applied cognitive technology* to reference the array of technology supports that are relevant to the lives of people with cognitive disabilities. Applied cognitive technology (ACT) refers to "technology supports that enable people with cognitive disabilities to successfully function in inclusive environments, to increase participation in tasks and activities in inclusive environments, and to promote social inclusion, self-determination, and quality of life" (Wehmeyer & Shogren, 2013, p. 92).

The difference between ACT and AT, at one level, is that AT is inward looking (e.g., what impairment does a person have that needs remediation or mitigation by technology), while ACT is outward looking (e.g., what technology supports someone to improve aspects of their lives, whether linked to an impairment or not). Many people use smartphones to navigate unfamiliar cities or countries or to get directions in their own community to a new restaurant. It's not that they could not do so without the technology, it is that the technology makes it all simpler and is a tool that can be used to improve access and participation. ACT allows for the differential use and application of technology to enhance overall well-being.

It is important to consider the issue of participation when considering ACT. The construct of 'participation' is important to existing and emerging models that emphasize that disability is best understood not as a fault within the person, but instead, as a function of the relationship between a person's capacities and the demands of typical environments in which they want to function. The World Health Organization's *International Classification of Functioning, Disability, and Health* ([ICF]; World Health Organization, 2001) suggests that impairments to health can result in limitations in activities and restricted participation, where activity refers to the execution of a task or action by a person and participation is defined as involvement in a life situation. Dean, Fisher, Shogren, and Wehmeyer (2016) defined participation as a person's self-determined involvement in a pattern of life where self-determined involvement refers to a person's active, intentional, volitional, goal-directed, sustained, and connected engagement in a pattern of life, and pattern of life represents the roles, life situations, and activities that comprise daily life.

Essentially, the ICF suggests that disability exists only in the gap between the person's abilities and capacities and the demands of the environment. To the degree that the environment can be designed to enable successful functioning and supports provided to enhance personal capacity and reduce or eliminate the gap between what a person can do and what is needed to function successfully in typical environments and contexts, then disability becomes, essentially, irrelevant (Buntinx, 2013). So, for example, in the past, working as a cashier required a person to have some math skills and the capacity to work a cash register. Now, of course, a person just has to scan the bar codes for each product and provide change indicated by the "point of sale computer" that has replaced cash registers.

By defining ACT as linked to participation, we are aligning technology access and use to strengths-based approaches to disability (rather than deficits-focused approaches) and referring to technology and information access that enables people to live full, rich, self-determined lives. This is not to abrogate the need for AT, but instead to shift the focus from deficits to strengths and participation.

Wehmeyer and Shogren (2013) identified some of the types of technology covered by ACT, including prompting and cueing technologies to assist in memory and organization functions, monitoring technologies, wayfinding and navigational supports, smart homes and smart technology, voice communication technologies, cloud and app-based technologies, and context aware and location-based learning (Wehmeyer & Shogren, 2013, p. 93). We will discuss how ACT can enable people with intellectual disability to function successfully in multiple environments and contexts in a subsequent section. First, though, it is important to discuss issues related to universal design and cognitive access.

9.1.3 Universal Design and Cognitive Access

Universal design (UD) emerged in the field of architecture in efforts to ensure that built environments were accessible to all people. An important element of UD is that environments be 'designed' in ways that everyone can use them without any needed modifications. Mace et al. (1997) at the Center for Universal Design proposed that the design of products and environments incorporate the following seven design principles:

1. *Equitable Use:* Products or environments should be useful to all people, avoid segregating or stigmatizing people, and ensure equity.
2. *Flexible Use*: Products or environments should provide choice in use, adapt to a user's pace, and accommodate an array of abilities.
3. *Simple and Intuitive Use:* Products or environments should be simple to understand and use, avoiding unnecessary complexity.
4. *Perceptible Information:* Products or environments should provide multiple modes to provide information for use.
5. *Tolerance for Error:* Products or environments should minimize negative consequences from inadvertent or unintended actions.
6. *Low Physical Effort:* Products or environments should be able to be used without fatigue and by a wide array of people. (Later versions of these principles included "cognitive" as part of principle 6 [e.g., Low physical and cognitive effort]).
7. *Size and Space for Approach and Use*: Products or environments should be accessible by people independent of body size, posture, or mobility.

In technology design and engineering, the term "born accessible" is used to describe the successful application of UD principles. These UD principles were soon applied to the development and use of AT, though, as we will discuss, often too infrequently. Also, the features that promoted cognitive access were often overlooked. In the late 1990s, there emerged a focus on features that enabled cognitive access for technology that was becoming important for participation, including computer, electronic, and information technologies.

Wehmeyer, Smith, Palmer, Davies, and Stock (2004) examined this emerging work and identified areas related to cognitive abilities that cognitively accessible technology would need to support. Such technology would need to be designed to support a wide array of abilities in memory and reasoning skills, language and literacy skills, learning skills, cognitive speed, and knowledge and achievement skills. Harkening to the focus of UD, the recommendation was all technology should incorporate features that account for the wide range of abilities in these cognitive areas. To address the diverse needs of people with cognitive disabilities, one must build agile, flexible, and customizable solutions. Wehmeyer and colleagues identified several UD features that would be particularly important to these efforts.

First, *flexibility in use* was identified as important for cognitively accessible technology. Technology designs should account for a wide range of users' accuracy and precision, and be able to adapt to a user's pace. As an example, Davies et al. (2015)

designed an interface to support more independent use of Facebook by people with intellectual disability. The difficulty for many users with intellectual disability was that the standard Facebook interfaces are complex, both visually and in their use, creating difficulties for people with intellectual disability as to where and how to respond and post. The cognitively accessible interface provided options for people to select which features they wanted to see (friends' lists, news feeds, groups, contacts, etc.) at any one time. Users could limit such features to those they wanted to see and could easily navigate.

Second, issues of *simplicity and intuitiveness of use* are important. Many devices are overly complex and operate counter to users' expectations (e.g., VCRs or many alarm clocks!). Universally designed devices also provide supports (prompting, graphic, visual, or audio directions) for use. Relatedly, the principle of *perceptible information* requires that information required to operate a device be easily seen, but also that such information be provided in multiple modalities, with redundant presentation of information. So, to ensure cognitive access, information needs to be available for use in ways that do not necessarily require high literacy skills. Work is currently being performed in the area of natural language processing and the need for language simplification for accessibility of content and meaning. Finally, the principle of *tolerance for error* is important to ensure cognitive access. Software that incorporates redundant features to minimize error provides cognitive access. For example, Davies, Stock, and Wehmeyer (2001) reported on an accessible web browser for use by people with intellectual disability. The browser design included audio cueing in which an audio message was played when a user clicked on certain icons that provided information to the user on the next step. Another error minimization feature involved linear navigation or consistent placement of familiar buttons from screen-to-screen.

These features form the basis for technology that is cognitively accessible. In the next section, we look at barriers to technology and information access and use for people with intellectual disability.

9.1.4 Barriers to Technology and Information Access and Use

There are several studies that looked at technology use by people with intellectual disability. Wehmeyer (1998) developed a survey examining technology use, need for technology, and barriers to use in five areas focusing on AT use for a specific purpose (i.e., mobility, hearing and vision, communication, home adaptation and access, environmental control, and independent living) and the use of personal computers. The study found that adults with intellectual disability underutilized AT devices and that in three of five categories, there were more people who needed access to technology but did not have it than there were people who needed such access and did have it. The barriers to technology access and use included lack of funding and/or high cost of devices, assessments/evaluations not available, device complexity, and unavailability of training and support.

Only about a third of the respondents had a computer at home, with another 23% having access to a computer at work or in another environment. Barriers to computer use included cost or lack of funds, lack of training, complexity of the device, lack of assessment, and a lack of information about what the computer could do to benefit the person.

In 2012, Tanis and colleagues repeated this study. Instead of mailing surveys, this study utilized a cognitively-accessible online survey so respondents with intellectual disability could more easily complete the survey. A total of 180 youth and young adults with intellectual disability involved in self-advocacy completed the survey, which included the AT use domains from Wehmeyer (1998) (home adaptations and environmental control were collapsed into a "daily living" category), questions about computer use, and questions about electronic and information technologies such as email and cell phones. Though more positive than the findings from the 1998 study, high percentages of respondents still reported a lack of access to AT from which they might benefit. As might be expected, a much higher percentage of respondents indicated they used a computer; however, current computer users cited lack of support to use the computer when faced with a problem as the most frequent barrier to computer use. For both AT and computer use, the barriers identified mirrored the previous study, including cost, maintenance, training, complexity, and support. Additionally, only 13% of respondents reported they owned or used a cell phone. The most recent survey, conducted by The Arc of the United States in 2017, determined that only 39% of people with intellectual disability used a smartphone. This survey found that fewer than half of respondents used a desktop or laptop computer, but two-thirds of the participants used a tablet device. Only 7% of respondents had smart home technology (The Arc, 2017).

In another study (Bryen, Cary, & Friedman, 2007), researchers determined that only 27% of people with intellectual disability owned or used a cell phone, compared to 60% of the general population at that time. These researchers found that a significant barrier to cell phone use by adults with intellectual disability pertained to issues of universal design. Barriers included the small size of the buttons needed to operate most cell phones as well as the cognitive complexity or confusing design of cell phones (e.g., in many cases, one pushes an "End" button to turn the phone both on and off).

Clearly, device complexity was a barrier identified by all of the above-cited studies. In a meta-analysis of single-subject design studies of technology use by people with intellectual disability, Wehmeyer, Palmer, Smith, Davies, and Stock (2008) found that only about a quarter of studies identified the application of any UD principles. Twenty-six percent of studies identified some element of flexibility of use, only 8% identified any features related to simple and intuitive use, and only 5% indicated any tolerance for error features.

The take-home message is that technology use is increasing by people with intellectual disability, but still remains unutilized and underutilized, and technology remains too complex to use, requiring more extensive supports for training, use, and long-term maintenance. The message of the Coleman Institute *Declaration* remains as relevant today as it was in 2013.

9.2 Technology Supports for Adaptive Behavior Across Life Domains

It is now the case that access to technology not only increases convenience in daily living, but is a gateway to a better life. In this section, we examine how technology can support adaptive behavior and participation in daily life.

9.2.1 Community Living and Access

That people with intellectual disability have the right to live, learn, work, and play in their communities has become a cornerstone of services and supports throughout the world. The potential of technology to enable people with intellectual disability to participate successfully in their community is significant. In this section, we consider technology supports to live more independently in one's community and to access one's community.

9.2.1.1 Independent Living Supports, Smart Homes, and Remote Supports

The most visible independent living supports today involve smart home features that, over the past few years, have become general consumer products. Early environmental control devices that facilitated independent living, such as lights that turned on and off with a hand clap, have now been replaced with commercially available products linked with conversational agents or assistants. Telling Alexa, Siri, or Google to turn on your lights, play the TV, answer the phone, provide the weather forecast, or a myriad of other tasks is commonplace. All of these benefit people with intellectual disability and will become more ubiquitous in time. Family members of people with cognitive disabilities are applying conversational agents to bridge information platforms for their loved ones using augmentative and alternative communication devices to engage with conversational agents. One issue that can make such technology less useful involves voice-recognition capacities of such devices. If a person with intellectual disability has difficulty enunciating, the voice-recognition process may fail. But, the voice-recognition capacity of these devices is continuing to improve specifically by addressing unique dialects of people with cognitive disabilities and allowing for customized language programming to eliminate that barrier.

Computers are important tools for independent living. From managing budgets to searching for restaurants to ordering clothes or supplies online, desktop and tablet computers (and smartphones with web browsers) are important for everyday activities. Ensuring that people with intellectual disability can use computers and mobile devices begins with ensuring that operating systems adhere to the cognitive accessibility design features previously discussed. Davies et al. (2001) showed that when such features were incorporated into a desktop computer operating system, people with intellectual disability could navigate to open their favorite programs and applications with minimal support. Stock, Davies, Davies, and Wehmeyer (2006) showed similar benefits to a cognitively accessible operating system on a mobile device.

Using the computer's operating system is, of course, only the first step in ensuring that people with intellectual disability can use computers. Accessibility and usability features of web content and web browsers remain an area of focus (Blanck, 2015). Design features that make websites accessible are those we have discussed for technology in general: paying attention to UD principles, cognitive load issues, focusing on simplicity and ease of use, and so forth. Blanck (2015) described how human-computer interaction researchers are developing analytic tools that will enable web designers to evaluate these accessibility factors as they build websites, making retrofitting of accessibility elements unnecessary. Further, efforts are underway to create standards that ensure web accessibility for people with disabilities (see W3C Initiative at https://www.w3.org/WAI/GL/task-forces/coga/).

As the *Internet of Things* (IoT) becomes a reality, such internet access will become more important to independent living. The IoT refers to the day when almost every device in one's home (not to mention one's automobile, work environment, and community) are connected to the web and to each other. The aforementioned smart speakers and personal agents, like Alexa and Siri, are examples of how everything is becoming connected. Amazon has begun selling microwaves with Alexa technology capacity. For people with cognitive disabilities for whom traditional appliances are too complex to operate, the interconnectedness of these elements will promote access and living supports. Ovens and microwaves will become automated to operate easily using voice commands or smartphone apps, and the risk associated with these appliances (e.g., leaving an oven on) can be dealt with through the technology. Just as clothes irons and coffee pots now turn off if left on, appliances and home devices will be able to be operated easily and safely. New smart mirrors, toilets, and closets provide unique supports to people with cognitive disabilities.

Cooking and meal preparation supports in smart homes can go beyond operating the appliances themselves. Smart home features, particularly the use of touchscreen monitors located in the kitchen, can enable people with intellectual disability to access recipes that include photos, videos, and audio information about ingredients and cooking procedures. Just as many people now use smartphone apps to plan menus, computer and mobile technology can similarly support these activities with people with intellectual disability. And, technology can assist in planning healthier meals. Ptomey et al. (2015) showed that using a tablet and health eating apps, people with intellectual disability were able to eat healthier and lost weight. Further, these participants also used the tablet to track exercise.

Of course, meal preparation is only one element of living more independently. One area in which people with intellectual disability experience difficulty is time management and scheduling. Davies, Stock, and Wehmeyer (2002) showed that people with intellectual disability could learn to use a cognitively-accessible time management/calendar/scheduling system. Davies, Stock, and Wehmeyer (2003a) showed that people with intellectual disability could use a computer to more independently manage their own budgets.

A final element of smart home technology involves the use of remote supports to ensure greater independence. There are privacy concerns associated with any technology that monitors a person, but in some cases (and if the person agrees), monitoring and sensing devices can support greater autonomy and self-determination. People with long-term health issues—susceptibility to seizures, heart ailments, or sleep apnea—can harness the power of sensors placed around a home that can detect vital health information and provide the opportunity for remote supports, either by collecting information to be reviewed by health care providers in the future or, if necessary, to notify support or emergency personnel. We will discuss health-related issues in more detail subsequently.

9.2.1.2 Community Navigation and Wayfinding

Transportation is a frequent barrier to community access and integration. Bodde and Seo (2009) reviewed studies looking at barriers for people with intellectual disability to engage in physical activity in the community. The top three barriers were transportation, financial limitations, and lack of awareness of options. Stock, Davies, Herold, and Wehmeyer (2019) identified literature supporting the fact that transportation barriers impact virtually every community participation and inclusion activity for people with intellectual disability, from physical activity and exercise to health care to religious participation.

Barriers to transportation access for people with intellectual disability typically include expense (automobiles are generally not an option for people with intellectual disability due to cost, and even ride-share options like Uber and Lyft tend to be too expensive), with safety an ongoing concern. Most communities have fixed route bus systems, but they are often complicated and confusing to use. Specialized paratransit systems often have problems with reliability and availability. As a result, people with intellectual disability often have to rely on friends and family members to provide rides (Bascom & Christensen, 2017).

Technology can provide solutions to these problems. Certainly, in the future, autonomous vehicles will provide options to people to get to where they want. But, they are expensive and it is likely that people with intellectual disability will not immediately benefit; however, more affordable personal technology can provide solutions. Wayfinding devices can reduce the complexity (and risk) associated with fixed route bus systems. Davies, Stock, Holloway, and Wehmeyer (2010) showed that the use of cognitively-accessible software on a GPS-enabled handheld computer enabled people with intellectual disability to navigate fixed-route bus transportation successfully with minimal support. Stock, Davies, Hoelzel, and Mullen (2013) conducted a study of a specialized transportation navigation app running on GPS-enabled using a smartphone. People with intellectual disability learned to use the system independently to use a fixed-route bus system and generalized the use of the smartphone across routes.

Smartphones have other support uses in transportation, allowing people with intellectual disability to get in touch with support personnel if something goes awry. Stock, Davies, Wehmeyer, and Palmer (2008) showed that a cognitively-accessible overlay on a mobile cellphone enabled people to more successfully place and receive calls. Planning for and mapping out a trip may be a barrier for people with intellectual disability. Stock and colleagues (2019) found that a 'smart' travel system using computer and GPS technologies to enable people with intellectual disability to assess travel needs, learn about and plan travel activities, and use public transportation resulted in greater independence in these activities.

Of course, community access involves more than transportation. When accessing the community, one must navigate through buildings, shopping malls, theaters, sports facilities, and so forth. Often, one does this using signage, kiosks, building directories, and other sources of information. Too often, these sources are only text-based. Such information can as easily be provided via digital formats using audio and video, often using smart devices connecting via Bluetooth or other sources, where users can receive the information in whatever format is best. Davies and Stock (2009) showed that people with intellectual disability could navigate a historic walking tour using a context-aware GPS system on a smartphone more independently than when using a paper guide. In another study, Davies, Stock, and Wehmeyer (2003b) used visual prompting on a smart handheld device to support people with intellectual disability to access a familiar Automated Teller Machine (ATM). Of course, as machines increasingly use facial recognition and fingerprint recognition software, ATMs, ticket machines, and other services will become more accessible to all.

Context-aware technology will become particularly important to assist people navigate around the community, as well as in grocery stores, shopping malls, and other community locations. For example, smartphones allow users to take photos and record audio easily, and prompting systems like that discussed by Davies et al. (2002) can be used to support community-based activities like shopping trips. Context-aware technology removes a step in the process needed to access information to participate in the community. For example, with context-aware devices, a person could be in a grocery store and receive a prompt from their phone asking if they would like to access a photo-list of items to purchase in that store.

A final community-based domain involves health-related supports. Health care systems are complex and health-related decisions may be equally complex. Haymes, Storey, Maldonado, Post, and Montgomery (2015) conducted a review of smart technology to meet the health-related needs of people with intellectual disability. Haymes and colleagues identified the role of smart devices to support a person with intellectual disability with diabetes in determining if blood sugar levels measured warrant immediate action, and provide recommendations for such action (eat certain foods immediately) or, if readings are more serious, notify emergency personnel. Further, smart technology can provide reminders for taking medications or for scheduling and keeping medical appointments.

Remote supports are equally relevant in health care. Information through monitoring devices can be collected when the person is home or in the community and can inform decisions about diet, exercise, etc. Smartphones and applications like Facetime or Skype can create better communication between people with intellectual disability and health care providers. Finally, accessible web browsers allow people with intellectual disability to get information about health conditions and become better informed health care consumers.

9.2.2 Employment

Technology supports such as computers, tablets, and smartphones will have the same function in employment supports as in community supports, so we will not revisit those. Wehmeyer et al. (2006) conducted a meta-analysis of single-subject design studies between 1977 and 2003 on the use of technology by people with intellectual disability in employment tasks. As with a larger single-subject design meta-analysis discussed previously (Wehmeyer et al., 2008), few of the papers studied technology incorporating UD features, with flexible use and simple intuitive use principles applied in only about one-quarter of the studies. Yet, there was evidence of the potential of technology to support enhanced performance in employment tasks. Damianidou, Arthur-Kelly, Lyons, and Wehmeyer (2019) updated this meta-analysis, examining studies from 2004 to 2016. This analysis also confirmed the utility of technology to improve performance and functioning in work environments. Damianidou, Foggett, Arthur-Kelly, Lyons, and Wehmeyer (2018) determined that technology incorporating UD features had greater efficacy in supporting successful performance of employment activities.

Another way technology impacts employment for people with intellectual disability is through job assessment and interest activities. Davies, Stock, Davies, and Wehmeyer (2018a) used a cloud-based app providing video and audio clips of jobs and work tasks to assist people with intellectual disability to identify interests and preferences in work environments. Stock, Davies, Secor, and Wehmeyer (2003) demonstrated the utility of computer-based simulations of work to determine career and vocational interests and aid in discovery. Stock, Davies, and Wehmeyer (2009) used computer-animated work tasks (using avatars) to teach vocational-related skills to young adults with intellectual disability.

It is worth noting that cloud-based technology (as used by Davies et al., 2018a) will become increasingly important. Most people are familiar with the cloud from, mainly, commercial sites like Amazon or streaming sites like Amazon Prime or Netflix. Currently, if someone needs accommodations to successfully use technology devices, those features reside on a specific device. If that person is using a different device, those accommodations are not available. In the near future, such customizations can be stored in the cloud and available for use on any device. Technology is also being applied to support job coaches for on-going and fading supports. The virtual job coach is emerging as a viable option to provide real time technology supports. Companies like Aira (https://aira.io/) are investigating the application of on-call supports for environmental navigation and employment task supports.

9.2.3 Recreation and Leisure

There are obvious ways that technology will support recreation and leisure activities for people with intellectual disability that mirror such supports for all people. Movie and television streaming technologies put favorite movies and shows at the reach of a remote control (or voice control!) in one's home. Computers themselves are sources for recreation and leisure activities. Many people enjoy playing solitaire or video games on a computer or a game on a smartphone, and people with intellectual disability share the same interests. Chan, Lambdin, Graham, Fragale, and Davis (2014) taught young people with intellectual disability to play *Angry Birds* on an iPad. Extended Realty (XR) has the potential to extend recreation activities to people with intellectual disability through various forms of computer-altered reality, including augmented reality (AR), mixed reality (MR) and virtual reality (VR). Weiss, Bialik, and Kizony (2004) used VR to enable five young men with cerebral palsy and intellectual disability to play games involving physical activities in which they would not otherwise have been able to engage.

Many people enjoy reading in their leisure time, and people with intellectual disability might enjoy this as well, if not for limited literacy skills. Davies, Davies, Stock, King, Woodard, and Wehmeyer (2008) evaluated the efficacy of a cognitively-accessible portable reading system (a digital talking book with cognitive access features) and found that people with intellectual disability could use the system and enjoyed reading audio books.

9.2.4 Social and Communication

Finally, technology can support the adaptive behavior of people with intellectual disability and improve participation by supporting social and communication activities. Obviously, many people with intellectual disability with speech impairments benefit from AAC. Increasingly, more mobile devices, like tablets, provide platforms for AAC. Apps like *Proloquo2go* provide increasingly powerful AAC support for people, and even symbol-based communication systems like PECS have migrated to tablets (Ganz, Hong, Goodwyn, Kite, & Gilliland, 2015). Keskinen, Heimonen, Turunen, Rajaniemi, and Kauppinen (2012) developed a multimodal communication application utilizing picture-based instant messaging (IM) capacities so people with intellectual disability could communicate by IM. Input could be text or speech. Now, most text and messaging apps allow both input options. Emails can be sent via voice recordings as well.

These days, much of what is 'social' is online. We mentioned a study showing that a cognitively-accessible overlay enabled people with intellectual disability to use Facebook (Davies et al., 2015). Davies, Stock, Davies, and Wehmeyer (2018b) evaluated a cognitively accessible tool for people with intellectual disability to communicate and share stories online. And, Davies, Stock, King, Wehmeyer, and Shogren (2017) evaluated a tool enabling people with intellectual disability to complete online forms and surveys, thus supporting them to communicate their opinions and requests in the ways that many people do today.

Finally, gaining social capital, defined as "the network and norms that allow people to work together, to resolve problems, and achieve common goals" (Partington, 2005, p. 241), is a means to a better life. Social capital has been connected to self-determination, civic tolerance, economic equality, happiness, goal achievement, and subjective well-being (Helliwell & Putnam, 1999; Leung, Kier, & Sproule, 2014). Investments in ensuring access to information and social media not only enhances social capital and provides access to formal supports but also provides opportunities to build lasting relationships among members of diverse communities (Bradley & Poppen, 2003).

9.3 Conclusion

There is not enough space in this chapter to discuss all of the ways technology will support the adaptive functioning and daily living of people with intellectual disability. As illustrated in the chapter, there is already technology available that can overcome barriers to full participation and the nature of technology is that it is forever changing. It is imperative that people who support people with intellectual disability remain aware of new technology and innovate by adopting technology solutions that promote and enhance participation and functioning.

References

Bascom, G. W., & Christensen, K. M. (2017). The impacts of limited transportation access on persons with disabilities' social participation. *Journal of Transport & Health, 7*, 227–234.

Blanck, P. (2015). eQuality: Web accessibility by people with cognitive disabilities. *Inclusion, 3*, 75–91.

Bodde, A. E., & Seo, D.-C. (2009). A review of social and environmental barriers to physical activity for adults with intellectual disabilities. *Disability and Health Journal, 2*, 57–66.

Braddock, D., Hoehl, J., Tanis, S., Ablowitz, E., & Haffer, L. (2013). The rights of people with cognitive disabilities to technology and information access. *Inclusion, 1*, 95–102.

Bradley, H., & Poppen, W. (2003). Assistive technology, computers, and Internet may decrease sense of isolation for homebound elderly and disabled persons. *Technology and Disability, 15*, 19–25.

Bryen, D.N., Carey, A., & Friedman, M. (2007). Cell phone use by adults with intellectual disabilities. *Intellectual and Developmental Disabilities, 45*(1), 1–9.

Buntinx, W. H. E. (2013). Understanding disability: A strengths-based approach. In M. L. Wehmeyer (Ed.), *The Oxford handbook on positive psychology and disability* (pp. 7–18). Oxford, UK: Oxford University Press.

Chan, J. M., Lambdin, L., Graham, K., Fragale, C., & Davis, T. (2014). A picture-based activity schedule to teach adults with mild intellectual disability to use an iPad during a leisure activity. *Journal of Behavioral Education, 23*, 247–257.

Damianidou, D., Arthur-Kelly, M., Lyons, G., & Wehmeyer, M. L. (2019). Technology use to support employment-related outcomes for people with intellectual and developmental disability: An updated meta-analysis. *International Journal of Developmental Disabilities, 65*(4), 220–230.

Damianidou, D., Foggett, J., Arthur-Kelly, M., Lyons, G., & Wehmeyer, M. L. (2018). Effectiveness of technology types in employment-related outcomes for people with intellectual and developmental disabilities: An extension meta-analysis. *Advances in Neurodevelopmental Disorders, 2*(3), 262–272.

Davies, D., Stock, S., Davies, C., & Wehmeyer, M. L. (2018a). A cloud-supported app for providing self-directed, localized job interest assessment and analysis for people with intellectual disability. *Advances in Neurodevelopmental Disabilities, 2*, 199–205.

Davies, D., Stock, S., Davies, C., & Wehmeyer, M. L. (2018b). A cognitively accessible digital storytelling tool for people with intellectual and other cognitive disabilities. *Global Journal of Intellectual & Developmental Disabilities, 5*(2), 1–6.

Davies, D., Stock, S., & Wehmeyer, M. (2003b). Application of computer simulation to teach ATM access to individuals with intellectual disabilities. *Education and Training in Developmental Disabilities, 38*, 451–456.

Davies, D., Stock, S., & Wehmeyer, M. L. (2001). Enhancing independent Internet access for individuals with mental retardation through the use of a specialized web browser: A pilot study. *Education and Training in Mental Retardation and Developmental Disabilities, 36*, 107–113.

Davies, D., Stock, S., & Wehmeyer, M. L. (2003a). Utilization of computer technology to facilitate money management by individuals with mental retardation. *Education and Training in Developmental Disabilities, 38*, 106–112.

Davies, D. K. & Stock, S. E. (2009). *Development and evaluation of a location based multimedia system for providing access to information in community settings for students and adults with intellectual disabilities*. Phase I final project report submitted to the US Department of Education, 31 Mar 2009.

Davies, D. K., Stock, S. E., Holloway, S., & Wehmeyer, M. L. (2010). Evaluating a GPS-based transportation device to support independent bus travel by people with intellectual disability. *Intellectual and Developmental Disabilities, 48*, 454–463.

Davies, D. K., Stock, S. E., King, L., Wehmeyer, M. L., & Shogren, K. A. (2017). An accessible testing, learning, and assessment system for people with intellectual disability. *International Journal of Developmental Disabilities, 63*(4), 201–210.

Davies, D. K., Stock, S. E., King, L., Woodard, J., & Wehmeyer, M. (2008). "Moby Dick is my favorite": Evaluating the use of a cognitively accessible portable reading system for audio books by people with intellectual disability. *Intellectual and Developmental Disabilities, 46*(4), 290–298.

Davies, D. K., Stock, S. E., King, L. R., Brown, B., Wehmeyer, M. L., & Shogren, K. A. (2015). An interface to support independent use of Facebook by people with intellectual disability. *Intellectual and Developmental Disabilities, 53*(1), 30–41.

Davies, D. M., Stock, S., & Wehmeyer, M. L. (2002). Enhancing independent time management and personal scheduling for individuals with mental retardation through use of a palmtop visual and audio prompting system. *Mental Retardation, 40*, 358–365.

Dean, E., Fisher, K., Shogren, K., & Wehmeyer, M. (2016). Participation and intellectual disability: A review of the literature. *Intellectual and Developmental Disabilities, 54*(6), 427–439.

Edyburn, D. L. (2004). Rethinking assistive technology. *Special Education Technology Practice, 5*(4), 16–23.

Ganz, J. B., Hong, E. R., Goodwyn, F., Kite, E., & Gilliland, W. (2015). Impact of PECS tablet computer app on receptive identification of pictures given a verbal stimulus. *Developmental Neurorehabilitation, 18*(2), 82–87.

Haymes, L. K., Storey, K., Maldonado, A., Post, M., & Montgomery, J. (2015). Using applied behavior analysis and smart technology for meeting the health needs of individuals with intellectual disabilities. *Developmental Neurorehabilitation, 18*, 407–419.

Helliwell, J. F., & Putnam, R. D. (1999). Economic growth and social capital in Italy. In I. P. Dasgupta & I. Sergeldin (Eds.), *Social capital: A multifaceted perspective* (pp. 253–269). Washington, DC: World Bank.

Keskinen, T., Heimonen, T., Turunen, M., Rajaniemi, J-P., Kauppinen, S. (2012). SymbolChat: A flexible picture-based communication platform for users with intellectual disabilities, Interacting with Computers, 24, 5, 374–386.

Leung, A., Kier, C., & Sproule, R. A. (2014). Happiness and social capital. In A. C. Michalos (Ed.), *Encyclopedia of quality of life and well-being research* (pp. 443–462). Dordrecht, The Netherlands: Springer.

Mace, R., Connell, B. R., Jones, M., Mueller, J., Mullick, A., Ostroff, E., … Vanderheiden, G. (1997). *The principals of universal design*. Raleigh, NC: Center for Universal Design. Accessed online at https://projects.ncsu.edu/ncsu/design/cud/about_ud/udprinciplestext.htm

Partington, K. (2005). What do we mean by our community? *Journal of Intellectual Disabilities, 9*(3), 241–251.

Ptomey, L. T., Sullivan, D. K., Lee, J., Goetz, J. R., Gibson, C., & Donnelly, J. E. (2015). The use of technology for delivering a weight loss program for adolescents with intellectual and developmental disabilities. *Journal of the Academy of Nutrition and Dietetics, 115*, 112–118.

Stock, S., Davies, D., Secor, R., & Wehmeyer, M. L. (2003). Self-directed career preference selection for individuals with intellectual disabilities: Using computer technology to enhance self-determination. *Journal of Vocational Rehabilitation, 19*, 95–104.

Stock, S., Davies, D., & Wehmeyer, M. L. (2009). Design and evaluation of a computer-animated simulation approach to support vocational social skills training for students and adults with intellectual disability. *Assistive Technology Outcomes and Benefits, 3*, 43–55.

Stock, S., Davies, D. K., Davies, K. R., & Wehmeyer, M. L. (2006). Evaluation of an application for making palmtop computers accessible to individuals with intellectual disabilities. *Journal of Intellectual and Developmental Disabilities, 31*, 39–46.

Stock, S. E., Davies, D. K., Herold, R. G., & Wehmeyer, M. L. (2019). Technology to support transportation needs assessment, training, and pre-trip planning by people with intellectual disability. *Advances in Neurodevelopmental Disorders, 3*(3), 319–324.

Stock, S. E., Davies, D. K., Hoelzel, L. A., & Mullen, R. J. (2013). Evaluation of a GPS-based system for supporting independent use of public transportation by adults with intellectual disability. *Inclusion, 1*, 133–144.

Stock, S. E., Davies, D. K., Wehmeyer, M. L., & Palmer, S. B. (2008). Evaluation of cognitively-accessible software to increase independent access to cell phone technology for people with intellectual disability. *Journal of Intellectual Disability Research, 52*(12), 1155–1164.

Stock, S.E., Davies, D.K., Herold, R.G., & Wehmeyer, M.L. (2019). Technology to support transportation needs assessment, training, and pre-trip planning by people with intellectual disability. *Advances in Neurodevelopmental Disorders, 3*(3), 319–324

Tanis, E. S., Palmer, S., Wehmeyer, M. L., Davies, D., Stock, S., Lobb, K., & Bishop, B. (2012). Self-report computer-based survey of technology use by people with intellectual and developmental disabilities. *Intellectual and Developmental Disabilities, 50*(1), 53–68.

The Arc. (2017). *FINDS survey community report data tables*. Minneapolis, MN: University of Minnesota. Accessed online at https://www.thearc.org/file/documents_finds/18_6_5-FINDS-Community-Report-Data-Tables.pdf

Walker, W. R., & Hermann, D. J. (2005). *Cognitive technology: Essays in the transformation of thought and society*. Jefferson, NC: McFarland & Co..

Wehmeyer, M. L. (1998). National survey of the use of assistive technology by adults with mental retardation. *Mental Retardation, 36*, 44–51.

Wehmeyer, M. L., Palmer, S., Smith, S., Parent, W., Davies, D., & Stock, S. (2006). Technology use by people with intellectual and developmental disabilities to support employment activities: A single-subject design meta-analysis. *Journal of Vocational Rehabilitation, 24*, 81–86.

Wehmeyer, M. L., Palmer, S., Smith, S. J., Davies, D., & Stock, S. (2008). The efficacy of technology use by people with intellectual disability: A single-subject design meta-analysis. *Journal of Special Education Technology, 23*(3), 21–30.

Wehmeyer, M. L., & Shogren, K. A. (2013). Establishing the field of applied cognitive technology. *Inclusion, 1*, 91–94.

Wehmeyer, M. L., Smith, S. J., Palmer, S. B., Davies, D. K., & Stock, S. (2004). Technology use and people with mental retardation. In L. M. Glidden (Ed.), *International review of research in mental retardation* (Vol. 29, pp. 293–337). San Diego, CA: Academic Press.

Weiss, P. L., Bialik, P., & Kizony, R. (2004). Virtual reality provides leisure time opportunities for young adults with physical and intellectual disabilities. *CyberPsychology and Behavior, 6*, 335–342.

World Health Organization. (2001). *International classification of functioning, disability, and health*. Geneva, Switzerland: World Health Organization.

Index

R. Lang, P. Sturmey (eds.), *Adaptive Behavior Strategies for Individuals with Intellectual and Developmental Disabilities*, Autism and Child Psychopathology Series, https://doi.org/10.1007/978-3-030-66441-1

The manufacturer's authorised representative in the EU is Springer Nature Customer Service Centre GmbH, Europaplatz 3, 69115 Heidelberg, Germany. If you have any concerns regarding our products, please contact ProductSafety@springernature.com

Printed and bound by CPI Group (UK) Ltd, Croydon, CR0 4YY
30/09/2026
02225325-0006